GEORGES GILLES DE LA TOURETTE

Georges Gilles de la Tourette

Beyond the Eponym

Olivier Walusinski

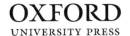

OXFORD
UNIVERSITY PRESS

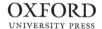

OXFORD
UNIVERSITY PRESS

Library of Congress Cataloging-in-Publication Data
Names: Walusinski, Olivier, author.
Title: Georges Gilles de la Tourette : beyond the eponym /
by Olivier Walusinski.
Description: New York, NY : Oxford University Press, [2019] |
Includes bibliographical references and index.
Identifiers: LCCN 2018011695 | ISBN 9780190636036 (alk. paper)
Subjects: | MESH: Gilles de la Tourette, Georges, 1857–1904. | Physicians |
Tourette Syndrome | Biography
Classification: LCC RC375 | NLM WZ 100 | DDC 616.8/3—dc23
LC record available at https://lccn.loc.gov/2018011695

9 8 7 6 5 4 3 2 1

Printed by Sheridan Books, Inc., United States of America

Contents

Foreword

THIS COMPREHENSIVE STUDY of Georges Gilles de la Tourette examines the rise and decline of a relatively obscure neurological figure, strategically placed in the halo of power and influence amid the vibrant atmosphere of Parisian neurology between the late nineteenth and early twentieth centuries. Gilles de la Tourette's close ties with the most celebrated neurologist of the nineteenth century, Jean-Martin Charcot, afforded his inclusion into the *cercle intime* of the Salpêtrière Hospital neurological service, where he profited from the national and international contacts that his mentor provided. Because of Charcot's special deference to his faithful students, Gilles de la Tourette's name became linked to the early definitive description of a neurological syndrome typified by motor and vocal tics, sometimes accompanied by bizarre and distinctive behaviors that drew particular attention, both medically and socially. This linkage remains in contemporary international neurological vocabulary, often misrepresented in a shortened surname adaptation as Tourette's syndrome. Gilles de la Tourette, himself, as a person, as a physician, as a scientific figure, did not distinguish himself particularly after Charcot's death, and his self-promoting ambition, foibles, and eventual neurological degenerative illness collectively led to a forced retirement and shameful end of his medical career. In spite of the importance of this period after Charcot's death in terms of burgeoning neurological knowledge and the struggle of the French Neurological School to remain preeminent internationally, no serious study of Gilles de la Tourette has ever been prepared for wide readership. This new biography, written by Olivier Walusinski, a serious and committed French physician with extensive historical credentials, studies this man and his era. The author has accessed archival materials heretofore never collected together. The result is a scholarly study and a dramatic rendering of one man's life in the context of an early career of luminance and then a gradual decline punctuated by scandal and misadventure, all unveiled amid the in-fighting of the French Neurological School and the sparkling ambience of Parisian society.

—Christopher G. Goetz, MD
Chicago, Illinois

Acknowledgments

I would like to express my sincere thanks to Dr. Gregory Duncan for his remarkable thesis[1] and Professor Jean-Philippe Neau (Poitiers) for setting me on the trail of the family archives. I am also indebted to the following people:

Anna Fitzgerald and Mary Malecek for their skillful translation into English. Craig Panner and Emily Samulski (Oxford University Press) for transforming this work into a published book.

Eglantine Desgraupes and Aude Lemercier for their patience and availability during my visits to the Charbonneau-Lassay Museum in Loudun.

Jean Leblanc and Soline Girard for their invaluable help in deciphering and transcribing the manuscripts.

Bernadette Molitor, Stéphanie Charreaux, Estelle Lambert, and Jean-François Vincent at the BIUS (interuniversities medical library) in Paris for their patience and their precious assistance with my bibliographic research.

Romain Tardy and Altea Swan for their help with my research at the Archives de l'Assistance Publique.

Professor Christopher Goetz, an internationally recognized specialist on the Salpêtrière School physicians, for the engaging foreword he spontaneously agreed to write.

Professor Jacques Poirier and Dr. Hubert Déchy for their multiple readings and their many corrections and suggestions.

Profs. Andreas Hartmann (Paris), Peter J. Koehler (Heerlen, NL), Paul Eling (Nijmegen, NL), and Howard I. Kushner (San Diego) for their advice and support.

Profs. German Berrios (Cambridge, UK), Martin Catala (Paris), Jacques Poirier (Paris), Jacques Philippon (Paris); Drs. Hubert Déchy (Versailles),

Michel Floris (Belgium), Jean-Pierre Luauté (Romans); Mrs. Soline Girard (France); Anna Fitzgerald (US); for their reviews and proofreading

Profs. Yves Agid (Paris), Claudio Bassetti (Bern), Julien Bogousslavsky (Montreux), François Boller (Washington), Marie-Germaine Bousser (Paris), Emmanuel Broussolle (Lyon), Andrea E. Cavanna (London), Stanley Finger (Saint-Louis), Axel Karenberg (Köln), Andrew Lees (London), Piero Salzarulo (Firenze), Frank W. Stanish (Calgary), Marie Vidailhet (Paris), and Drs. Laura Bossi (Paris), Paul B. Foley (Sydney), Heinz Krestel (Bern), Douglas Lanska (Tomah), Boleslav L. Lichterman (Moscow), Lorenzo Lorusso (Chiari), Jean-Pierre Luauté (Romans), Vincent Ould Aoudia (Nantes), Jacques Paillot (Chartres), Bradley S. Peterson (New York), Paul Raymond (Nozay), Wolter Seuntjens (Erfurt), and Cristiano Termine (Varese), and Andrew Waclawik (Madison) for their friendship and their generous encouragement.

Note

1. Duncan G. *Gilles de la Tourette: Aspects connus et méconnus de sa vie et de son œuvre.* Thèse Poitiers 95POIT1044. 1995.

Note on Terms

Externe. Nonresident student at a teaching hospital. The *externes* did
   not live at the hospital and had neither diagnostic nor therapeutic
   responsibilities.
Interne. House physician or house officer. The internes lived at the
   hospital and had diagnostic and therapeutic responsibilities.
Chef de Clinique. Senior house officer or resident.
Internat. House officership, internship, or residency.
Assistance Publique. The manager of the Parisian public hospital system.

French daily newspapers quoted: *L'Action française, L'Aurore, Le Figaro, Le
Gaulois, Gil Blas, L'Éclair, Le Petit Journal, La Patrie, Le Journal*
Each chapter of the book can be read independently.

Introduction

Gilles de la Tourette

A Familiar Name, a Misunderstood Illness,
a Forgotten Man

Some, to the fascination of a name, suspend judgement.

Why a Biography?

The name Gilles de la Tourette is recognizable for many people. They intuitively think of the disease while remaining unaware of its clinical picture or reducing it to tics alone. The name is more familiar to physicians and well known to neurologists. But who was Georges Gilles de la Tourette (1857–1904; Figure I.1)? Scholarly, exhaustive biographies have been written about his teacher, Jean-Martin Charcot (1825–1893; Figure I.2), and his most famous colleague, Joseph Babiński (1857–1932). And lesser-known students of Charcot have had the honor of a biography, for example Désiré-Magloire Bourneville (1840–1909), Charles Féré (1852–1907), Edouard Brissaud (1852–1909), and Henri Parinaud (1844–1905). And yet, very little has been written about the life of Georges Gilles de la Tourette.

Certain historians take the slightly condescending view that biography is a hybrid form, blending all of the "different lives" of an individual—intellectual, social, and professional—without any pretension of literature, the result being nothing beyond a minor record of history. However, biographies are

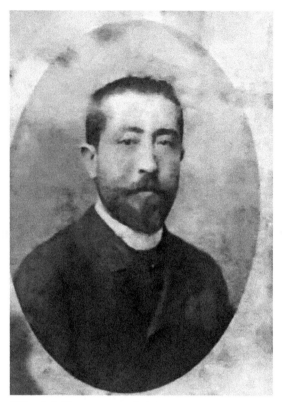

FIGURE I.I Georges Gilles de la Tourette around 1893.
Copyright, Musée Charbonneau-Lassay. Ville de Loudun, with kind permission.

essential. We take our memories with us when we go, and the only way to collect them—and to recollect them—for today and for tomorrow, is through narratives that put a life and a life's work into perspective.

Made Famous by an Eponym

Gilles de la Tourette's posthumous fame is recent. The 1936 edition of a leading French encyclopedia, the *Larousse*, contains a dozen lines on Gilles de la Tourette, whereas the 1960 edition makes no mention of him at all. Medical fame is evanescent; it comes and goes, and, by dint of circumstances, it may return. Gilles de la Tourette once again gained prominence in the 1960s as interest grew in the syndrome that bears his name. As the English author MacDonald Critchley (1900–1997) wrote: "The Malady of Gilles de la Tourette: what a compelling and grandiloquent choice of words! As a matter of fact, it is a fragment of poetry with its iambus following a dactyl. More than

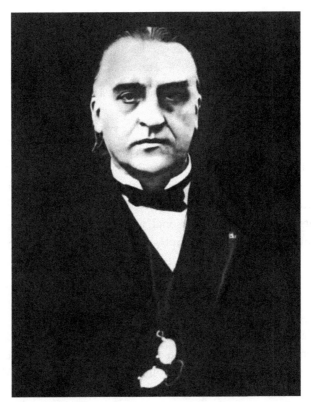

FIGURE I.2 Jean-Martin Charcot around 1890.
Postcard, private collection of the author.

that, it is a musical theme which reverberates in one's imagery. Little wonder that the eponym fixates itself in the mind of every student at the outset of his career in neurology, there to remain throughout his life like a limpet."

The eponym's pretty ring has thus played a role in Gilles de la Tourette's fame. There is a touch of exoticism for English-speakers, as well as an evocation of onomastic and nobiliary pride. One patient's mother reportedly told Arthur K. Shapiro (1923–1995), "What a pretty name for such a terrible disease," indicating that those familiar with the syndrome are much more ambivalent about the eponym.

The affection Charcot had for Gilles de la Tourette stands in stark contrast to the slanderous remarks made by many of their contemporaries, and this paradox alone may justify examining Gilles de la Tourette's life. But, in delving into previously unpublished documentary sources, acquired through the Gilles de la Tourette family archive and a delight for any historian, one finds even further reasons to resuscitate this physician, writer, historian, and theater critic who worked in one of the world's largest centers for neurology at the end of the nineteenth century, the Hôpital La Salpêtrière.

Previously Unpublished Family Archives

After their mother's death (September 10, 1979, in Saint-Fargeau-Ponthierry), the children of Jeanne Dalpeyrat (1890–1979) decided to donate the family archives she had maintained to Loudun's Charbonneau-Lassay Museum. Two crates in the museum's attic contain numerous letters from Gilles de la Tourette's correspondence with friends and colleagues, administrative documents concerning his personal and professional affairs, and unpublished family photos. This biography draws on these previously unpublished archives.

Gilles de la Tourette's Personality

Gilles de la Tourette's passion and diligence, so appreciated by Charcot, led to a very high output; he published in all of the fields that interested him: medicine, history, journalism, and theater. Intensely ambitious, Gilles de la Tourette also completed the obstacle course of competitive exams that structure the medical and university professions in France. As he climbed his career ladder, Gilles de la Tourette met men for whom he developed deep admiration and staunch attachment, especially Charcot and Paul Brouardel (1837–1906).

His loyalty as a friend was only matched by his loyalty to his roots, in Poitou and the town of Loudun. His first historical works centered on characters who gave Loudun its place in history, namely, Théophraste Renaudot, the father of journalism and advertising and an important source of personal inspiration for Gilles de la Tourette in his own journalistic pursuits. Later books focused on Urbain Grandier and an Ursuline Mother Superior, Sister Jeanne des Anges, the protagonists in the town's legendary confrontation with demonic forces. These two figures, emblematic of intolerance and superstition, provided material to which he could apply the neuropsychological knowledge gained at La Salpêtrière, along with his republican, progressive, and anti-clerical ideals.

Aided by his friend Bourneville, a physician and politician who held similar views, he was able to start publishing his medical writings at a very early age, even before his doctorate. His first articles appeared in Bourneville's journal *Le Progrès Médical*, then in *Les Archives de Neurologie*. He would later be involved in founding *La Nouvelle Iconographie de La Salpêtrière*.

French National Archives and Library

When Georges Montorgueil (1857–1933), editor-in-chief of the major evening newspaper *Le Temps*, died, all of his correspondence was entrusted to the French National Archives, including the numerous letters he received from Gilles de la Tourette. Their correspondence, from 1892 to 1901, sheds light on hidden and perhaps secret aspects of Gilles de la Tourette's quest for notoriety. For example, the letters reveal Gilles de la Tourette's constant need for recognition and all of the subterfuge he engaged in to attain it. The mainstream press of his day features prominently, as it often reported on the work carried out at La Salpêtrière and by Gilles de la Tourette in particular. But, of course, avidly seeking media attention has its disadvantages, which Gilles de la Tourette learned when journalists highlighted stories, some of them scandalous, in which he found himself involved against his wishes. For the first time, these events will be examined based on several sources from the French National Library and the family archives.

The Journalist

Jules Claretie (1840–1913), novelist and chronicler of late nineteenth-century Parisian life, was a close friend of Gilles de la Tourette, and their epistolary exchange provides a window on the artistic life in which they actively participated, including theater. Gilles de la Tourette wrote regularly in the cultural periodical *La Revue Hebdomadaire* under the pen name of Paracelsus whose articles focused on psychiatry, hygiene, theater productions, and so on. On the whole, Gilles de la Tourette's writings are characterized by an elegant literary style with occasional flights of lyricism, but they also bear the mark of his work method, which at times bordered on plagiarism. The emblematic example is his first book, the biography of Théophraste Renaudot, published in 1884. His mastery of the subject matter is surprising for such a young man, but, in fact, he drew much inspiration from the book by Eugène Hatin (1809–1893) and omitted to credit him.

The Eponymous Disease

When Gilles de la Tourette was still a medical student, he translated English articles on various types of abnormal behavior for *Les Archives de Neurologie*, a journal founded by Charcot, who took an interest in the articles as well as their precocious translator. Shortly thereafter, Charcot accorded Gilles de la Tourette the task of publishing observations of patients that Charcot had treated and for whom the diagnosis of chorea left him unsatisfied. Charcot quickly realized that the article initially published by Gilles de la Tourette was incomplete and its title misleading. Yet, because of the esteem and friendship he felt for Gilles de la Tourette, whose name was so melodious, Charcot named the disorder after him. He did, however, task Georges Guinon (1859–1932), the *interne* who replaced Gilles de la Tourette, with adding the psychopathological elements in a second publication.

Given how attached Gilles de la Tourette was to many of his other publications, it is curious that he took little pride in this seminal paper. It should be noted, however, that the article generated little interest at the time.

The Author

The two books that Gilles de la Tourette considered to be his magnum opus— *L'hypnotisme et les états analogues* and *Traité de l'Hystérie*—were rapidly outdated and have today lost all of their significance. Nonetheless, analyzing them gives some measure of the difficulties that nineteenth-century physicians faced in making well-founded diagnoses and ensuring truly curative treatment at a time when their only tool, clinical medicine, was in its infancy and treatment methods were often more iatrogenic than therapeutic. These works also reveal the unspeakable suffering endured by some of the patients and their stupefying resignation. Evoking the treatments they were subjected to is a sort of homage to these patients and a way of thanking them for the medical progress we currently enjoy.

A Man of Acclaim

Gilles de la Tourette's brazen ambition, born of a need for recognition and fame, was gratified when he was appointed to the sought-after post of Chief Physician for the 1900 World's Fair in Paris, entailing four years of preparatory construction. The effusive and unanimous praise he garnered in this role are proof of his skills and talents as an organizer, even though he had obtained his position through opportunistic tactics.

The Fatal Kiss of Aphrodite

Arx Tarpeia Capitoli proxima ("the Tarpeian Rock stands close to the Capitol"). In other words, a fall from grace is always possible. Gilles de la Tourette's life was haunted by a disease that, unknown to him, was insidiously undermining his health: general paralysis. The condition was clearly in evidence by 1893. Some of his writings reveal a flight of ideas resulting from a delirious megalomania, which reached its height in 1901. It is pathetically illustrated in the hitherto unpublished cover letter, presented in this volume, of Gilles de la Tourette's candidacy for the Chair of History of Medicine—the last rung in the university career ladder before full professorship, which Gilles de la Tourette never achieved. After three years of progressive mental deterioration, Gilles de la Tourette succumbed; he was only forty-seven years old.

Justification

This brief summation of such a productive, intense existence should suffice to demonstrate that Gilles de la Tourette is deserving of a biography. The famous historian and professor Jean Tulard often told his students, "Never write the biography of a man you don't like!" Indeed, it may very well be the biographer's role to share with readers the affection inspired by his or her subject.

About This Book

This book is divided into four parts. The first part explores the name of Gilles de la Tourette and the family's origins, the basis for establishing the family tree; a family that produced no fewer than twelve physicians in four generations. Georges Gilles de la Tourette's brilliant academic career as an adolescent and, later, as a medical student is recounted in detail. Previously unpublished documents are used to elucidate the murder attempt that Gilles de la Tourette was victim to in 1893. His nomination as Chief Physician for the 1900 World's Fair in Paris provides an opportunity to disprove the scandalous rumors targeting him at the time and to enumerate the many duties and responsibilities he successfully managed. While the few existing biographies of Gilles de la Tourette offer little information about his unfortunate demise, the discovery of new documents make it possible to present the final three years of his life in detail.

The second part of this book analyzes the works and medical publications of Gilles de la Tourette. After a short first chapter on his doctoral thesis, a longer chapter addresses the eponymous syndrome in depth, including the origins of this seminal work, the initial errors, and the essential role played by Jean-Martin Charcot. The various books published by Gilles de la Tourette are analyzed within the framework of their historical context, with a special emphasis on *Le Traité de l'Hystérie*, a source of insight concerning the controversies that have developed since its publication with regard to this area of Charcot's work.

The third part of this book examines the works that Gilles de la Tourette published as a historian and his polemic pieces as a journalist. Some of these articles are not well known, given that he wrote under the pen name Paracelsus. Gilles de la Tourette was also friends with a high-profile journalist at the time, Georges Montorgueil. Their friendship lasted many years and was motivated in part by self-interest. The chapter on their correspondence, which is held by the Archives Nationales in Paris, analyzes their exchange and reveals hidden aspects of Gilles de la Tourette's personality. This biographical sketch is followed by a brief and surprising chapter consisting of two poems that Gilles de la Tourette wrote while traveling.

The fourth and final part of this book consists of an annotated summary of all Gilles de la Tourette's publications, useful as a historical research tool.

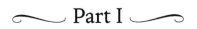

Part I

Life

1

Georges Gilles de la Tourette
(1857–1904)

Origins and Family Life

G ILLES DE LA Tourette is an agreeable-sounding name, both in French and in English. Unfortunately, the eponym, which explains Gilles de la Tourette's lasting fame, is too often reduced to "Tourette," even though, as the origins of his name indicate, "Gilles" is preferable if simplification is indeed necessary. This chapter presents the key events in his personal and family life together, giving some idea of how the provincial bourgeoisie lived in France during the nineteenth century.

The Birth in Saint-Gervais les Trois Clochers

Georges Gilles de la Tourette (1857–1904; Figure 1.1) was born on October 30, 1857, in the village of Saint-Gervais, near the city of Chatellerault in the region of Poitou in western France. The birth took place at the home of Brutus Gilles de la Tourette (1794–1861), probably because he was a physician and the uncle of Georges's father, Théodore-Edouard Gilles de la Tourette (1827–1902). A declaration of birth was made to the mayor of Saint-Gervais, Anacharsis Chasteau, but the record contains errors, despite Chasteau's having previously served as the village notary. The child's registered name was Gilles Georges Albert Brutus de la Tourette and was only

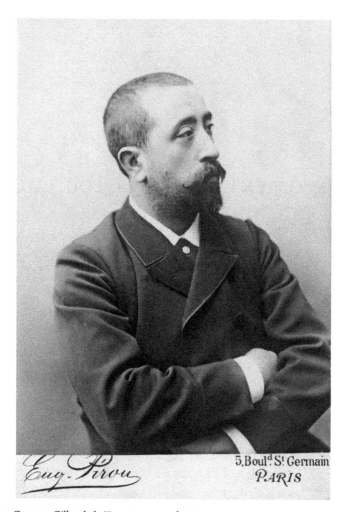

FIGURE I.I Georges Gilles de la Tourette around 1890.
BIU santé, Paris with kind permission.

corrected administratively some thirty years later. His family and given names thus caused confusion throughout his life. Gilles de la Tourette is indeed his family name.

Georges's father, aged thirty when Georges was born, was a shopkeeper on the Rue Bourbon in Chatellerault, the prefectural seat of the Vienne administrative district. His mother, Marie-Françoise Augry des Effes (1831–1902), aged twenty-five at the time, was a housewife (Figure 1.2). Georges was the eldest of four children. His siblings included three sisters: Marie-Albertine (1859–?), Marie-Marguerite (1862–1953), and finally, Laetitia-Anne (1866–?).

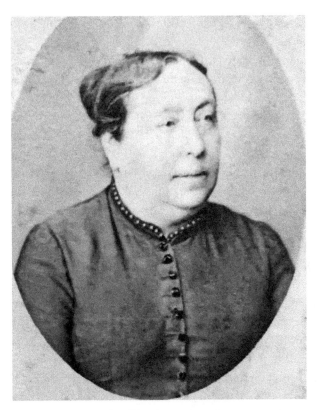

FIGURE 1.2 Marie-Françoise Augry des Effes, Georges's mother.
Copyright Musée Charbonneau-Lassay, Ville de Loudun, with kind permission.

Family Legend

According to documents at the Charbonneau-Lassay Museum in Loudun, where the family archives were found, one of the family's ancestors was apparently an Armenian who, forced to leave the Shah's court in Persia following a revolution around 1200, came to settle in what is now the Poitou-Charentes region, where he married the daughter of a merchant from the town of Niort. The foreigner took the name of Gilles Gifray. His third son took part in the Crusades and distinguished himself through his bravery. In an accolade ceremony, the French King Saint-Louis (1214–1270) is said to have declared: *"I hereby ennoble you and your descendants."* Upon his return from Palestine, Gilles Gifray founded the chapter of Faye-la-Vineuse, a village not far from Saint-Gervais, where he is buried. Until 1793, around the time of the French Revolution, the chapter's canons always included a Gilles, indicating that the family availed itself of simony.[1]

Ancestors, from Gilles to Gilles de la Tourette

Other documents indicate that Jean Gilles, Lord of La Guyonnière and a native of the Vendômois in north-central France, was granted the position of Receiver General of Finances in Poitiers on April 11, 1573. He appears to have founded a large family of "Gilles" in Poitou that includes at least five branches: Gilles de la Coudre, Gilles de la Tourette, Gilles du Vigneau, Gilles de la Veau, and Gilles de Perrière or Gilles des Perrières in the towns and villages of Poitiers, Chatellerault, Loudun, Saint-Gervais, and Faye-la-Vineuse, respectively. Nicolas Gilles, Sieur of Vigneau (1662–1725) (see the family tree in Figure 1.3), born in Faye-la-Vineuse, married Marguerite Pion (1671–1726) on February 8, 1694. The first of their eight children, baptized Joseph (Joseph-Charles I), Sieur of La Tourette (1694–1771), married Françoise Métaier (1707–1781). One of the nine children from their union was Joseph-Charles Gilles de la Tourette (Joseph-Charles II), a merchant married to Marie-Françoise Mercieul and also a salt-tax collector. Georges Gilles de la Tourette was the great-grandson of their eldest son Joseph-Charles (1756–1798; aka Joseph-Charles III), named after his father and grandfather. The sixth of their eight children, Pierre-Clément Gilles de la Tourette (1766–1840), would have a great-granddaughter named Marie Detrois, Georges's future wife; they were fourth cousins.[2]

De la Tourette, a Toponymic Reference

"La Tourette" shows up in the family's archival documents starting in the eighteenth century; until then, they had simply been the Gilles family. Where did this addition come from? Family records of the French nobility show that there were several noblemen with the title "Marquis de la Tourette," particularly in Poitou and Dordogne. But was this a sign of true nobility or simply a toponymic reference? In 1697, an extract of *"the register of the council of Marie de Rochechouart, abbess of Fontevrault"* documented *"a request for an exemption concerning a rent of 6 livres given to the Eglise Saint-Jacques for a house situated on its fief of La Tourette"*; the abbey of Fontevrault is located twenty kilometers north of Loudun. In a register listing conferments and requests for offices and documenting the taking possession of canonries, curacies, and chapels, the "deliberations of the Faye-la-Vineuse chapter" held between 1741 and 1789 are included, as well as the activities of a "Pierre-Michel-Nicolas Gilles, Sieur of La Tourette." A bundle of papers dating from 1714–1765 also contains documents concerning a *"legal proceeding between Antoine Gilles, Sieur of La Tourette, weekly priest of the chapter of Faye, and chaplain*

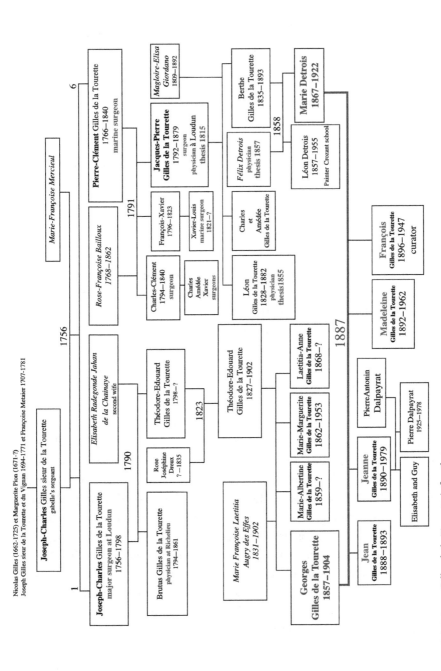

Nicolas Gilles (1662–1725) et Marguerite Pion (1671–?)
Joseph Gilles sieur de la Tourette et du Vignau 1694–1771 et Françoise Metaier 1707–1781

FIGURE 1.3 Gilles de la Tourette's family tree.
Prepared by the author.

of Notre-Dame, defendant; and Gabriel Jamet, fiscal prosecutor of Champigny, seeking to obligate the chaplain to manifest feudal obedience toward said seigniory."[3] This suggests that, as the large Gilles family grew in the Poitou region, place-names were added in the early eighteenth century as an identifying toponymic detail.

While Georges Gilles de la Tourette always expressed his attachment to Loudun, where several members of his family lived, his family's "historic" roots in the eighteenth century were in the place known as "La Tourette," in Faye-la-Vineuse, twenty-five kilometers from Loudun. This is where his great-grandfather, Joseph-Charles Gilles de la Tourette, was born in 1756.

Loudun became the family's village when Joseph-Charles Gilles de la Tourette moved there to practice as a surgeon.

A Family of Physicians

This large family counted no fewer than twelve physicians and surgeons in four generations, and Georges followed in their distinguished footsteps. Joseph-Charles III studied surgery in Paris and practiced in Loudun, as noted earlier, where he was a royal demonstrator in the medical arts of pregnancy and childbirth. He was also *prévôt*, the head of the region's brotherhood of obstetricians. In 1787, he published *"an educational work, also intended for those wishing to learn methods of relieving humanity of its sufferings."* The subject was childbirth and the title *L'art des accouchements*. Its author described it as *"suitable for basic instruction of surgery students, necessary to midwives for distinguishing between those cases in which they may intervene, and those which they must turn over to the Men of the Art."*[4] The Wellcome Library in London also holds an unpublished two-volume text written by Joseph-Charles III entitled *L'Hygiène moderne ou l'art de vivre en santé et de prolonger la vie* (Loudun, 1787).[5] This treatise on health and diet, which contains numerous cross-outs, corrections, and inserts, was clearly prepared for publication, as both volumes include hand-drawn frontispieces. Figure 1.4 shows a leaflet that Joseph-Charles III himself printed in 1790 to advertise the book he planned to publish. However, as the French Revolution was ongoing, he was probably never able to see his project through to completion. Joseph-Charles was the grandfather of Théodore-Edouard Gilles de la Tourette (1827–1902), Georges Gilles de la Tourette's father.

Pierre-Clément Gilles de la Tourette (1766–1840) was a French Navy surgeon in Rochefort in southwestern France; he later set up as a physician in Loudun. The most famous of Pierre-Clément's sons was Jacques-Pierre Gilles de la Tourette (1792–1879; Figure 1.5), a high-ranking military surgeon for the imperial army. During the siege of Torgau in Saxony from October 18 to

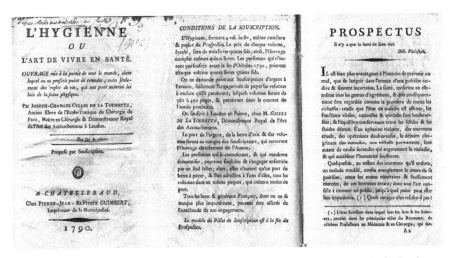

FIGURE I.4 The leaflet printed in 1790 by Joseph-Charles Gilles de la Tourette for his book.
Private collection of the author.

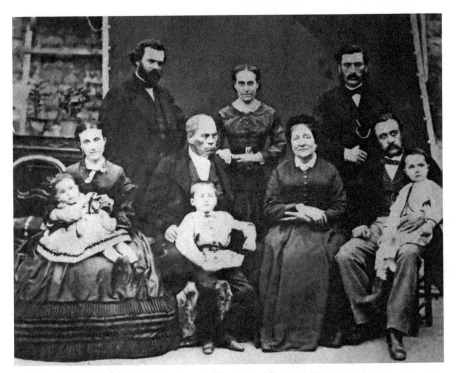

FIGURE I.5 Jacques-Pierre Gilles de la Tourette and his wife Magloire Giordano. *Bottom left, seated*: Berthe Gilles de la Tourette and her baby daughter, Marie.
Copyright Musée Charbonneau-Lassay, Ville de Loudun, with kind permission.

December 26, 1813, by the Prussian forces under the General Bogislav von Tauentzien (1760–1824), Jacques-Pierre cared for some of the 10,000 injured soldiers in Napoleon's army. He remained in Torgau until March 1814 due to a serious typhus epidemic. On March 10, 1814, he was decorated by the Emperor (médaille des Frères d'Armes).

Drawing on what he had learned from combating typhus, Jacques-Pierre prepared a doctoral thesis that he defended in Paris, a year later, on March 17, 1815: *Remarques et observations sur le typhus contagieux qui a régné épidémiquement à Torgau en Saxe, depuis le mois de septembre 1813, jusqu'au mois de mars 1814* (Remarks and observations on the contagious typhus epidemic in Torgau, Saxony, that lasted from September 1813, to March 1814).[6] This thesis is still considered relevant by historians studying the epidemics that plagued Napoleon's campaigns across Europe.[7] After the war, Jacques-Pierre Gilles de la Tourette pursued his medical career in Loudun, where he also took an active interest in local archaeology and history. On November 4, 1826, he married Magloire Elisa Giordano (1809–1892). Their fourth child, Berthe Gilles de la Tourette (1835–1893), was the mother of Marie Detrois, who will marry Georges Gilles de la Tourette in 1887.

The youngest brother of Jacques-Pierre Gilles de la Tourette, named Charles-Clément Gilles de la Tourette (1794–1840), was also a surgeon, and, in keeping with family tradition, his three sons became physicians as well. The youngest, Xavier, lived and practiced in New York.[2] The eldest, Léon Gilles de la Tourette (1828–1882; Figure 1.6), served as a high-ranking military surgeon during the Franco-Prussian War of 1870–1871 (Figure 1.7). He then had a civil career as a physician for state railroad employees, based in Loudun. People remembered him as a devoted doctor who wore a large cape and always traveled on a legendary white horse. Also a historian and archaeologist, he assembled a motley assortment of remarkable stones and Gallo-Roman vestiges that would form the initial collection at the Loudun museum, and he instructed Louis Charbonneau-Lassay (1871–1946) in the techniques of archaeological field research. At the place known as *La Bâtie*, between Loudun and Thouars, he uncovered a sarcophagus containing the remains of a knight known as "Frétard," which since that time have been kept in the Eglise Saint-Pierre in Loudun. On August 15, 1868, Léon was the delegate for the physicians of Vienne at the inauguration of a statue erected in Quimper (Brittany) in honor of René Théophile Hyacinthe Laënnec (1781–1826).[8]

Finally, it should be noted that Léon wrote his doctoral thesis (defended on June 23, 1855, in Paris) on pernicious fever in the district of Loudun. Although he refers to the miasmas thought to cause malaria, it is likely that the cases

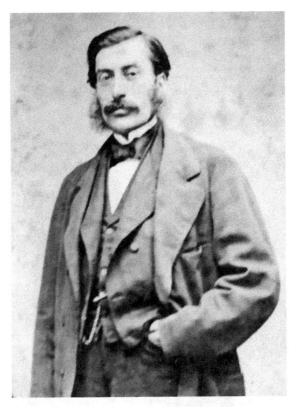

FIGURE I.6 Léon Gilles de la Tourette (1828–1882).
Copyright Musée Charbonneau-Lassay, Ville de Loudun, with kind permission.

described, for which he recommended quinquina, were typhoid fever. The cause of the outbreak was attributed to sewage ponds around the city.[8]

Naming Troubles

The problems with the spelling of the family name were apparently recurrent. In a letter probably addressed to Jacques-Pierre Gilles de la Tourette, dated April 30, 1869, his niece, daughter of Charles-Clément, described her own difficulties with her records, similar to those Georges faced. The confusion around the family name gave rise to multiple variants, nearly untraceable. Here are some examples included in this long letter:

"His marriage certificate shows Charles-Clément Gilles de Latourette, and he signed as C. C. de la Tourette. You signed as Gilles de la Tourette. . . . Joseph signed as Joseph O. G. Latourette and Xavier's father, as Gilles de la Tourette II. On my father's birth

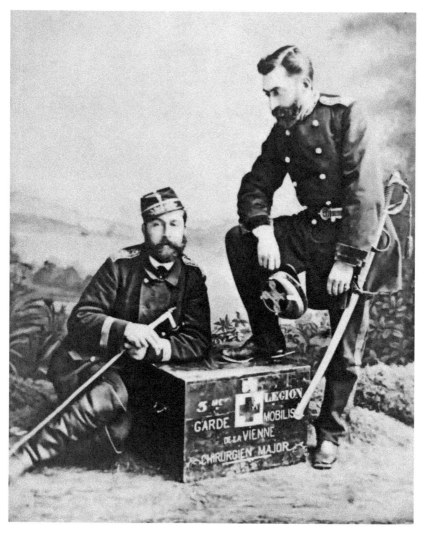

FIGURE 1.7 On the right, Léon Gilles de la Tourette, surgeon during the Franco-Prussian War in 1870.
Copyright Musée Charbonneau-Lassay, Ville de Loudun, with kind permission.

certificate, the times perfectly explain the reserve shown; the declarant was the citizen Gilles de la Tourette and the signature is G. Latourette (Year 2 of the Republic)."

Another signed as Gilles Delatourette in a single word, and so forth. The variants are numerous and confusing, but, in all documents found concerning Georges, Gilles de la Tourette is correctly spelled and not linked in any way to the French nobility.

As the name became more widely known, the confusion persisted. An association of patients with Gilles de la Tourette syndrome and their families was created in 1971 in New York under the name "Gilles de la Tourette Syndrome Association, Inc.," but, in April 1975, Marjorie Guthrie, founder and president of the local committee for the prevention of Huntington's disease and a generous donor to the Gilles de la Tourette Syndrome Association, suggested that the name was too long and difficult to pronounce for English speakers. A decision was made to shorten it, and, unfortunately, the association has since been known as the Tourette Syndrome Association. Today, international publications refer to the illness using the regrettable abbreviation of "Tourette syndrome."[9]

The errors continued after Georges's death. In the obituary section of *La Vie Médicale*, on May 25, 1904, a certain Michaut submitted a slanderous diatribe against Georges Gilles de la Tourette, rather than the usual eulogy. Of course, he did not check the accuracy of what he wrote: *"A victim of medical ambition recently died in a rest home in Lausanne. Gilles La Tourette (he dressed up his name with an article), who lost his mind five years ago, recently passed away at the age of forty-seven."*[10] In a 1948 memoir, Julien Besançon (1862–1952) made similarly ludicrous remarks: *"Gilles de la Tourette tried to excuse the nobility of his 'de la' name by a fanatical anticlericalism that often lacked refinement. He had learned from a master, Charcot, and from his alter ego, the secularist Bourneville."*[11] It bears restating that the name Gilles de la Tourette does not have any actual ties with the French nobility, and by no means did Georges himself try to refashion his name. Nonetheless, he was repeatedly the victim of this sort of caustic slander, especially after his death. Those who criticized him represented a clerical, right-leaning faction with which Gilles de la Tourette, Désiré-Magloire Bourneville (1840–1909), and Jean-Martin Charcot (1825–1893) were frequently at odds (the following chapters provide numerous examples of their conflicts).

Marriage with Marie Destrois

Gilles de la Tourette's marriage to his cousin Marie Detrois (1867–1922) (Figure 1.8) meant that the family name was now on both sides of their family tree. The ceremony took place on August 2, 1887, in Loudun. His teachers Paul Brouardel (1837–1906), François Damaschino (1840–1889), and Charcot served as his witnesses. Marie Detrois, a Gilles de la Tourette on her mother's side of the family, thus picked up the family name again. A card from the family's archives indicates that Georges and Marie were in Scotland for their honeymoon.

When Marie became a Gilles de la Tourette, her family heritage had to live up to the medical legend of her husband's name. In this respect, she

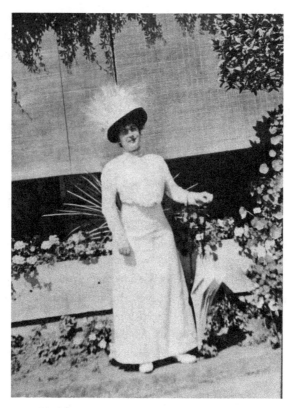

FIGURE I.8 Marie Detrois (1867–1922) married to Georges on August 2, 1887.
Copyright Musée Charbonneau-Lassay, Ville de Loudun, with kind permission.

did not disappoint. Marie's great-grandfather Pierre-Clément Gilles de la Tourette, her grandfather Jacques-Pierre Gilles de la Tourette, and her father Félix Detrois were all physicians, following the family tradition. Félix Detrois defended his thesis on June 24, 1857, in Paris: *De l'hyperémie chronique de l'estomac.* After his marriage on April 25, 1858, with Berthe Gilles de la Tourette (1835–1893), the fourth child of Jacques-Pierre Gilles de la Tourette, he spent his entire career in Chinon, a city renowned for its wines. Whereas Marie Gilles de la Tourette married a physician, her brother Léon Detrois (1857–1955) forged his own path as a well-known painter who signed his works "Léon Detroy."

Children of Georges and Marie

Georges and Marie Gilles de la Tourette had four children. The eldest, Jean (1888–1893), died of meningitis on July 11, 1893, at the age of five (Figure 1.9).

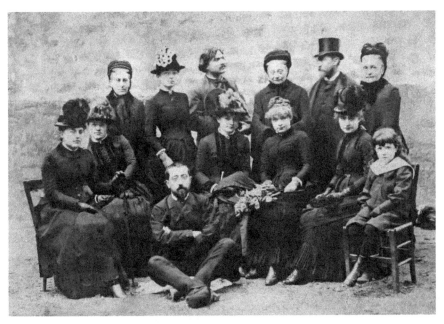

FIGURE I.9 Georges, seated. Marie and Jean seated on the right, a few weeks before Jean's death in July 1893. At the back right, standing, Félix and Berthe Detrois, Marie's parents.
Copyright Musée Charbonneau-Lassay, Ville de Loudun, with kind permission.

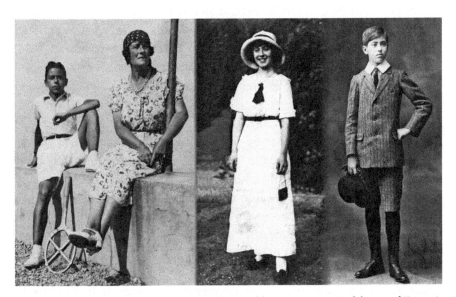

FIGURE I.10 From left to right, Jeanne Dalpeyrat and her son, Pierre; Madeleine and François Gilles de la Tourette.
Copyright Musée Charbonneau-Lassay, Ville de Loudun, with kind permission.

Their daughter, Jeanne (1890–1979), married Antonin Dalpeyrat in Paris on January 10, 1923. She kept the family archives that are now part of the collection at the Loudun museum (Figure 1.10). One of her sons, Pierre Dalpeyrat (1925–1978), was supposedly a gangster in the 1950s and went by the name of "Pierrot les Rouflaquettes," a reference to his sideburns, according to a collateral descendant. Georges Gilles de la Tourette had an outlaw for a grandson!

Their second daughter, Madeleine Gilles de la Tourette (1892–1962), did not marry and had no children. Finally, the fourth child, François Gilles de la Tourette (1896–1947), was an art critic, author of several books, and curator at the Petit Palais and later the Musée National d'Art Moderne, in Paris (Figure 1.10). *L'Orient et les peintres de Venise* (*The Orient and the Painters of Venice*), his first book, was published in 1923, followed by books on Nicolas Poussin, Lautrec, and Robert Delaunay, among others. Today, the family name of Gilles de la Tourette is no longer in use.

A Parisian Life

Georges Gilles de la Tourette grew up in Chatellerault, where he attended primary and secondary school. He began his medical studies in Poitiers and then pursued them in Paris, where he lived at 36 Rue Bonaparte in 1878, and at 43 Rue Monge in 1879. According to his military records, he had been conscripted while a medical student in 1875 and served as a nurse from November 8, 1876, to November 8, 1877. At his initial medical exam, on October 27, 1876, he measured 1.66 meters tall. His eyes were reported as blue and his hair and eyebrows as light brown.

The year before his marriage, on February 6, 1886, he moved to 14 Rue de Beaune, where he set up his first medical office. This is where the couple was living when their first three children were born. In 1893, after Jean's death, undoubtedly to distance unhappy memories, the family moved one street away, to 39 Rue de l'Université, where they lived in a ground-level apartment. Three years later, François Gilles de la Tourette was born. A photo of the Rue de l'Université office exists (Figure 1.11), and, although the quality is poor, it suggests the era's taste for heavy decoration and calls to mind Charcot's interior on Boulevard Saint-Germain. There appears to be a painting of Jacques-Pierre Gilles de la Tourette in the background.

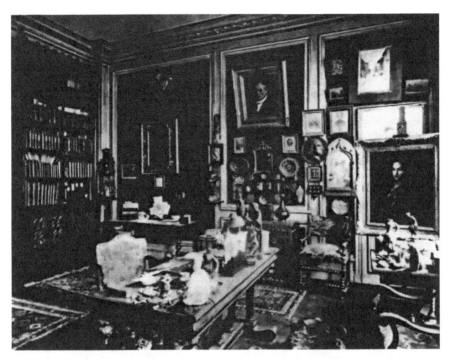

FIGURE I.II Gilles de la Tourette's interior on 39 rue de l'Uniersité Paris VII, around 1900.
Private collection of the author.

The following chapter introduces young Gilles de la Tourette, first the brilliant but unruly student and later the ambitious young physician making his way within the hospital and university hierarchies.

Notes

1. For Catholics, simony is the buying and selling of spiritual goods, in particular of sacraments, but also of ecclesiastical offices.
2. Beauchet-Filleau H & P. *Dictionnaire historique et généalogique des familles du Poitou*. Poitiers: Imprimerie Ourdin. 1891.
3. Beauchet-Filleau H, De Chergé Ch. *Dictionnaire historique et généalogique des familles du Poitou*. Fontenay le Comte: Lussaud frères. 1963.
4. Gilles de la Tourette JC. *L'Art des accouchemens: propre aux instructions élémentaires des élèves en chirurgie, nécessaire aux sages-femmes pour leur indiquer les cas où elles peuvent opérer, et ceux où elles doivent mander les hommes de l'art: ouvrage didactique, également fait pour les personnes qui désirent s'instruire des moyens de soulager l'humanité souffrante*. A Paris, chez Le Clerc et à Angers, chez Pavie, 1787.

5. Wellcome Library. GB. References MS8570/1 and MS8570/2. Translation of title: *Modern Hygiene or the Art of Healthy Living and Longevity*.

6. Gilles de La Tourette JP. Remarques et observations sur le typhus contagieux qui a régné épidémiquement à Torgau en Saxe, depuis le mois de septembre 1813 jusqu'au mois de mars 1814. Thèse no. 71. Paris: Imprimerie Didot jeune. 1815.

7. Ducoulombier H. L'aigle et le pou: le typhus dans la Grande Armée. *Histoire des Sciences Médicales*. 2014;48(3):351–360.

8. Galbrun M. Léon Gilles de la Tourette, un précurseur de notre musée. La Voix du Loudunais du 28 novembre 1948.

9. Kushner H. *A Cursing Brain, the Histories of Tourette Syndrome*. Cambridge, MA: Harvard University Press. 1999.

10. Michaut. Varia, nécrologie. *La Vie Médicale*. 1904;13(516):333.

11. Besançon J. *La pie borgne*. Paris: La Clé d'Or. 1948.

2

Education, Medical Studies, Medical Practice

Early Education

At the lower secondary school in Chatellerault, Georges Gilles de la Tourette was a brilliant student, although disruptive and undisciplined. He would always have an impulsive personality. By the age of sixteen, he had finished his secondary school education, having obtained both the literary and scientific baccalaureates since, at that time, the two diplomas were necessary to enter medical school.

Gilles de la Tourette's precocity in school was at times a handicap, resulting in a lack of maturity in his daily life. According to Paul Le Gendre (1854–1936), Gilles de la Tourette's mother was aware of the problem and had carefully considered it; she *"thought he was too young for the risks of the Latin Quarter in Paris and thus moved him to Poitiers, where he remained for around four years."*[1] Le Gendre was an *interne* (medical student living and working in the hospital) at the same time as Gilles de la Tourette, becoming a close friend and later his biographer. Le Gendre wrote: *"At a time when students in Paris had no direction whatsoever in their studies, starting in a provincial school was an excellent approach. The danger for Gilles, had he come to Paris too young, would not have been, I believe, giving in to easy pleasures at the brasseries of Boulevard Saint-Michel; he was as hard working as he was curious. But his curiosity would have been a danger. With his taste for history and literature, he might have been tempted to abandon his classes at the Faculté de Médecine and the hospitals for the classes at the Sorbonne and the Collège de*

France. Or he may have slipped into one of the literary or mainstream newspapers and ended up exclusively a journalist, rather than finding in journalism a pastime that provided diversion from his medical career." At the Ecole de Médecine de Poitiers, Gilles de la Tourette studied with Pierre-Ernest Guignard (1817–1882) in 1875, and, in 1876, with Jean Guérineau, a physician with a scientific mind who sought to apply the laws of physics to physiology.

Competitive Examinations

From the beginning of the nineteenth century to the present, competitive exams have dominated both university life and hospital life. They are a French peculiarity, the purpose of which is to select an "elite" based on a series of challenging tests. The so-called *externat, internat, and médicat* examinations in Paris hospitals were established by the statutes of the Health Service in 1804, while the *agrégation* examination for academic positions dates from 1823. Paris hospital examinations, completely independent from university examinations, were overseen by the managing entity of the Parisian public hospitals, the "Assistance Publique." In French medicine, these examinations are the most prestigious and difficult to pass.

From the time of his arrival in Paris in 1877, Gilles de la Tourette began to prepare for the *externe* exam required to work and study in the Paris hospitals. For his first attempt at the exam, he did not return after the initial component on Wednesday, October 24, 1877; the subject was *"bones of the orbital cavity."* Joseph Babiński (1857–1932) passed the exam that year. Gilles de la Tourette would pass it in 1878, ranking 195th out of 231 candidates. Le Gendre also passed the exam in 1878. The tests were completed orally, and the subjects were selected at random. The candidate had five minutes to prepare, then five minutes for the presentation. The jury included Fulgence Raymond (1844–1910), who would succeed Jean-Martin Charcot (1825–1893) as chair of neurology at the Faculty of Medicine in 1894. Not surprisingly, Georges was listed as "Latourette" on the registration papers, with the inconsistent spelling of his name following him even to medical school. On Saturday, October 26, 1878, the twenty-three candidates were given the subject *"varicose veins in the lower limbs."* Sixth in the line-up of candidates, Georges received a grade of 9/20. For the second component, held on Tuesday, November 26, 1878, he was the first candidate to present on *"erysipelas"* and received a grade of 13/20.[2] With these results he passed the exam and qualified as an *externe* in the Paris hospitals. In his day, nearly two-thirds of the candidates passed the test.

His first year of *externat* took place in 1879, at Hôpital des Enfants Malades (children's hospital) with Dr. Jacques-Louis Molland (1826–1879), known for his description of the different modes of progression in pneumonia. In 1880, at Hôpital Saint-Louis, Gilles de la Tourette divided his second year between dermatology, with Professor Jean-Baptiste Hillairet (1815–1882), and surgery with Professor Auguste Le Dentu (1841–1926), an ardent advocate of emergency appendectomies and a pioneer of urological surgery and surgery on the adrenal glands. On Gilles de la Tourette's administrative evaluation,[3] Hillairet complimented his student: *"High level of knowledge, very hard-working, full of enthusiasm in his duties."* Le Dentu's assessment was also favorable: *"Distinguished and knowledgeable student, likely to succeed."*

All *externes* prepared for the competitive exam to advance to the next level: the *internat*. Relatively few students passed this exam; they were an elite, not only because the exam was difficult, but also because the *internat* was a comprehensive four-year training program during which students had hospital duties overseen by expert teachers, some of whom were famous. To replace *internes* obligated to give up their positions between two exam sessions (military obligations, disease, and death were not uncommon), the hospital administration appointed the best among those who had failed the last exam as "temporary" *internes*.[4]

In 1881, Georges was a temporary *interne* and had the opportunity to study with Louis Landouzy (1845–1917), the first to attribute an infectious origin to herpes in 1884. Gilles de la Tourette passed the *interne* exam for the Paris hospitals in December 1881. Charcot was a member of the jury chaired by Léon Labbé (1832–1916). Gilles de la Tourette received a grade of 15/20, ranking twenty-eight of the fifty-two who had passed.[5] Their class included several young men who would rise to prominence: Antonin Marfan (1858–1942), Eugène Doyen (1859–1926), Louis Thoinot (1858–1915), and Georges's friend, Le Gendre.

Meeting Charcot as an *Interne*

Gilles de la Tourette began his *internat* at the Hôpital du Midi with Zozime Désiré Simonet (1823–1884), who wrote in his evaluation: *"Carried out his duties as well as could be expected given his numerous personal activities and the frequent leaves he took during the year. Did not perform on-call or night duties."* This assessment suggests that his superior did not approve of him, which may explain why Gilles de la Tourette spent the second part of 1882 with Achille Gougenheim (1839–1901), at Hôpital de Lourcine. Gougenheim is known for having defended the first thesis on aneurysms in the arteries of the brain. In 1883, Gilles de la Tourette continued his training in what is now known as "internal medicine" at Hôpital Laënnec, under the Professor Damaschino (1840–1889), with whom he would form a lasting friendship (Figure 2.1). Damaschino would be one of the witnesses at his wedding, and Gilles de la Tourette would write Damaschino's eulogy when he died prematurely at age forty-nine.[6] Damaschino evaluated his student very favorably: *"Hard-working, knowledgeable, ambitious, and capable of pursuing an enviable scientific career."*

In 1884, Gilles de la Tourette moved to Charcot's department at La Salpêtrière. Charcot described him as *"very knowledgeable, very devoted to the department, first-class interne."* At the time, Charcot was at the summit of his neurological career. He was fifty-nine and famous throughout the world. He had been studying hysteria for fifteen years. From that point forward, he would concentrate his attention on this condition, for which his research method, the anatomical-clinical method, had failed, as it had for epilepsy; both pathologies were neurological in appearance but had no appreciable anatomical correlate in terms of lesions in the nervous system. Except for two articles in English

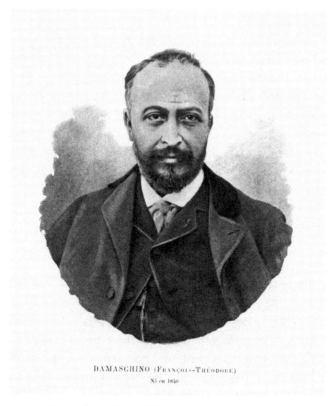

DAMASCHINO (François-Théodore)
Né en 1840

FIGURE 2.1 François Damaschino (1840–1889).
Private collection of the author.

published in the New York journal *Forum*, Charcot would no longer publish after 1884 under his own name, choosing instead to promote the publications of his favorite students.

Le Gendre wrote unequivocally of Gilles de la Tourette's relationship with Charcot: *"From this day forward, his vocation was set. There were other teachers, such as Damaschino, Brouardel, and Alfred Fournier, for whom he would always express his gratitude in the warmest terms, but Charcot would be his veritable god. As soon as he started working with Charcot, he made sure to carefully note everything his teacher said or merely suggested day after day."* Charcot himself paid tribute to the patient historiographical transcription of his own thoughts over eight years, when he wrote in the preface of *Traité de l'Hystérie*: *'While reading the work of Gilles de la Tourette before it was printed, I was surprised on several occasions to find ideas of mine I considered absolutely personal, ideas I thought I never talked about, which, in any case, had never been published.'* From the beginning of his career, Gilles de la Tourette always sought to promote and protect Charcot's ideas. He revered the Master, never questioned him, and adopted all of his positions uncritically.

In 1831, the hospital administration instituted a competitive exam followed by a jury selection to award a medal to the *interne* with the most favorable record of service. The medal winner would then have the opportunity to complete a research project in the hospital of his choice.

Gilles de la Tourette enrolled to compete for this *internat* medal in 1883 but did not submit his project. He competed in 1885 but was not awarded the medal[7] (Figure 2.2). The seminal article describing the disease that would be named for him was written in 1884, during his *internat* year under Charcot, and was published in January 1885, in *Les Archives de Neurologie*.[8] In his 1893 homage to the Master, Gilles de la Tourette described how Charcot worked: *"Possessing a keen knowledge of his students, he divided the tasks between them and knew both how to inspire each one in his work and leave him the honor of its completion."*[9] The 1885 article, written by a young physician still in training, perfectly illustrates Charcot's approach: he suggested a topic, discreetly oversaw all phases of the work, then had his student publish it under his own name. Charcot knew how to leverage the specific strengths of each of his students, and he guided their work without seeking his own fame or claiming the results for himself. Gilles de la Tourette was particularly reverential, feeling intellectually indebted to the Master throughout his life.

A Portrait of an Interne

What sort of personality did Gilles de la Tourette have? Why did Charcot take a liking to him and accord him the task of writing the Salpêtrière summary reports on hysteria in addition to the article that led to the eponym? As Le

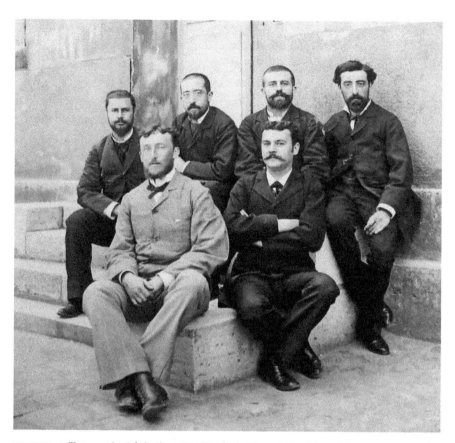

FIGURE 2.2 "Internat La Salpêtrière, 1884." In the bright suit, René Semelaigne (1855–1934), the grandson of Philippe Pinel (1745–1826). Georges is seated behind him.
Private collection of the author.

Gendre portrayed Gilles de la Tourette at the time, he was *"a jovial and exuberant boy, with the gift of the gab and a presumptuous tone. Unfortunately, his voice was gruff and a little hoarse. Very enthusiastic, but rather impatient, he wasn't one to let opponents exhaust their arguments little by little, then refute them point by point; he flew to defend himself from the first contradiction. His many adversaries did not lessen his impetuosity, and the husky strains of his voice could be heard bursting forth in the middle of even the noisiest discussions."* This portrait should be read alongside that penned by Léon Daudet (1867–1942) in 1915, its caustic tone very different. Léon Daudet was the son of the famous writer Alphonse Daudet (1840–1897), who was a close friend of Charcot. Léon, also a talented writer, became a famous journalist and a vocal critic of the French Republic, the Dreyfusard camp, and democracy in general. *"Gilles de la Tourette was ugly, like a Papuan idol covered with patches of hair. He was neither good nor bad, neither studious nor lazy, neither intelligent nor stupid, and he oscillated, either dull or malicious, between any number of strengths and weaknesses, never embodying any one for long. He had a raspy and scorched voice, abrupt gestures, and a grotesque demeanor. He was seen as unusual. He would broach an interesting subject, then let it drop in favor of another. He disconcerted his teachers with quirks that became increasingly frequent and less and less amusing.*"[10] Daudet struck again in 1922: *"Another puppet, who had a sad end, was the poor Gilles de la Tourette. This bouncy name did not match his hairy and rough appearance, that of a guignol carved in yellow wood. He affected the artist's macabre air, joking as he chuckled, chuckling as he joked, and when he guffawed he spread an odor of carbolated liver."*[11] Gilles de la Tourette is portrayed here as repulsive, which is how Daudet highlighted his personal and ideological dislike of the young physician. Daudet was known for never hesitating to defame, especially when doing so added color to his diatribes. Despite its exaggeration and bias, this depiction captures some aspects of Gilles de la Tourette's appearance and behavior.

Arsène Arnaud Claretie, known as Jules Claretie (1840–1913), was a novelist, theater critic, and chronicler of Parisian life (Figure 2.3). Inspired by the socialist ideals of politicians such as Jules Ferry (1832–1893), Emile Combes (1835–1921), and Jean Jaurès (1859–1914), Claretie was an active Dreyfusard Republican—and a convincing one. There is no doubt that Gilles de la Tourette shared the same progressive and anticlerical stance. Claretie,

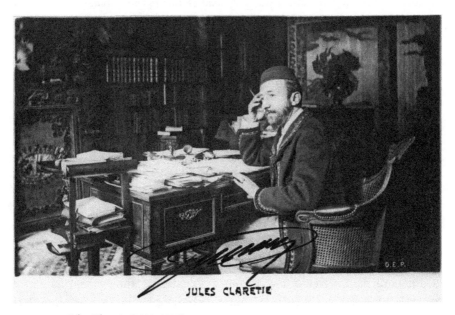

JULES CLARETIE

FIGURE 2.3 Jules Claretie (1840–1913).
Postcard, private collection of the author.

a regular at the Tuesday evening gatherings in the Charcot's home, paints an entirely different picture of Georges in this 1904 portrait: *"This man that science has just lost, I can still see him as a young* interne, *gay and charming. Under the large tree in the courtyard, near the old buildings of the hospital, where the fictional Manon Lescaut and the historical Théroigne once strolled, we dined and confabulated, enjoying the fresh air, drinking the Touraine wine that Gilles de la Tourette had brought from a vineyard once belonging to Rabelais. He had a keen intelligence, an alert mind, he championed political causes, took an interest in literature, he adored Charcot and was esteemed by him in turn, as was the eminent Professor Gilbert Ballet, a native of Haute-Vienne like myself to whom I am indebted for my novel* Les Amours d'un Interne. *Gilles de la Tourette, a lover of journalism who dreamed of a statue to honor Théophraste Renaudot, developed his theories and shared his hopes."*[12]

Thesis

Gilles de la Tourette spent his last and fourth year as an *interne*, in 1885, at Hôpital de La Pitié, in the department of Paul Brouardel (1837–1906) (Figure 2.4), who found him to be *"an excellent* interne, *very knowledgeable, dedicated, excellent relations with others; has a brilliant career ahead of him."* As Le Gendre writes, *"Mr. Brouardel was very fond of this talented student who was so ardent in his work and had literary as well as medical abilities; in 1885, he made him his assistant for his forensic medicine classes."*

It was during his time as an *interne* under Charcot in 1884, and under Brouardel in 1885, that Gilles de la Tourette researched and wrote his thesis, which he defended on December 28, 1885. Charcot presided over the jury, which also included Damaschino, Landouzy, and Alix Joffroy (1844–1908). The work was entitled: *"Etudes cliniques et physiologiques sur la marche; la marche dans les maladies du système nerveux étudiée par la méthode des empreintes"* (Clinical and physiological studies of gait; walking in patients with nervous system diseases, studied by the footprint tracing method); we cover Gilles de la Tourette's thesis in Chapter 8. Parallel to his training at the hospital, and like many La Salpêtrière students at that time, Gilles de la Tourette took histology and histopathology courses with Louis Ranvier (1835–1922) and Louis Malassez (1849–1909) at the Collège de France.

Edouard de Lavarenne (1855?–1907), founder of the journal *La Presse Médicale*, summed up Gilles de la Tourette's biography this way in 1893: *"It is true that Gilles de la Tourette was prodigiously active, his activity sometimes verging on agitation, and one wonders if this state didn't become, before long, an unhealthy*

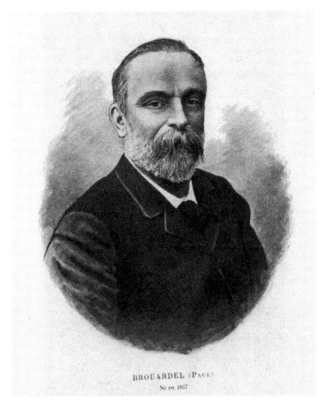

BROUARDEL (Paul)
Né en 1837

FIGURE 2.4 Paul Brouardel (1837–1906).
Private collection of the author.

one."[13] Gilles de la Tourette's hyperactivity was deeply ingrained, a cardinal trait of his personality that made an impression on everyone around him.

Chef de Clinique

Charcot chose Gilles de la Tourette to replace Babiński as *chef de clinique* starting in November 1887; these duties would last two years. It was at the start of his *clinicat* that André Brouillet (1857–1914) presented his famous painting, *Une leçon clinique à la Salpêtrière,* at the 1887 Salon des Indépendants. The painting shows Gilles de la Tourette in the foreground, wearing a large white apron, his gaze focused on Marie "Blanche" Wittmann (1859–1913) (Figure 2.5). Wittmann was a laundress who had entered the hospital ten years earlier, on May 6, 1877, at the age of eighteen, for hysteria. In the painting, she is supported by Babiński, as the head nurse Marguerite Bottard (1822–1906) looks on.[14]

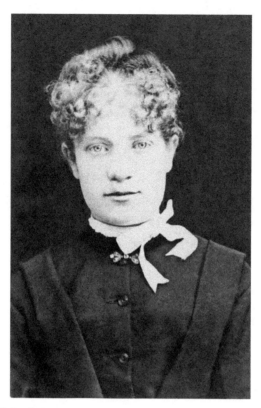

FIGURE 2.5 Marie "Blanche" Wittmann (1859–1913).
Private collection of the author.

Blanche W., as Gilles de la Tourette referred to her in his writings, was one
of the patients with whom he spent long days on hypnosis experiments, which
were in progress as Brouillet was working on his painting. In his account of
the 1887 Salon, Louis de Fourcaud (1851–1914)[15] wrote: *"The subject of Mr.
Brouillet's remarkable painting is a lesson by Prof. Charcot at Hôpital La Salpêtrière.
In the bright room, its large windows forming the painting's background, the Master
of nervous diseases faces a poor woman suffering from hysterical phenomena. She is
upright but supported by an interne, and accompanied by two nurses, one of them
older. Her wrists are contracted, her eyes adrift. The patient is young, even pretty—
what a shame! The great doctor is about to begin his experiments, and with measure
and benevolence, standing near the patient, he leads into his explanations. One can
see the attention on every face. There are internes, students taking notes, specialist
physicians, such as Gilles de la Tourette, who wrote an excellent book on the subject;
there are chemists such as Mr. Floquet, writers such as Mr. Philippe Burty[16] and Mr.
Jules Claretie, and even a priest.[17] Light is subtly captured in the various parts of the
room. The scene is striking and sure to retain its virtue, given the skill with which it*

has been rendered."[18] To avoid anachronism, we must imagine ourselves in the timeframe of the 1887 Salon. Fourcaud had probably never met the physicians painted by Brouillet, except for Charcot, and was unable to put names to faces. Those who became major names in neurology, Babiński and Pierre Marie (1853 –1940), for example, had yet to publish the work that would make them famous. Only Gilles de la Tourette was known for his publications, including his biography of Théophraste Renaudot, and that of Sœur Jeanne des Anges in Bourneville's "Bibliothèque diabolique" collection, along with his recently released book on hypnotism (we return to this in later chapters). Brouillet's painting is currently on display near the entrance to the medical history museum, at the Faculté de Médecine on Rue de l'Ecole de Médecine in Paris. The plaque naming the people in the painting contains an error, frequently reproduced. Georges is identified as the bearded man on Charcot's right, behind the man with the pencil, who is Paul Richer (1849–1933). The bearded man scratching his face is, in fact, another former Charcot *interne*, Charles Féré (1852–1907).

Gilles de la Tourette was also known for his political engagement during his time as *chef de clinique*. On July 11, 1889, in the paper *Le Gaulois*, the journalist known by the pen name of Saint Real reported the following: *"A very touching display of support for the former Prime Minister of Greece (whose dignified resignation caused a stir during the 1885 blockade) took place yesterday, Wednesday, at three o'clock. A delegation of thirty students made its way to the Hôtel Continental, led by Mr. Gilles de la Tourette, chef de clinique at the Faculté de Médecine. Mr. Delyannis*[19] *welcomed the students with rare affability. Speaking on behalf of young people in universities, Mr. Gilles de la Tourette expressed their deep admiration for the great patriot and son of a hero who, in response to legitimate claims, preferred to step down from power rather than perpetuate the barbaric notion that force is above and beyond the law."*[20]

According to Le Gendre, in addition to caring for hospitalized patients, the *chef de clinique* had to *"prepare the lessons of a professor, such as Prof. Charcot at La Salpêtrière, and reconcile initiative with obedience. Overseeing every detail of a vast department was an exhausting task. But Gilles not only found every means to complete his work; he also developed excellent friendships. In 1888, collaborating with the skillful artist P. Richer and with Londe, he helped to launch the publication La Nouvelle Iconographie de La Salpêtrière."* The first issue of this new journal, dated January–February 1888, featured an article by Gilles de la Tourette—"L'attitude et la marche dans l'hémiplégie hystérique" (Attitude and gait in hysterical hemiplegia)—an opportunity to refer to his thesis and to reproduce two of the footprint drawings it contained (see Chapter 8).

Gilles de la Tourette's primary activity remained his work for the Master at La Salpêtrière. Charcot was the head of a school in the most rigorous sense and knew how to impose discipline on his students, according to Georges Guinon (1859–1932): *"Charcot exercised his intransigent authority first and foremost over his students, none of whom would ever dare to defy him."*[21] Charcot, a demanding teacher, could not have produced a body of internationally known work while he was still alive without the help and enthusiasm of numerous colleagues, especially those *internes* and *chefs de clinique* who became his faithful disciples. It was this subtle alchemy that led Babiński to remark, at the 100-year anniversary celebration of Charcot's birth: *"Charcot knew how to create close bonds with those who, like myself, lived and worked with him. His genius alone earned him unanimous esteem."*[22]

Charcot's talent consisted in identifying the strengths and the potential of his students according to each man's personality. He encouraged them to pursue the path best suited to their abilities. Without claiming their results for himself, he used their findings to further his own work and publications. In the case of Bourneville, he provided Charcot with a link to the progressive political world and was his preferred publisher. Another example is Albert Gombault (1844–1904), Charcot's *interne* for 1872. The Master soon noticed Gombault's meticulous attention to detail and had him carry out microscopic examination of anatomical parts from the autopsies of patients who died in the department. For twenty-five years, his work behind the scenes allowed Charcot to consolidate his anatomical-clinical method. Gombault, a shy and reserved man, thus became a recognized expert in anatomical pathology of the nervous system.

Paul Richer, an *interne* with artistic talents who illustrated his own thesis on hysteria, accompanied Charcot to museums. As for Gilles de la Tourette, there can be no doubt that Charcot thought highly of his enthusiasm and capacity for hard work as well as his writing abilities. Charcot paid him the honor of choosing him to be his private secretary from 1887 to 1888 (see Chapter 3). And Gilles de la Tourette held Charcot in high esteem: *"Aside from the joys of family life, aside from the keen and constant interest he took in his students, Charcot only cared for science, the arts, and philosophy. Those who lived close to him on a daily basis can attest to the fact that he never partook in futile conversations."*

Meeting Sigmund Freud at La Salpêtrière

One function of the *chef de clinique* was to orient students and to welcome guests and foreign physicians visiting the department. In this way, Gilles de la Tourette served as a guide for Sigmund Freud (1856–1939), who stayed in Paris from October 20, 1885, to February 28, 1886. Freud described the people he met, in particular Gilles de la Tourette, in the numerous letters he sent to his fiancée in Vienna, Martha Bernays (1861–1951).[23] On January 18, 1886, he wrote: *"He* [Charcot] *has invited me, along with Richetti, to visit him at his home tomorrow, Tuesday, after dinner. 'Many people will be in attendance.' I'm sure you can imagine my apprehension mixed with curiosity and pride. White gloves, white tie, and even a new shirt, a visit to the barber's for what little hair I have left. And a little cocaine to loosen my tongue."* During another evening, on January 20, 1886, he met Gilles de la Tourette: *"We were the first to arrive and had to wait for the diners to leave the dining room. In the meantime, we admired the marvelous salons. But then the guests arrived and we were under fire. Mr. and Mrs. Charcot, Miss Jeanne Charcot, Mr. Léon Charcot, a young Mr. Daudet, son of Alphonse Daudet; Prof. Brouardel, a medical examiner with an energetic and intelligent face; Mr. Strauss, Pasteur's assistant and well known for his work on cholera; Prof. Lépine of Lyon, one of the most eminent French clinicians; a sickly little man and an authentic southerner, Mr. Gilles de la Tourette. . . . I approached Lépine whose work I know and had a long conversation with him, then I spoke with Strauss and Gilles de la Tourette."* Freud had seen Gilles de la Tourette at La Salpêtrière before that evening and was already familiar with the man and his manners. It was his noisy hyperactivity, his hypomanic logorrhea that Freud associated with southern ways.

On February 2, 1886, Freud was once again Charcot's guest: *"It was deathly boring and my little dose of cocaine saved me. If you can imagine, this time there were forty or fifty people and I only knew three or four. . . . The Chief was not at his best and remained seated almost the entire time; he looked very tired to me. Naturally, he didn't fail to invite me here and there, to offer me food and drink, but that's all I got from him. . . . It was only toward the end of the evening that I began a political conversation with Gilles de la Tourette in which he, of course, prophesized the most terrible of wars with Germany. I immediately let him know that I was neither German nor Austrian but Jewish. This kind of conversation I always find very disagreeable because it stirs up something German in me that I decided long ago to stifle."* What Freud related perfectly illustrates the spirit of revenge that was palpable at all levels of French society after France's defeat in the 1870 Franco-Prussian War. Gilles de la Tourette's premonition was neither extraordinary nor specific to him alone. On Wednesday, February 10, 1886, Freud continued with the description of another evening: *"I once again spoke at length with Charcot himself, from whom I also borrowed a book and one issue of a journal. . . . I left with Mr. Gilles de la Tourette; even though it was half past midnight, he invited me into his home to give me a paper he had promised me. The following day I couldn't help but think myself an ass to be leaving Paris now, as spring approaches and Notre Dame is so beautiful in the sun. I would only have to ask Charcot to be allowed to treat the patients as I see fit. But I am neither courageous nor carefree enough to prolong my stay here."* It is well known that Freud held Charcot in high esteem, and the feeling was apparently mutual; their correspondence, however, reveals more about Charcot than Freud.[24] Unfortunately, no documents written by Gilles de la Tourette have been found that mention Freud, and apparently they did not keep in touch after Freud's departure from Paris. We will return to Freud's explanations of convulsive tics in Chapter 9, on Tourette syndrome.

"Médecin des Hôpitaux" and University Career

In Gilles de la Tourette's day, the function and title of "physician in the Paris hospitals" entailed passing a competitive exam that included a written component, an oral component, and a "patient" component. The administration usually organized two exams per year and recruited three physicians from each exam. There were around seventy candidate physicians, with only around ten physicians taking the exam for the first time at each session. The successful applicants became "Central Office Physicians," a status shared by numerous doctors who were not yet assigned to a specific hospital department. The "Central Office," created on 24 Nivôse An X (January 14, 1802), was in operation until October 1895 and was located Place du Parvis-Notre-Dame, next to the Hôpital de l'Hôtel-Dieu. Its role was to receive patients who, after having been examined, were either sent to the hospital within the Paris system that had room for them, depending on their pathology, or were sent home with treatment. When a hospital position was vacated, it was assigned to the Central Office Physician who had been waiting the longest. Central Office Physicians also replaced the *chefs de service* (chief physicians) during their vacations or other absences.

Gilles de la Tourette had already made seven attempts when he registered for the hospital physician exam on Monday, February 27, 1893. There were seventy-one other candidates, including sixty-three "veterans" like himself. The members of the jury, presided over by Labbé, were Albert Robin (1847–1928), Joffroy, Eugène d'Heilly (1832–1902), Charles Fernet (1838–1919), Albert Brault (1852–1939), and Jean-Joseph Peyrot (1843–1917). The subject of the first three-hour written component was *"acute non-tuberculous cerebral meningitis; clinical, anatomical-pathological, and bacteriological diagnosis."* Gilles de la Tourette read his response on Friday, March 3, 1893, and obtained a grade of 29 out of 30. For the patient component that took place at Hôpital de l'Hôtel-Dieu, he was randomly assigned the case of a patient in the Saint Thomas ward, bed No. 11, who was suffering from *"acute rheumatoid arthritis of the joints, heart murmur, with prior perityphlitis and slight alcoholism."* He obtained 20/20. Gilles de la Tourette's anxiety, if any, over his results was soon allayed; he passed the 1893 exam with the best grade.[25] He was officially named Hospital Physician on May 15, 1893, and *chef de service* on January 1, 1896.

The main dates of Gilles de la Tourette hospital career are listed in the table at the end of this chapter. His frequent absences beginning in the 1901 were due to his failing health; he was obligated to stop working entirely in the summer of 1901. In 1902, Gilles de la Tourette's name was barred as *chef de service* at Hôpital Saint-Antoine with the note: *"Leave of absence as of December 26."* He was replaced the same day in his department by Doctor Paul-Louis Le Noir (1863–1945). In accordance with Article 53 of the general employee health regulations, when a *chef de service* had a well-documented illness that prevented him from carrying out his duties, the Director of the Administration, based on a previous opinion of the Board of Supervision, could replace him and grant a leave of absence rather than requiring him to resign. The Board of Supervision advised a leave of absence for Gilles de la Tourette at its October 23, 1902 session.[26] He was hospitalized around this time in Lausanne, Switzerland.

University Career: A Setback in 1892

After a physician had served as a *chef de clinique*, he could embark on a university career by taking the *agrégation* exam. If he passed, he became an assistant to a chair-holding professor, replacing him when needed and helping him with his classes. The rank of professor, generally associated with that of *chef de service* in a hospital, was accorded by the board of the Faculté de Médecine. This board, composed of chair-holding professors, would deliberate then vote until a majority had been reached.

Passing the national *agrégation* exam conferred the status of *agrégé*, created in 1823. The president of the jury was named by the French Ministry of Public Instruction; he submitted a list of jury members to be approved by the minister. An unfortunate incident biased the examination the year of Gilles de la Tourette's first attempt. The reasons for this are related to Charcot and his School: *"At the end of 1891, the Ministry of Public Instruction has selected Charles Bouchard to preside over the next* agrégation *exam. Bouchard was one of the first* internes *under Charcot and his teacher was a potent force in helping him advance his brilliant career. He went on to become a hospital physician, then an* agrégé *in 1869, and in 1879 he was accorded the Chair of General Pathology. But Bouchard went his own way, creating his own school, and showed clear signs of independence. Although Charcot never spoke of a real break in relations, the conflict with Bouchard was visible and the two men made veiled criticisms of each other, their comments remaining draped in official politeness."*[27] The Minister of Public Instruction at that time was Léon Bourgeois (1851–1925). The nomination of Charles Bouchard (1837–1915), who was envious of his former teacher's prestige and well-connected in the French ministries, was a sign of his growing power and something of a challenge to Charcot's authority. The jury was mainly composed of professors from provincial medical schools who had to assess sixteen candidates. Charcot had no influence over most of the jury members.

On Thursday, January 14, 1892, Gilles de la Tourette completed the oral components: *"purulent pleurisy"* then *"paroxysmic hemoglobinuria."*[28] *"The candidates for the five available positions in Paris included the students of Charcot and Bouchard, along with several others having no ties to either teacher. Babiński and Gilles de la Tourette, representing the Salpêtrière School, were the most eminent candidates. When the exam results were announced, three of the five successful candidates were students of Bouchard; neither of Charcot's two candidates passed."* Among the unsuccessful candidates, Brault, Babiński, Henri Richardière (1857–1940), Charles Achard (1860–1945), and Robert Wurtz (1858–1919) initiated a procedure to have the exam annulled due to irregularities, but Gilles de la Tourette[29,30] did not join them, even though the situation must have been difficult for him and slowed his own career. Here is what Gilles de la Tourette said in his 1893 homage to Charcot: *"Two years ago, one of them [Bouchard], who had conquered the greatest heights thanks to Charcot's powerful influence, suddenly separated from him. Charcot was deeply hurt, certainly more than he acknowledged. He perhaps took consolation in the fact that his other students remained faithful to him, joining together to dress the wound he had suffered."* Babiński, who had already failed in 1889,[31] would never make another attempt and would never become a professor.

University Career: Success in 1895

When Bourneville presented the list of candidates for the 1895 exam in his journal *Le Progrès Médical*, he added: *"Our readers will remark as we have, and with regret, that many of our very distinguished physician colleagues did not enroll for the examination of the Faculté de Médecine de Paris. Is it a case of 'once bitten, twice shy?' We certainly doubt it. But the jury must not be to their liking."*[32] Bourneville was clearly referring to Babiński. Gilles de la Tourette passed the 1895 *agrégation* with the top grade for the internal pathology and legal medicine category; the other candidates included Achard, Thoinot, Fernand Widal

(1862–1929), and Wurtz. Le Gendre noted: *"He certainly had many of the qual-ities required of a future professor: the ardor of his convictions, the desire to share them, and an indefatigable drive. And then one of his former students, today our col-league, paid him no small tribute with the following: 'He believed passionately in what he was doing, not only in medicine, where his confidence inspired his students and made disciples of them, but also in every other endeavor. He was first and foremost a man of action: his daring, his initiative, his triumph over the instinctive laziness that keeps us from expressing our ideas, were already extraordinary. But he went further by extending his audacity to those around him, somehow instilling it in his students' souls! For this, I am profoundly grateful. So many teachers, even the most illustrious, leave what germinates timidly in each of us to dry up prematurely!'"*

Professor of Neurology

There is no written account of Gilles de la Tourette's legal medicine classes at the Faculté. Surprisingly, he did not use his teaching materials for any books. However, there can be no doubt that he adored the first semester of the 1899–1900 university year, when Fulgence Raymond (1844–1910), Charcot's first successor to the Chair of Nervous System Diseases, asked him to fill in during his sick leave. As reported in *Le Progrès Médical*: "Mr. *Gilles de la Tourette, professeur agrégé, started his classes on nervous diseases at La Salpêtrière on November 24, at 10 am. He thanked Prof. Raymond, who holds the great Chair of Nervous System Diseases; Gilles de la Tourette will replace him this semester during his sick leave. . . . Gilles de la Tourette's lessons will primarily draw on the Master's method to clearly delineate, without dogma, the clinical types that emerge from pa-tient observation of symptoms and lesions. Starting these lessons with a subject that was particularly dear to Charcot—hysteria—is a tribute to his memory."*[33] Gilles de la Tourette sent the following invitation to his friend, the journalist Georges Montorgueil (1857–1933): *"My dear friend, I stopped by to say hello and invite you, Friday the 24th at 10 am, to my first lesson, if this is not too early for a professional night-bird like yourself. Raymond, the professor who holds the Chair is not well & as an agrégé I must replace him and climb . . . into the seat, for a time, that once belonged to my Master Charcot. Affectionately yours."* Although we do not have Montorgueil's written response, here is a brief note from Gilles de la Tourette dated November 12, 1899: *". . . I am enclosing a little note that you might publish in your* Echos *a few days before the 27th or even right away. I would be very pleased to see you that day. . . ."*[34] Gilles de la Tourette did not neglect to inform the public via the press that he would be occupying the prestigious Chair—a good way to keep his name known!

For several years already, Gilles de la Tourette had been giving neurology lessons in the successive departments he directed. His *Leçons de clinique thérapeutique sur les maladies du système nerveux*, published in 1898, gives us a sense of what he taught while occupying the medical school chair: *"Treating nervous system diseases is difficult; the relevant chapters in pedagogical treatises are often neglected by readers, who quickly realize that the author has focused more intently on the illness, rather than the patient to be treated. My purpose is to help readers become familiar with the patient and to guide them in the therapies for treating his illness."*[35] For example, to treat *"hysterical anorexia,"* Gilles de la Tourette *"required absolute isolation of the patient; once removed from her usual milieu and subjected to a foreign will, she will quickly recover her normal gastric functioning and thus be able to regain both weight and strength."*

Unlike Charcot, Gilles de la Tourette did not introduce any new ideas with his lessons. Nevertheless, from time to time, the press reported on Gilles de la Tourette's teaching, probably hoping to achieve the same effect as with Charcot. Jean Ciseaux, journalist at *Gil Blas*, gave a pertinent account on May 22, 1895: *"What is happening at present with the hysterical acrobats at Hôpital Cochin is very curious indeed! It is in the department of Gilles de la Tourette, the brilliant student and successor of Charcot, that these exceptional subjects are currently being treated. . . . But first, a portrait of Gilles de la Tourette, whose work is better known than the man himself. A professor from head to toe, his speech is full and encompassing, his thinking clear and brilliant. He knows what he means and says it the way he means to, his language giving shape to ideas in vigorous, cogent aphorisms. His tone is conversational, with moments that reveal his literary and artistic side, but he remains unaffected and relaxed, still showing something of the student with his spiritual gayety, and this puts his audience at ease."* Gilles de la Tourette then presented a young man with what Charcot called hysterical stigmata, currently considered a form of hives known as dermographism: *"Gilles de la Tourette applied a blunted point and wrote "Louis," the subject's name. His skin retained the details of this barely perceptible contact, swelling and reddening, gangrenous and shiny as in a case of hives. The scarcely traced name remained visible throughout the entire lesson. . . . Doctor Gilles de la Tourette's experiments have revealed that the acrobats are sometimes hysterics, relying on their nervous affection to perform their feats. They use tricks, but their tricks resemble an exact science. They are not stupid, but their lot is not a happy one."*[36]

Gilles de la Tourette also gave classes at the nursing schools founded by Bourneville: *"Yesterday, Dr. Bourneville gave his first classes at the municipal nursing school at Hôpital de la Pitié. Today, the classes at La Salpêtrière will begin, which are exclusively for women. . . . The aim is to raise the moral and professional level of hospital personnel and to teach the students the necessary foundations for caring for the sick and wounded.*"[37]

On September 12, 1900, Gilles de la Tourette was very proud to invite Claretie, who used to attend Charcot's lessons, to a public consultation: *"My Dear Master,* [38] *I am only passing through Paris, as I shall return to Poitou from the 16th to the 19th to be with my dear old father. . . . Would you be so kind as to set aside a morning for me, as you are accustomed to doing so graciously every year? We will meet at La Salpêtrière, as always, to enjoy the memory of our old master, Charcot. Would you like to attend a public consultation (you who attended so assiduously his Lessons), on Tuesday the 25th, for example?"* Like his master, Gilles de la Tourette always invited writers to his public events with a view to advancing his personal projects.

Private Practice

Until the 1958 law that created university hospital centers and "full-time" hospital physicians, hospital work in France was a part-time occupation, allowing for private practice on the side. So, like other hospital physicians, Gilles de la Tourette saw patients at his home, first at 14 Rue de Beaune, then at 39 Rue de l'Université, in the Seventh Arrondissement of Paris.

The Loudun archives contain letters indicating the sorts of cases Gilles de la Tourette handled in his private practice. For example, this letter written by Aurore Sand, granddaughter of the writer George Sand (1804–1876):

Dear Doctor, I am writing to request that you send a recommendation to the Director of the Hospital/Sanatorium de Hendaye [Pyrenees region] where a tubercular child of a poor abandoned girl was recently brought. The child is greatly in need of care, I do believe, but perhaps they will cure him there. I am sending you his name in the hope that a note from you will do much to help. Thank you with all of my heart. Aurore Sand.

This woman's request is indicative of Gilles de la Tourette's fame and authority.

In the correspondence exchanged with Claretie, there is a series of letters which also shed light on Gilles de la Tourette's private practice. Like Charcot, though to a lesser degree, he saw patients from around the world. The Brazilian patient referred to in the following letter is one example whose pathology is also of interest:

April 5, 1900, My Dear Master, I read the letter from the Commander Moreno del Christo. True, I think he has beriberi. It exists in his country; I have seen several cases among his compatriots and from neighboring tropical countries and these cases are always cured when the patients leave their place of origin. But given the lack of detailed information in the letter, it is very difficult to be sure. I am nonetheless enclosing a prescription, if you would be so kind as to forward it to its destination.

Then, one month later, on June 5, 1900:

My Dear Master, I am enclosing the letter I have just received from Commander Gabriel B. Moreno del Christo. He has decided to come to Paris for treatment of his impotent legs. He should have his head examined as well, I do believe, because he has a fair case of megalomania. It must be the sun in Saint-Domingue. . . . Gilles de la Tourette.

One month later, on July 5, 1900:

My Dear Master, This morning I examined Mgr. Moreno del Christo. As well I thought from a distance, he is suffering from beriberi. I have often seen such cases, sent to me from the mouth of the Amazon by a friend that, alas, is no longer of this world! The poor bishop is almost incapable of moving his paralyzed legs, which are swollen and atrophied. But beriberi patients transported from the place of origin to Europe are always cured and I am very hopeful. The climate alone, as well as removal from the infected location and 2 or 3 hours of electricity are supremely beneficial. Our client is over 70 but he is vigorous. I have handed him over to Doctor Comar, who will provide very good care; naturally, I shall oversee the treatment. Unfortunately, it will take several months. . . . Gilles de la Tourette.

In this case, the clinical description is entirely compatible with Gilles de la Tourette's diagnosis. As vitamins were unknown in 1900, he does not mention the deficiency causing the condition.[39] His reasoning reflects what was known at the time, as indicated in the beriberi article in the 1907 *Pratique Médico-chiurgicale* of Brissaud, Pinard, and Reclus.

Gilles de la Tourette counted among his patients many members of Parisian high society. Like Charcot, he was a well-known physician called on for serious cases, regardless of whether the causes were neurological. He benefited indirectly from Charcot's fame and that of his school, a link Gilles de la Tourette never failed to highlight in his frequent public appearances and his press interviews. An example can be found in this excerpt from the literary periodical *Gil Blas* reporting on the illness of Charles Floquet (1828–1896), a former Président du Conseil (head of the French government under the Third Republic): *"The health of Mr. Charles Floquet, former* Président du Conseil, *senator for the Seine district, has left his family and friends extremely worried. Mr. Floquet is suffering from pulmonary congestion, the first symptoms of which appeared three days ago. . . . After examining the patient, Drs. Millard*[40] *and Gilles de la Tourette declared that the situation was serious and prescribed vigorous treatment. The physicians examine the patient three times a day and have written the following note for visitors: 'Pulmonary congestion brought on by flu, serious condition,*

Drs. Millard and Gilles de la Tourette.' "[41] Gilles de la Tourette sent this telegram to his friend Montorgueil, a journalist at *L'Eclair:* "*My dear friend. . . . His condition is still serious (very serious). At 7 am, Millard and I shall examine him again and the bulletin will most likely be the same. If there is anything in particular, I shall let you know if I can. Kind regards.*"[42] And, two days later: "*Drs. Millard and Gilles de la Tourette, who are treating Mr. Charles Floquet, did not write any bulletins. They only issued a laconic note indicating that the honorable senator's condition was serious. Dr. Gilles de la Tourette, whom we met leaving the residence at Rue de Lille, told us that the situation was hopeless. The fatal outcome is imminent. Mr. Paul Doumer went to see the former* Président de la Chambre *in the evening. Mr. Floquet, close to death, did not recognize him.*" [43] Gilles de la Tourette's pride in his connections with those in power may have intensified the megalomaniacal tendencies which had already started to disturb his thinking.

Gilles de la Tourette was also called upon by the family of Alphonse Daudet, whom Charcot had considered a friend and treated for tabes. Daudet died on December 16, 1897, at his home, 41 Rue de l'Université. His last moments were recounted in the December 18 edition of the periodical *L'Aurore* by Philippe Dubois, who started by explaining that his sons realized he was slipping away and laid him out on his bed. "*The servants were in a panic to find a physician. Dr. Gilles de la Tourette lives in a neighboring building; there was also Dr. Potain.*[44] *Alas, when the doctors arrived, the man in the bed was moribund and it was only to appease the distraught family that they attempted the impossible. Mr. Gilles de la Tourette and Mr. Potain first tried to induce artificial respiration by means of rhythmical tractions of the tongue.*[45] *Finally, they tried faradizing the diaphragm. Their efforts were in vain. The master passed away gently without suffering, like a lamp that has run out of oil.*"[46]

In Summary

After his brilliant studies, Gilles de la Tourette quickly became famous as Charcot's former student and disciple. His personal aim was to imitate the master's practices both as a physician and teacher. His international clientele and the famous public figures who called on him are indicative of his social success as well as the ambition by which he attained it. His capacity for hard work and his exuberance, traits that Charcot noticed and came to value so highly, were gradually exaggerated, starting in 1893, by megalomania, a symptom of the general paralysis that would destroy his health. Although brief, Gilles de la Tourette's protean career involved him in all aspects of hospital and academic life.

The Key Dates in His Career

1878 externe
1881 interne
1885 doctoral thesis
1887 chef de Clinique (senior house officer)
1893–1895 physician at the Central Office.

> June 22–July 19, 1893 *Chef de service* of the isolation ward at
> Hôpital Saint-Antoine
> October 1, 1893, to March 1, 1894 *Chef de service* at
> Hôpital Cochin
> April 1–May 1; June 9–July 25 *Chef de service* at Hôpital de
> l'Hôtel-Dieu
> July 25–August 20; September 1–17 *Chef de service* at Hôpital de
> l'Hôtel-Dieu
> November 15–December 26, 1894 *Chef de service* at Hôpital de La
> Charité
> 1895 *Chef de service* at Hôpital Cochin

1896–1897 *chef de service* with tenure at Hôpital Hérold, one year
after this hospital was created
1898–1901 *chef de service* at Hôpital Saint-Antoine
1900–1901 Serving as Chief Physician for the World's Fair in Paris

He was on leave January 1 to 11, then from June 1 to July 1 1901, then
again from August 10 to September 1, 1901. He requested a leave from
April 7 to 14, which was "rescinded." He was absent from May 26 to June
3, then from June 4 to September 4, due to illness.
1902 *chef de service* at Hôpital Saint-Antoine. Gilles de la Tourette's
name was barred as *chef de service* with the note: *"Leave of absence as
of December 26."* He was replaced the same day in his department by
Doctor Paul-Louis Le Noir (1863–1945). In accordance with Article
53 of the general employee health regulations, when a *chef de service*
had a well-documented illness that prevented him from carrying out
his duties, the Director of the Administration, based on a previous
opinion of the Board of Supervision, could replace him and grant a
leave of absence rather than requiring him to resign. The Board of
Supervision advised a leave of absence for Gilles de la Tourette at its
October 23, 1902 session.[47] He was hospitalized around this time in
Lausanne, Switzerland.

Notes

1. Le Gendre P. Gilles de la Tourette 1857–1904. *Bulletins et Mémoires de la Société Médicale des Hôpitaux de Paris.* 1905;21(3):1298–1311.

2. Archives AP-HP 761FOSS10. Service des archives de l'Assistance publique-Hôpitaux de Paris, 7, rue des Minimes, 75003 Paris.

3. Gilles de la Tourette G. Fiche d'évaluation des personnels, externat et internat. Registre 774 FOSSEYEUX. Fiche 774 Foss13. Service des Archives de l'Assistance Publique, Hôpitaux de Paris. 7 Rue des Minimes 75003 Paris.

4. In the French healthcare system an *interne* was a house physician or house officer. The *internes* lived at the hospital and had diagnostic and therapeutic responsibilities. By contrast, an *externe* was a nonresident student at a teaching hospital. The *externes* did not live at the hospital and had neither diagnostic nor therapeutic responsibilities.

5. Archives AP-HP 761FOSS17 et 761FOSS39. Service des archives de l'Assistance publique-Hôpitaux de Paris, 7, rue des Minimes, 75003 Paris

6. Gilles de la Tourette G. François Damaschino. *Le Progrès Médical.* 1889;17-2(52):592–594.

7. Archives AP-HP 761FOSS56. Service des archives de l'Assistance publique-Hôpitaux de Paris, 7, rue des Minimes, 75003 Paris.

8. Gilles de la Tourette G. Etude sur une affection nerveuse caractérisée par de l'incoordination motrice accompagnée d'écholalie et de coprolalie. *Archives de Neurologie.* 1885;9(25):19–42.

9. Gilles de la Tourette G. Le Professeur J.-M. Charcot. *La Revue Hebdomadaire.* 1893;2(8, n°66):608–622. / Gilles de la Tourette G. J.-M. Charcot. *Nouvelle Iconographie de La Salpêtrière.* 1893;6(3):240–250.

10. Daudet L. *Devant la douleur, souvenirs des milieux littéraires, politiques, artistiques et médicaux de 1880 à 1905.* Paris: Nouvelle Librairie Nationale. 1915.

11. Daudet L. *Les œuvres dans les hommes.* Paris: Nouvelle Librairie Nationale. 1922.

12. Claretie J. La Vie à Paris. *Le Temps.* 1904;44(15 885):2–3.

13. de Lavarenne E. Gilles de la Tourette. *La Presse Médicale.* 1893;1(45):353–354.

14. Signoret JL. Une leçon clinique à La Salpêtrière (1887) par André Brouillet. *La Revue Neurologique (Paris).* 1983;139(12):687–701.

15. Louis de Fourcaud was an art, music, and literary critic. He was also a professor at the Beaux-arts school in Paris.

16. Philippe Burty (1830–1890).

17. There is no priest in the painting, but Henry Berbez (1862–?), an *externe* at the time, situated just behind Gilles de la Tourette, was wearing a clergyman's collar.

18. Fourcaud. Le Salon de 1887. *Le Gaulois.* 30 avril 1887;21(1705):4.

19. Theódhoros Dhilighiánnis or Theódhoros Delyannis (1820–1905), a Greek politician who represented Greece at the 1878 Congress of Berlin, was obligated to resign when Greece was blockaded in response to its threats against Turkey. Mouÿ Ch. Souvenirs d'une diplomate, le blocus d'Athènes. *Revue des deux Mondes.* 1901;2:280–313.

20. Saint Real. Les étudiants français chez Son Excellence Delyannis. *Le Gaulois.* Jeudi 11 juillet 1889;23(2500):2.

21. Guinon G. Charcot intime. *Paris Médical.* 1925;56:511–516.

22. Babiński J. Eloge de J.M. Charcot. *La Revue Neurologique.* 1925;32(6):746–756.

23. Freud S. *Correspondance: 1873–1939. Lettres choisies et présentées par Ernst Freud; traduit de l'allemand par Anne Berman, avec la collaboration de Jean-Pierre Grossein.* Paris: Gallimard. 1966.

24. Gelfand T. "Mon cher docteur Freud": Charcot's unpublished correspondance to Freud, 1888–1893. *Bull Hist Med.* 1988;62:563–588.

25. Archives AP-HP 761FOSS56. Service des archives de l'Assistance publique-Hôpitaux de Paris, 7, rue des Minimes, 75003 Paris.

26. Archives AP-HP 1L 38. (point n° 6, p. 23). Service des archives de l'Assistance publique-Hôpitaux de Paris, 7, rue des Minimes, 75003 Paris.

27. Bonduelle M, Gelfand T, Goetz CG. *Charcot, un grand médecin dans son siècle.* Paris: Michalon. 1996.

28. Anonyme. Faculté de Médecine. Concours d'agrégation en médecine. *Le Progrès Médical.* 1892;15(2):33/61.

29. Philippon J, Poirier J. *Joseph Babiński, A Biography.* New York: Oxford University Press. 2009.

30. Bourneville DM. Les concours d'agrégation: une série de citations. *Le Progrès Médical.* 1892;20(22):421–423

31. Poirier J. La première agrégation de Joseph Babiński. *Neurologie Libérale.* 2015;1(1):27–32.

32. Bourneville DM. Concours d'agrégation en médecine. *Le Progrès Médical.* 1894;20(49):453.

33. Bourneville DM. Clinique des maladies nerveuses: M. le Dr Gilles de la Tourette, agrégé. *Le Progrès Médical.* 1895;10(48):436.

34. Archives Nationales 428AP/2 Correspondance Montorgueil-Gilles de la Tourette.

35. Gilles de la Tourette G. *Leçons de clinique thérapeutique sur les maladies du système nerveux.* Paris: E. Plon-Nourrit et Cie. 1898.

36. Ciseaux J. Journaux & Revues. *Gil Blas.* Mercredi 22 mai 1895;17(5634):3.

37. Jacques J. Nouvelles. *Gil Blas.* Jeudi 4 octobre 1894;16(5424):2.

38. This form of address in French is a sign of deference to someone carrying a title; Claretie was a member of the Académie Française.

39. In 1911, Casimir Funk (1884–1967), a Polish biochemist (who emigrated to the United States in 1915), isolated a few centigrams of a substance from 100 kilograms of rice that could cure beriberi in pigeons fed with polished rice. He called it a vitamin because it contained an amine compound. He suggested that scurvy, pellagra, and rickets could also be due to deficiencies in substances of the same type. His conclusions were not accepted at the time by the scientific community, which was looking for an infectious cause for these pathologies.

40. Dr. Auguste Millard (1830–1915).

41. Anonyme. Notes & informations. *Gil Blas.* Vendredi 17 janvier 1896;18(5904):2.

42. Archives Nationales 428AP/2.Correspondance Montorgueil-Gilles de la Tourette.

43. Anonyme. Notes & informations. *Gil Blas.* Dimanche 19 janvier 1896;18(5906):2.

44. Prof. Carl Pierre Édouard Potain (1825–1901), Bouillaud's student and Vaquez's teacher. Professor of medical pathology and clinical medicine.

45. Technique invented by Jean-Baptiste Vincent Laborde (1830–1903) in 1892. Poirirer J. Le docteur Jean-Baptiste Vincent Laborde, neurologue et neurophysiologiste oublié. *Geriatr Pyschol Neuropsychiatr Vieil.* 2015;13(1):73–82.

46. Dubois Ph. A la maison mortuaire. *L'Aurore.* Samedi 18 décembre 1897;1(61):1–2.

47. Archives AP-HP 1L 38. (point n° 6, p. 23). Service des archives de l'Assistance publique-Hôpitaux de Paris, 7, rue des Minimes, 75003 Paris.

3

Secretary, Colleague, and Friend of Jean-Martin Charcot

An Assistant and Colleague

In 1881, at the height of his career, Charcot engaged a secretary to help him in his practice. After Charles Féré (1852–1907) and Pierre Marie (1853–1940), he selected Gilles de la Tourette for this coveted post (1887–1888) and, finally, Georges Guinon (1859–1932) in the last years of his life. Among other things, the secretary prepared the Master's consultations at La Salpêtrière, but also at his home on Boulevard Saint-Germain. He also collated articles and observations and wrote summary reports for Charcot, who used them to prepare his lessons. Gilles de la Tourette described Charcot's working habits as follows: *"Every morning, even during vacations (he allowed himself no more than one month of vacation per year), at exactly 9.30 he would go to his department, where he could still be found at noon. . . . A punctual man, he required the same regularity of his chefs de clinique; everything had to be ready for his classes. Every Tuesday morning, prior to the big lesson (on Fridays, he gave another extemporaneous clinical lesson), he would see for the last time the patients on whom he was to speak, and if one of them was absent, Charcot would become extraordinarily angry, especially around the first of January. The young internes who had just arrived quickly understood, and the next time, no one was missing. He never gave a lesson that was not prepared well in advance and excessively documented. Leaving the lecture hall, when he wished the lesson to be published, he would say to one of his students: 'Here are my notes, write*

them up'; the entire lesson had been written by hand, with nothing superfluous, in a
firm, vigorous style whose precision and clarity we all admired."

Another indicator of Gilles de la Tourette's intense activity during this period was his involvement with learned societies. From May 10, 1884, to January
22, 1889, he attended all weekly sessions of the Société de Biologie and wrote
a summary report for each meeting for the journal *Le Progrès Médical*, taking
over the task from his friend Fernand Bottey (1858–1900) (Figure 3.1). Also
during this time, from May 14, 1884, to December 26, 1888, he attended
meetings of the Société de Thérapeutique and published summaries, once or
twice a month, in *Le Progrès Médical*, as Bottey had done before him. All of
these writings were in addition to his numerous personal publications. At the
Société de Médecine Légale,[1] which elected him a member on February 13,
1888, he participated with great passion in the debates; for example, on April
9, 1888, when he challenged Charles-Albert Vibert (1854–1918), head of the
legal medicine laboratory at the Faculté de Médecine. Vibert was addressing
the effects of railroad accidents but omitted to cite Charcot's work on their
psychological consequences.[2]

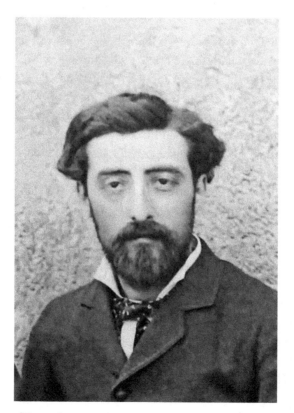

FIGURE 3.I Fernand Bottey (1858–1900).
Private collection of the author.

The following unpublished letters from the Loudun archives were sent to Georges by Charcot. They bear witness to the close ties between the two men and offer a behind-the-scenes look at Charcot's La Salpêtrière lessons. Each of these letters describes the tasks performed by Gilles de la Tourette as secretary to Charcot: stepping in during Charcot's absence, research and preparation for Charcot's lessons, and sharing professional worries about the rivalry between the La Salpêtrière and Nancy Schools. Hippolyte Bernheim (1840–1919), who headed the Nancy School, contested Charcot's theories of hysteria. The letter about their rivalry is indicative of the discussions between Charcot and Gilles de la Tourette in the beginning of the 1890s on the medical-legal consequences of hypnotism.

Each letter from Charcot is presented in extenso along with any necessary explanations.

Charcot and Gilles de la Tourette: Somnambulism

The first letter, undated, reveals the collaborative relationship between the two men (Figure 3.2). It also sheds new light on Charcot's personality. While one tends to imagine the Master always confident and sure of himself, here he seems doubtful and turns to his secretary and student for reassurance that the data he was to present at his next lesson were reliable:

My dear Gilles de la T.

I shall probably give a lesson in a week from tomorrow on spontaneous somnambulism, in particular the delirious somnambulic attack (in which there is a danger for the patient and for others), with regard to a case I have at La Salpêtrière. I would like you to provide me with:

1) the "Men . . ." report that I sent you,

2) concerning this report, a summary of all cases you have collected on the subject, with a brief observation and the bibliographic information.

At the same time, formulate an opinion, if you have one, on the following:

1) the possibility of suicide in hysterics,

2) the possibility of committing murder in delirious somnambulism, or actual cases established by fact,

3) minor crimes or less serious accidents, thefts, etc., in spontaneous somnambulism—that is, use the texts to show that you were the first, if I am not mistaken, to clearly propose that natural somnambulism is nothing other than a +/− automatic delirious hysterical attack, unless it is epilepsy. And on this subject, probability that a delirious or automatic epileptic attack could initiate the hystero-epileptic attack; probability of committing a crime, a homicide, suicide, real or apparent. Is there, in

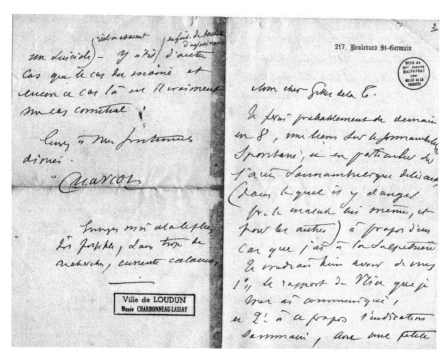

FIGURE 3.2 Charcot's letter to Georges Gilles de la Tourette: *"I shall probably give a lesson in a week from tomorrow on spontaneous somnambulism."*
Copyright Musée Charbonneau-Lassay, Ville de Loudun, with kind permission.

fact, attempted murder in other cases than that of the monk, and is this really a case of epilepsy?

Yours truly, Charcot.

Send this to me as soon as possible, without too much research, *currente calamo*.[3]

The lesson took place on Tuesday, January 31, 1888: *"Epileptic Crisis— Ambulatory Automatism."* Charcot interrogated a thirty-seven-year-old man, the victim of amnesic episodes in which he would travel for one or two days and not know where he was when he "woke up." Charcot explained: *"You will not find many stories like this one in books. It centers on a pathological phenomenon that departs from the ordinary and merits a bit of discussion. . . . We asked ourselves what this meant, what this singular state of unconsciousness was that, all of a sudden, for a few hours or a few days, could plunge this man's life into a state of obscurity. We told ourselves that if we could prevent this good man from walking through fields or cities, with no advantage to himself, we would have achieved something useful. I have thought this through and will try to justify this opinion, that the condition from which he suffers is epileptic in nature. It is an ambulatory automatism, to employ an expression I have already used for a situation*

*whereby one walks automatically, and no exterior characteristic reveals this au-
tomatism to the individual walking. Note that we have a very good understanding
of post-epileptic madness in epilepsy: an individual has an epileptic attack and
under the influence of a terrifying dream, he becomes violent, he breaks everything
around him, and then he begins to walk, but not in a calm manner. At his first false
move, the police arrest him and he finds himself in prison. That sort of epileptic
could very well murder someone, commit suicide, whereas this good man, if he
hadn't known how to swim, he probably wouldn't have jumped into the water. In
his case, there is no trace of over-excitement or violence. In general, an extremely
violent attack is one of the characteristics of post-epileptic madness and, clearly,
does not apply to our case. But this is probably the same series of phenomena, only
with another appearance."*[4]

Charcot's interpretation is surprising, as what he describes in no way
resembles epilepsy as it is currently defined. Today's nosologies classify "epileptic psychoses" into three groups according to when they occur in time: (1)
psychiatric phenomena simultaneous with status epilepticus involving complex partial temporal seizures, (2) postictal psychoses, and (3) intercurrent
psychoses. Visual or auditory hallucinations are the most frequent manifestation, with or without confusion and agitation. The somatoform disorders
or dissociative disorders have a prolonged duration and manifest themselves
by the violence of their "convulsive" symptoms, rather than ambulation
with amnesia.[5] To return to the second half of the nineteenth century, the
porosity of neurological and psychiatric concepts reflected how society and
physicians viewed disease and behavior. Whereas Charcot had shown that
hysteria could exist in both sexes, he believed that in male hysterics, generally
laborers or craftsmen, it only occurred after traumatic events, particularly
work accidents. However, from 1870 to 1893, his analysis evolved, and he
came to consider that the attack was only dangerous when the patient profile
involved "movement pathology," as in the case of vagabonds and irrepress-
ible travelers.

Certain men and women who were forced to leave rural areas by the economic crisis following the 1870 Franco-Prussian War and by other political
or societal situations were considered victim to *"hystero-neurasthenic attacks."*
This is how the "wandering Jew" became a stigmatized figure throughout
Europe, after the pogroms in Poland and Russia in 1881.[6] The first medical text
mentioning vagabondage appeared in 1875 and was written by Achille Foville,
the younger (1831–1887). He presented fourteen cases of vagabonds described
as *"traveling or migrating lunatics."*[7] Traveling is an act that is *"usually thought
out and rationally motivated, but it may also result from delirious thinking."* Most
"migrating lunatics" suffered from hallucinatory persecutions, which was the

basis for Foville's conclusion that all vagabonds were mentally ill.[8] Charcot seemed to subscribe to this dominant idea, related to the concepts of degeneration, early-onset dementia, and psychopathological heredity developed by nineteenth-century alienists, the first of whom was Bénédict-Augustin Morel (1809–1873).[9,10] As for Gilles de la Tourette, he employed the term "delirious states" for what were considered *"somnambulic states of hysteria,"*[11] although he wrote that *"noctambulism or dream enactment fall within physiological bounds."* Other descriptions were added by Charcot's disciples in Bordeaux, for example Philippe Tissié (1852–1935)[12] or Emmanuel Régis (1855–1918), who, with his student Victor-Charles Dubourdieu (1867–?), created the term *"dromomania."*[13] Their teacher, Albert Pitres (1848–1928), wrote of *"impulsive vagabondage."*[14] Henry Meige (1866–1940) wrote his thesis on the subject in 1893[15] and published his findings in *La Nouvelle Iconographie de La Salpêtrière* the same year[16] (Figure 3.3). Today, these descriptions are recognized under the term "dissociative fugue" or "dreamy state" and do not involve epileptic phenomena.[17,18] Pathophysiological explanations are starting to emerge, implicating the activation of certain default mode neuronal networks (DMN) in the active waking state.[19]

For Gilles de la Tourette, *"somnambulism is the most well-known and well-studied of all hypnotic states."* Paul Richer (1849–1933) provided an approach to the concept developed by Charcot in 1881: *"Somnambulism appears to be mixed with the passionate attitudes of the* grande attaque hystérique *or to replace them completely."*[20] In his book, *L'hypnotisme et les états analogues au point de vue médico-légal,* on hypnotism and legal medicine, Gilles de la Tourette partially answered the questions raised in Charcot's brief note: *"Somnambulists may commit criminal acts during their sleep and claim immunity from legal responsibility."*[21] Gilles de la Tourette drew on examples from the medical literature, in particular from Daniel Hack Tuke (1827–1895), who only described clinical cases that he had personally observed.[22] Charcot gave another lesson on the same theme on Tuesday, February 21, 1889: *"Case of epileptic ambulatory automatism";*[23] that day, he presented the case of Men . . . mentioned in the note to Gilles de la Tourette. Work on this topic at La Salpêtrière was ongoing. In 1891 and 1892, Guinon replaced Gilles de la Tourette as Charcot's secretary and transcribed other lessons on hysterical somnambulism.[24,25] In 1909, a book entitled *Fugues et vagabondages: Etude clinique et psychologique* was published that covered all clinical forms and summarized the concepts associated with fugues. Alix Joffroy (1844–1908), former *interne* under Charcot, had begun the book just before his death, and his *interne* Roger Dupouy completed it (1877–?).[26]

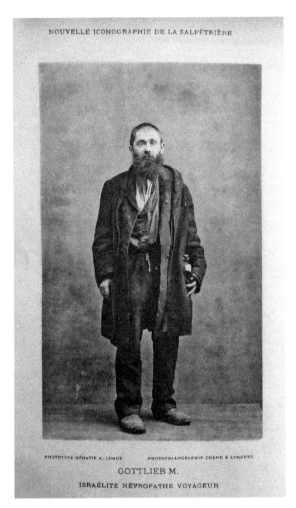

NOUVELLE ICONOGRAPHIE DE LA SALPÊTRIÈRE

PHOTOTYPE NÉGATIF A. LONDE   PHOTOCOLLOGRAPHIE CHÉNE & LONGUET

GOTTLIEB M.
ISRAÉLITE NÉVROPATHE VOYAGEUR

FIGURE 3.3 Illustration of the chapter by Henry Meige in *La Nouvelle Iconographie de la Salpêtrière*, 1893: *"Traveling Jewish Lunatic."*
Private collection of the author.

Charcot and Gilles de la Tourette: Case of *"La Dormeuse"*

In a letter dated Sunday, November 27, 1887, Charcot informed Gilles de la Tourette that he had been called away (Figure 3.4):

Sunday

My dear Gilles de la Tourette,

I have to leave tonight. I shall not be back for the Tuesday lesson. Have the patients come back Friday, I shall have returned by then and since I have no time to

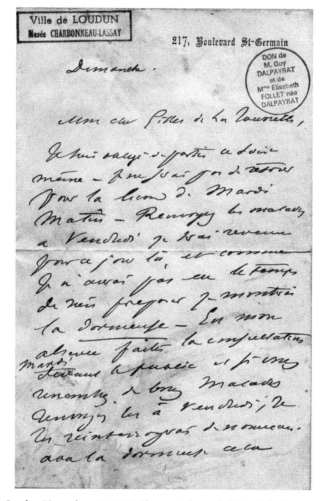

FIGURE 3.4 Sunday, November 27, 1887, Charcot informed Gilles de la Tourette that he had been called away.
Copyright Musée Charbonneau-Lassay, Ville de Loudun, with kind permission.

prepare anything, I shall talk about "la dormeuse" [the sleeping woman]. During my absence, take charge of the public consultation on Tuesday, and if you come across any good patients, tell them to come back Friday. I shall interrogate them; with "la dormeuse," that will be enough for the lesson. Tell the audience that I was called away suddenly and very much regret my absence. Sincerely yours, Charcot. November 27, 1887.

Gilles de la Tourette added a note: *"Monsieur Charcot leaving for a trip to Nice or Cannes or Marseille for a consultation with Don Pedro d'Alcântara, Emperor of Brazil."* Charcot trusted Gilles de la Tourette and felt comfortable leaving him with the responsibility of his practice and his department while he attended to the world's major figures, being the famous physician that he was. The Emperor of Brazil, who was visiting the Côte d'Azur, was accustomed to the Tuesday night dinners at Boulevard Saint-Germain and wanted his friend Charcot to examine a medical problem. Before leaving, Charcot made arrangements with his secretary so as not to miss any interesting cases.

When he got back, Charcot decided to present Eudoxie, admitted at age twenty-seven to La Salpêtrière in 1862, the year Charcot took his position at the hospital. Bourneville had been treating her since 1870, when he was an *interne* with Louis Delasiauve (1804–1893). The department eventually closed due to the dilapidated state of the building, and, at the end of 1870, Eudoxie was among the epileptic and hysteric patients that the administration asked Charcot to care for. She had thus been under his care for seventeen years when he wrote his letter to Gilles de la Tourette. He undoubtedly knew her well, and the lesson would be easy to prepare after his unexpected voyage. Bourneville and Paul Regnard (1850–1927) prepared the observation of this patient in 1879, for *L'Iconographie photographique de La Salpêtrière*.[27] Eudoxie, *"remarkably stout"* and suffering from complete paraplegia since the age of twenty-two, frequently vomited. Her abdomen was distended: *"On the left side, there is bogginess and a dull percussion note; exploration is painful; the test for ascites does not appear positive. Whether this is an old bout of circumscribed peritonitis or an ovarian cyst, we are unable to tell; the patient's obesity and pain make a complete examination impossible."*

Bourneville saw these manifestations (which strike today's reader as organic and serious) along with the paralysis as arguments in favor of a hysteria diagnosis. He essentially focused on the recurrent episodes of excessive sleep, each one lasting several days. While she was "sleeping," Eudoxie's upper limbs were contracted in a semi-flexed position, and her eyelids fluttered and could not be forced apart. She did not snore. Attempts to wake her, even forcefully, were futile. Charcot had already discussed her case during a lesson in 1883. His detailed, semiological presentation had a clear pedagogical purpose: to distinguish hysterical sleep from physiological sleep. As for Gilles de la Tourette, in January 1888, he published an article on sleeping episodes attributed to hysteria, beginning with a long section that drew on descriptions by earlier authors.[28]

A lesson by the Master on the same patient, given Tuesday, November 13, 1888, was transcribed and published in the second volume of his Tuesday Lessons for that year. The patient had been sleeping for twelve days.[29] Charcot probably gave a lesson on hysterical sleep or "lethargic sleep," as he termed it, on several different occasions. By today's diagnostic standards, in addition to the diagnosis of hysteria which remains a possibility, schizophrenic psychosis is more likely than a recurring hypersomnia such as Kleine-Levin syndrome. During the latter, prolonged sleep episodes are associated with hyperphagia and with sexual and social disinhibition accompanied by hallucinosis and a feeling of derealization; none of these symptoms was mentioned in the writings of Bourneville, Charcot, or Gilles de la Tourette.

Charcot and Gilles de la Tourette: One Hysteria

Charcot sent another hastily written note dated December 29, 1890. He once again needed to prepare a lesson. Once again, he called on his secretary (Figure 3.5):

My dear Gilles de la Tourette,

On December 17, 1887, you published a short piece on hysteria and syphilis in Le Progrès Médical and announced you would publish the complete observation in the Milan journal Morgagni. Do you have this issue of Morgagni? If so, please be so kind as to send it to me today, it would be helpful for tomorrow's lesson. Yours, Charcot.

This is the only letter written by Charcot on paper with the medical school's letterhead (*Faculté de Médecine—Clinique des maladies du système nerveux—Hospice de La Salpêtrière*); all other letters are marked with Charcot's home address (*217 Boulevard St-Germain*). Gilles de la Tourette did indeed publish an article in 1888 in the Milan journal *Il Morgagni*,[30] previously published in *Le Progrès Médical* on December 17, 1887[31]; its title translates as "Hysteria and Syphilis: The Influence of an Earlier Disease or Poisoning on the Mode of Localization and on the Form of Hysteria Attacks." Gilles de la Tourette had transcribed a lesson in which Charcot clarified his interpretation of hysteria: anesthesia and paralysis could appear during disease or poisoning, such as typhoid fever, saturnism, alcoholism, or, in the case of this lesson, during the progression of syphilis. However, *"regardless of its context, hysteria remains essentially the same; there is no saturnine hysteria, no alcoholic hysteria, no typhoidal hysteria—there is not even a traumatic hysteria, at least in the strict sense of the word. There are only manifestations of hysteria in patients with saturnism, in alcoholics, in traumatized patients, and so forth. The seed sprouts more or less effectively, puts out shoots in one direction or another, according to the soil, but it always remains itself, which is to say one thing, and if the soil sometimes gives it a certain character, it nonetheless always keeps its own specific physiognomy, which those who look closely will always know how to identify."[32]*

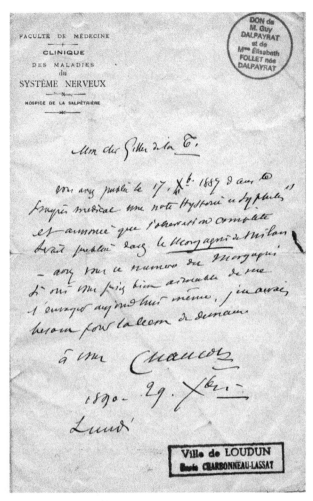

FIGURE 3.5 The only letter written by Charcot on paper with the medical school's letterhead.
Copyright Musée Charbonneau-Lassay, Ville de Loudun, with kind permission.

Charcot and Gilles de la Tourette: a "Tuesday Lessons" Publication

Charcot's Tuesday Lessons were famous for incorporating transcribed dialogues between the master and his patients from all sorts of consultations at La Salpêtrière. Unlike the traditional professorial lessons in Charcot's other books, they reflected the spontaneity and candor of real-life interactions. As Pierre Marie recalled in 1925: "*The Tuesday Lessons took place where the outpatient clinic was located. Patients waiting for a consultation would be presented one after the other. Charcot questioned them himself. The medical nature of these representations did not overshadow their conviviality, and one learned from the questions and answers, a sort of Socratic method Charcot supplemented with observations from his long clinical experience, how to arrive at a diagnosis."[33]* The note addressed to Gilles de la Tourette on August 17, 1889, is technical and concerns the printing of Tuesday Lessons transcribed in books by Edouard-Emmery Blin (1863–1930), Jean-Baptiste Charcot (1867–1936), and Henri Colin (1860–1930).

My dear Gilles de la Tourette,

I have the proofs and am quite pleased. Let me know whether Colin, who is taking care of the printing of my lessons, could take the electros. My lesson will be ready in around ten days. Also, let me know where the Berliner issue is. Is it with you or with me? Please do not leave without telling me; I shall be in trouble otherwise. Yours sincerely, Charcot.

PS: I saw that you drew a very fitting picture of Bernheim.

Charcot was pleased with the illustrations in the second volume of his Lessons. The word "electro" is an abbreviation for "electrotype."[34] Charcot could read German and took an interest in foreign publications; he was probably speaking of *Berliner klinische Wochenschrift: Organ für pracktische Aerzte*, published by A. Hirschwald from 1864 to 1921. He needed a recent issue to prepare the proofs and counted on his secretary to find it. The postscript is more mysterious. Had Gilles de la Tourette drawn a caricature of Hippolyte Bernheim (Figure 3.6) from Nancy? Bernheim opposed Charcot's views on hysteria, maintaining that the capacity for hypnosis was not physiologically specific and represented only a generalized process of suggestibility. One of Charcot's main principles was that the capacity for hypnosis was necessarily linked to hysteria and that both were different aspects of the same neurological state. Relations between the Nancy and Salpêtrière Schools were always tense; beyond the scientific conflict, Charcot had little regard for Bernheim, who nonetheless made a point of contradicting him. The following letter reveals the repercussions of an important chapter in this confrontation of opinions and personalities.

Charcot and Gilles de la Tourette: Gouffé Affair and Dispute with the Nancy School

This letter has an uncharacteristic tone. Charcot comes across as less distant than usual, but a sense of worry and doubt is perceptible (Figure 3.7).

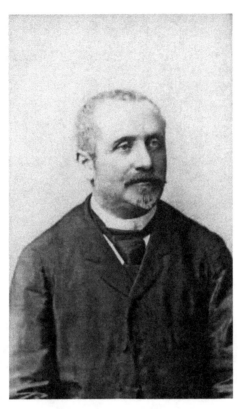

FIGURE 3.6 Hippolyte Bernheim (1840–1919).
Private collection of the author.

My dear Gilles de la Tourette,

I am very worried.

Bernheim did not know and I have the proofs of your epilogue.

Did he change his mind, and what to do now that we can no longer mention Le Temps anymore? Couldn't you find out from Taleur [Caleur?] where things stand?

Yours, Charcot. Tuesday night.

Though undated, the letter refers to what became known as the "Gouffé affair" or "Eyraud-Bompard affair" and can thus be situated at the beginning of 1891. It also reveals the personal impact the affair had on the two men. Guinon had replaced Gilles de la Tourette as Charcot's secretary. During his *internat* with Paul Brouardel (1837–1906), Gilles de la Tourette had developed an expertise in legal medicine. In addition, he had already published a legal medicine book in 1887 entitled *L'hypnotisme et les états analogues au point de*

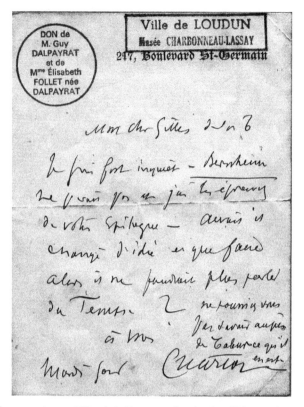

FIGURE 3.7 Charcot writes to Gilles de la Tourette after the Gouffé/Eyraud-Bompard affair.
Copyright Musée Charbonneau-Lassay, Ville de Loudun, with kind permission.

vue médico-légal,[35] prefaced by Brouardel[36] (Charcot wrote the preface to the German translation).[37] Although he wasn't directly involved in the legal proceedings, Gilles de la Tourette followed this affair with the utmost interest. He had just finished the first volume of his *Traité clinique et thérapeutique de l'hystérie*, and it was about to be published. In it, he described experiments on hypnotic suggestion that he had conducted at La Salpêtrière with Blanche Wittmann (1859–1913) in 1888. Despite initial resistance, the patient carried out a simulated poisoning in a lucid state, after suggestion by Gilles de la Tourette under hypnosis. However, when the press took hold of the Gouffé affair, Gilles de la Tourette, a key player in the vehement controversy between La Salpêtrière School and Bernheim's Nancy School, expressed an opposing view in the medical press, echoed by the mainstream press. No crime can be committed in a hypnotic state, he claimed. Here is how Gilles de la Tourette wished his own contradictions to be understood: *"In hypnotism, one cannot be logical in every situation, and there is a significant difference between laboratory experiments, for example, and practical investigations with a specific medical-legal purpose."* The position defended by Gilles de la Tourette, which is to say by La Salpêtrière School, was clear: *"The hypnotic somnambulist is not a pure automaton, a simple machine that can be turned in any direction the winds of the mind may blow. He possesses a personality, and although it is reduced, to use general terms, it remains persistently whole in certain cases and affirms itself clearly through a resistance to suggested ideas."*[38]

The key facts of the Gouffé affair are as follows. On July 26, 1889, a bailiff in the faubourg of Montmartre, Toussaint-Augustin Gouffé, aged forty-seven, was reported missing to the police. Two weeks later, a road worker discovered human remains in a ditch, along with remnants of a trunk, in Millery, near Lyon. Thus began the story of the "mysterious trunk" which would capture the public's imagination. Professor Alexandre Lacassagne (1843–1924) from Lyon, performing one of the first scientific forensic analyses, identified the remains as those of Gouffé.[39] The investigation revealed that Gouffé had met Gabrielle Bompard (1868–1920) in a café. Coaxed by Bompard, Gouffé went to see her in a Parisian apartment that her accomplice, Michel Eyraud (1843–1891), had rented (Figure 3.8). After inviting Gouffé to sit on the sofa, she wrapped her bathrobe sash around his neck; Eyraud, hidden behind a curtain, grabbed the sash, attached it to a rope on a pulley fastened to the ceiling, and pulled. Gouffé was hanged to death. When he saw that the bailiff was not carrying any money, Eyraud took the victim's keys and went alone to his office, but he did not find the loot he was hoping for. The murderers, who had premeditated their crime, placed the body in a trunk that they had purchased ahead of time in London and abandoned it on the road to Millery before embarking for England, then America. Weary of being on the run with the swaggering Eyraud, Gabrielle Bompard left him in January 1890 and returned to France, where she discovered she was a media sensation. Flattered by this celebrity and naïvely hoping to enhance it by telling her version of the facts, she went to the police and turned herself in. Police finally apprehended Eyraud in June 1890, in Cuba, after he had confounded them several times.

The French public was intrigued by this denouement in the tropics and by Eyraud himself, a picaresque, polyglot bandit who lived under different identities throughout North and South America, thumbing his nose at the detectives sent to find him. Newspapers, recognizing a lucrative opportunity, increased their print runs and offered readers new angles on the enigma every day, along with side stories about Bompard's *libertinage*, or the minor trafficking that was part of daily life on the big Parisian boulevards. After this murder, *"motivated by greed and with debauchery for a lure,"* nearly 20,000 onlookers followed Gouffé's funeral procession, fascinated by the idea that the coffin contained a dismembered body with only the torso intact.

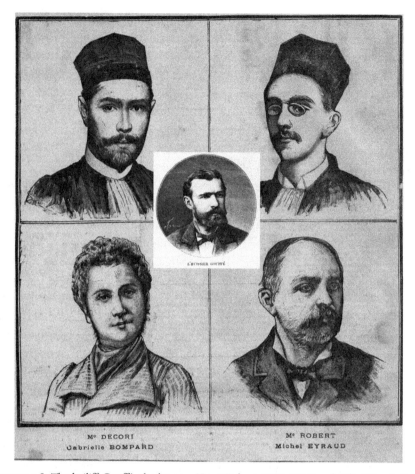

M⁰ DECORI
Gabrielle BOMPARD

M⁰ ROBERT
Michel EYRAUD

FIGURE 3.8 The bailiff Gouffé, the lawyers Henri-Robert (1863–1936) and Félix Décori, Gabrielle Bompard, and Michel Eyraud in *L'Intransigeant Illustré,* Thursday, December 18, 1890. Private collection of the author.

Before the trial, Gabrielle Bompard's behavior was very strange. According to the investigation documents, she described the details *"with complete indifference and without remorse,"* and seemed *"unaware of the moral significance of the acts she had been witness to."* Judge Paul Dopffer (1844–1922) ordered Brouardel, Gilbert Ballet (1853–1916), and Auguste Mottet (1832–1909) to evaluate the mental state of the accused. They concluded that no mental alienation existed and that *"while she could not be considered immune from liability for the acts imputed to her, she does have a mild form of hysteria."*[40] Bernheim, without having examined her, wrote an opinion piece in *La Revue de l'Hypnotisme* in which he maintained that Gabrielle Bompard acted under hypnosis, by suggestion, which entailed *"any idea accepted by the brain, whatever the origin of this idea."*[41] Her lawyer, Mr. Henri-Robert (1863–1936) (Figure 3.8), used this

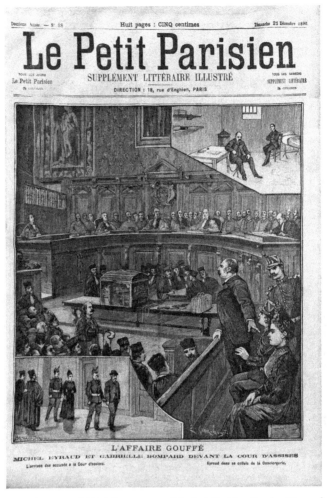

FIGURE 3.9 Eyraud-Bompard Trial, front cover of *Le Petit Parisien*, Sunday, December 21, 1890. Private collection of the author.

argument, claiming that his psychically fragile client was under Eyraud's control and that he had transformed her into an involuntary accomplice. During the trial (Figure 3.9), the legal specialist Jules Liégeois (1833–1908) (Figure 3.10) replaced Bernheim, who had broken his leg.

The prosecutor, Jules Quesnay de Beaurepaire (1834–1923), made the following argument: *"During his deposition yesterday (one could almost speak of a lecture), a witness took pains to develop new theories and defended a presumption of suggestion and a presumption of immunity from liability; I am speaking of Mr. Liégeois, Professor of Law in Nancy. . . . Several physicians, along with Mr. Liégeois, attribute an unprecedented significance to suggestion. The physicians did not come to debate the issue with our physicians; Professor Liégeois spoke on their behalf. . . . The*

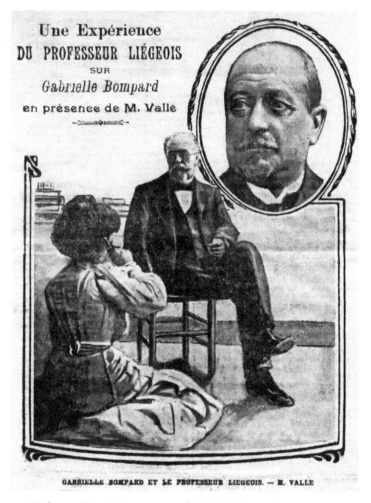

FIGURE 3.10 Professeur Liégeois's assessment of Gabrielle Bompard.
Private collection of the author.

innovators from Nancy do not proceed scientifically, by linking together the observed facts, as does the well-established Paris School; they proceed by affirmation. . . . Directly contradicting our learned men, they posit that suggestion can be established with the eyes alone, without relying on speech, and that suggestion can occur outside of hypnotic sleep; this is what is known as 'mental suggestion in the waking state.' "[42] For Liégeois, a subject who committed a misdemeanor or crime under hypnosis was immune from liability.[43] On the contrary, the prosecutor adopted La Salpêtrière School's position and rejected that of the Nancy School as unscientific. A woman could be raped under hypnosis but could not be an involuntary murderer.

Gilles de la Tourette noted: *"The hypnotized person always remains an individual who can manifest his or her will by resisting suggestions. This resistance can manifest itself in different ways, with a high degree of variability, depending on the subject. One of the most basic is the pure and simple refusal to carry out the order or answer the questions asked."*[44] Gilles de la Tourette shared Brissaud's view that if the crime or misdemeanor was the result of an action carried out *"under the influence of an imperative and premeditated suggestion, the hypnotizer must be punished and not the hypnotized person."*[45] Bompard, condemned to twenty years of forced labor and deemed *"morally blind,"* declared to the courtroom audience: *"I made a humane gesture towards a creature who only took up arms to realize the generous idea of eliminating bailiffs."* Her puerility was disconcerting: *"Sometimes she smiled like a girl about to receive an award for good behavior. Sometimes she took on the glum expression of a boarder forbidden to leave the convent. Sometimes she burst into laughter; sometimes she pouted and turned her back on the proceedings."*[46] Eyraud was condemned to death and executed.

Gilles de la Tourette had already excoriated Liégeois's book on suggestion and somnambulism in 1889, notably the idea that *"it is not necessary to be a physician to study hypnotism in a legitimate way."*[47] Unknown to Liégeois when he wrote his book, he foresaw how his adversaries would be proven right: *"To make our opponents take suggestion seriously, is it necessary to provide them with a real crime, an actual cadaver? This we obviously cannot do, so we hasten to triumph in this debate."* [48]

Gilles de la Tourette hastened to publish what he entitled an "epilogue" to the famous trial, which appeared in *Le Progrès Médical* of January 24, 1891: *"We readily admit that we are pleased to be involved in this case, as it gives us the opportunity to proclaim victory, definitive victory this time, we hope, for the ideas of our two Masters, Prof. Charcot and Prof. Brouardel, whom we have spent many years and considerable energy defending. . . . The doctrines of the Nancy School have suffered a defeat in the legal realm, which is all the more regrettable since nothing in this case justified going into battle."* Gilles de la Tourette sent Charcot the proofs for his article *"L'épilogue d'un procès célèbre,"* but several weeks passed between its writing and publication. During this interval, Bernheim published an article in the newspaper *Le Temps*, justifying his point of view on suggestion and criminality. Gilles de la Tourette then made an addition to *Le Progrès Médical* article after his exchange with Charcot, as evidenced by a cross-reference: *"In his article in* Le Temps *(January 29, 1891), published after this Bulletin was prepared, Mr. Bernheim, assessing the opinions of La Salpêtrière School on the subject of hypnotism, says somewhat scornfully: 'It is a set of experimental facts rather than a doctrine, because the facts are presented without theoretical interpretation.'"* Bernheim's text had been published in the newspaper's supplement,[49] and Bernheim himself continued to defend his thesis of "crime by suggestion," using the case of Gabrielle Bompard, among others, in his 1910 book, *Hypnotisme et Suggestion*[50]; he also referred to the case of rape followed by pregnancy that Augustin-René Bellanger (1810–1854) reported in 1854.[51]

As for Gilles de la Tourette, he summed up his point of view in his 1892 *Exposé des titres et travaux scientifiques* (written for the *agrégation* examination): "*Criminal suggestion cannot be a dangerous instrument outside of 'laboratory crimes,' where it is controlled; rape is the only crime associated with hypnotism, and it is committed against and not by the hypnotized person.*"[52] As early as 1786, a disciple of Franz Anton Mesmer (1734–1815) known as the Marquis de Puységur, born Amand Marc Chastenet (1751–1825),[53] defended the same position: "*All of the questions I have examined in this area have finally confirmed that the practice of animal magnetism, in the hands of honest people, is but another method to do as much good as possible. In the hands of unscrupulous people, no abuse can result, because patients cannot be brought into a state of absolute dependence, or if they can, they can only be tricked at the risk of causing incalculable harm to their health, making any scheme impossible to carry out.*"[54]

During the first international conference on experimental and therapeutic hypnotism, held in Paris from August 8 to 12, 1889, and thus prior to the Gouffé affair, a memorable showdown took place when Gilles de la Tourette severely criticized Bernheim's presentation. Neither was willing to concede anything on the definition of hypnotism, its practice, or the medical-legal consequences. As he had in the past, Bernheim invited Gilles de la Tourette to return to Nancy and criticized him for only having made a half-day's visit to his hospital.[55] Two days later, a similar scenario pitted Liégeois against Gilles de la Tourette, who declared: "*I assumed that the organizing committee, by allowing a law professor to examine how hypnotism relates to jurisprudence and legal medicine, had asked the rapporteur to mainly consider the legal side of the question, but I see that I was wrong.*" As this comment suggests, the conference was like a rehearsal, laying the groundwork for the oratory jousting of the Eyraud-Bompard trial. Gilles de la Tourette concluded his presentation this way: "*At La Salpêtrière, we have made it a rule to only use hypnotism in serious cases of hysteria, where there is everything to gain and nothing to lose. In Nancy, Mr. Bernheim puts his entire department to sleep; he claims he can hypnotize nine tuberculosis patients out of ten. In this case, while I know what they have to lose, I do not see what they have to gain.*"[56]

Auguste Voisin (1829–1898) explained the ideas of Gilles de la Tourette and Brouardel at the criminal anthropology conference in Brussels in 1892: "*Suggestion can, in certain cases, cause partial amnesia, thereby taking away the individual's idea of his real personality, and leading to a psychic hallucination that, standing in for the 'Me,' plays the role of a new personality. . . . The abolition of moral freedom is fictitious. The hypnotized person examines within himself the significance and severity of the suggested act; he remains in control of resisting or carrying out that act under his own free will, which means that he remains entirely responsible.*"[57]

Salvatore Ottolenghi (1861–1934), a professor of psychiatry and legal medicine in Turin, summarized the issue in 1900: "*Although the influence of hypnosis on criminal behavior often seems entirely theoretical, and the search for a crime perpetrated under hypnosis has always been in vain, these efforts have clearly shown that the influence of suggestion on criminal acts is greater than one would have imagined. Research on hypnosis has been highly beneficial in that it has drawn the attention of learned men to suggestion: a psychic force, one of the most important for intellectual and moral life, whether or not it is well intended. One can make use of suggestion not only in hypnotic states, but also in a more or less normal state of wakefulness.*"[58] This type of "suggestion," which plays an important role in establishing dominance in cults and sects, is not the only type currently studied. The issue of crime committed under hypnosis periodically resurfaces and is still the object of scientific research.[59]

The Gouffé affair inspired several French novelists. Eyraud's evasion of capture and his worldliness are evident in certain aspects of Arsène Lupin, created by writer Maurice Leblanc (1864–1941).[60] The first to make the affair into a novel was Jules Hippolyte Beaujoint (1830–1892) (pseudonym Jules de Grandpré), an author of popular fiction who was used to large print runs. *La malle sanglante* (literally, the bloody trunk) was published as soon as the case was closed.[61] The physician Emile Laurent (1861–1904) wrote another book from a medical-scientific perspective that also drew on the psychology of emotions.[62]

Many years later, in 1934, Edmond Locard (1877–1966), physician and director of the forensics laboratory in Lyon, published *La malle sanglante de Millery, affaire Gabrielle Bompard-Eyraud*.[63] He dedicated the book to "*My revered teacher, Professor A. Lacassagne.*" Lacassagne had created the field of "criminalistics," in which the scientific principles of legal medicine (ballistics, toxicology, etc.) are applied to the problems of police investigations.

Pierre Bouchardon (1870–1950), the famous prosecutor in the Joseph Caillaux and Mata Hari affairs, wrote a number of books on criminal cases. His *Malle mystérieuse*, published in 1933,[64] is a highly detailed novel inspired by the investigation. It is undoubtedly the best book for those wanting to delve into this case and its medical-legal consequences from a factual perspective. Liégeois's deposition is recounted in detail: "*Professor Liégeois did not attain the desired goal. . . . He entertained, instead of convincing.*" First Bouchardon cites

Babiński: "*The mind's critical faculties are not abolished during hypnotic sleep; the subject does not become passive and can make choices between various suggestions. The will is so insignificantly negated that the subject has the ability to keep secrets, even unimportant ones, from someone trying to find out what they are.*"[65] Then Bouchardon cites a contradictory passage by Liégeois: "*Any person placed in a state of somnambulism becomes a pure automaton in the experimenter's hands, both morally and physically.*"[66] The book also contains the grandiloquent arguments of Bompard's lawyer, Mr. Henri-Robert (1863–1936): "*Today hypnotism has made its triumphal entry into the criminal court.*" Bouchardon highlights Henri-Robert's conclusion: "*Gabriel Bompard is sick. We should provide the sick with treatment, cure them if possible. We should not send them to prison, and we should not send them to the scaffold.*"[67]

Finally, a parallel can be drawn with the work of Jules Barbey d'Aurevilly (1808–1889), known as the "*Connétable des lettres*" ("high officer of literature"). Barbey d'Aurevilly is famous for describing a case of anemia caused by self-induced hemorrhaging in his novel *Une histoire sans nom*, published in 1882. Paradoxically, this "nameless story" would provide a name to some unusual conditions involving self-mutilation, for which Jean Bernard (1907–2006) proposed the eponym of Lasthénie de Ferjol syndrome in 1967.[68] The novel's heroine is left pregnant and mute after being raped by a priest, Father Riculf, while she is in a somnambulic state. Although he does not explicitly acknowledge it, Gilles de la Tourette must have been influenced by this story: "*It was a profound dilemma between two souls, protracted and mysterious, and the mystery of it had to be amplified, so that even Agathe would not learn of this ignominious pregnancy that Mme de Ferjol intended to keep deep underground, even more than Lasthénie did, for Lasthénie, at that time, did not believe in her pregnancy. Overcome by new sensations, she believed she had an unknown illness, with deceptive symptoms, and that her mother had made a monstrous mistake. This error outraged her. She struggled painfully against her mother's affront. . . . But she did not lower her head under the degrading slap of her criticisms. She had the sublime stubbornness of innocence. . . . And because she was unlike this passionate, despotic, and hot-headed mother, who would have roared like a lioness had she been in Lasthénie's place, she often said to her: 'How you will one day regret making me suffer so, Mother!' with the meekness of a lamb that does not resist its own slaughter.*"[69]

These various letters clearly show the close friendship that developed between Gilles de la Tourette and Charcot; Charcot's esteem for and trust in Gilles de la Tourette are evident. In turn, Gilles de la Tourette not only devoted himself to facilitating the Master's daily work, but also used his knowledge of legal medicine to defend La Salpêtrière School. Having adopted Charcot's opinions, expertise, and ideas, Gilles de la Tourette became his unwavering advocate, during his lifetime and even after his death. Their collaboration conferred on Gilles de la Tourette the status of a learned disciple, which he took advantage of throughout his hospital career and in his private practice.

Another relationship that underscores the ties between Master and student is the relationship between Gilles de la Tourette and Charcot's son, Jean-Baptiste Charcot (1867–1936).

Close Friendship with Jean-Baptiste Charcot

As one of Charcot's favorite pupils, Gilles de la Tourette gained access to the Master's inner circles and became a close, lifelong friend of Charcot's son. Their friendship would prove decisive as Gilles de la Tourette's health declined (see Chapter 7), and Jean-Baptiste Charcot's aid became invaluable to Marie Gilles de la Tourette, not only for her husband's admission to the hospital, but throughout their long stay in Switzerland.

A letter written by Jean-Baptiste to his father, dated August 17, 1889, shows these close personal ties between the Charcot and Gilles de la Tourette families:

Dear Father, I have just dined at Hôpital de la Charité with Gilles de la Tourette and Dr. Leguay. After dinner, I accompanied them to Rue de Beaune where Gilles resides. The two of them are collaborating on a long work concerning possession. They have already written 551 pages, *grand aigle* or *petit aigle*; I am not sure, perhaps *moyen aigle*. Before they settled down to work, Gilles walked me through his rooms. He has beautiful curios, especially two superb Tournemine drawings that he paid 5 F for at the Hôtel Drouot. Every great man has his weakness. He also showed me a new photograph he will present to you next Sunday. If he is not sent to the city of Toulon by Dr. Brouardel to welcome the troops from Tonkin, he will take the express train Sunday morning with Dr. Leguay and myself. Dr. Leguay discovered the authentic manuscript of the Ursuline Mother Superior. This precious book is at the library in Tours, under the protection of Mr. Dubost. Nothing is more touching than sentiment to Dubost (a weak-minded man). Mr. Leguay approaches literature like Pathouter [?—difficult to decipher] approaches china and he is a wonder with dates, knows all of the holy and profane scriptures, knows Albert Wolff and Lambardemont, along with Father Mignon and Baschet. He will give me one devil of a recommendation. A good person to know; I did not waste my evening. Unfortunately, I could not stay with my two companions, who wrote twelve medium-format pages that evening. They must be happy; as for the rest of us, writing a single page over a lifetime seems an achievement. We will arrive in Chinon around four o'clock. Mr. Gilles de la Tourette and Mr. Leguay will leave in the evening. As for me, I shall stay with you for a while. My men and I are in need of rest. I dismissed my model today. Georges is doing his twenty-eight days in Tours and must make his way to Chinon.

Another event indicative of this friendship was related ten years later, on June 30, 1898, in the "Courtroom Gazette" section of the newspaper *Le Figaro*, by Albert Bataille (1856–1899). The article described how an altercation, in which J-B. Charcot slapped Georges Hugo (1868–1925) during an evening gathering in May 1898 at the Odéon Théâtre, ended up as a court case. Since Charcot declined the duel proposed by Hugo, Hugo turned the matter over to the police and Charcot was summoned to appear before a correctional court. Here is a brief version of the back-story: On February 12, 1891, Léon Daudet married Jeanne Hugo, Victor Hugo's granddaughter (immortalized by Hugo in *L'art d'être grand-père—The Art of Being a Grandfather*) and the sister of his best friend, Georges Hugo. However, the marriage was not a happy one and a divorce was pronounced in 1896. Jeanne Hugo married again, this time to J-B. Charcot. At the theater that evening, Georges Hugo apparently provoked J-B. Charcot by making a show of standing beside Daudet, and this on the heels of a long series of disagreements between the two protagonists. Gilles de la Tourette, in attendance at the Odéon that evening with J-B. Charcot, testified in court: *"Georges Hugo made as if he was going to lift his cane. At that moment, Mr. Jean Charcot slapped him, quite splendidly, I might add."* Bataille recounted how Gilles de la Tourette defended his friend J-B. Charcot: *"Dr. Gilles de la Tourette stated that he had the greatest esteem for Mr. Jean Charcot, who epitomizes loyalty and gentlemanliness, who has never picked a fight with anyone. 'It was,' he added, 'his brother-in-law who provoked him! For some time, Mr. Georges Hugo had made a point of appearing in public with Mr. Léon Daudet, the divorced husband of his sister. Mrs. Jean Charcot looked on the continual presence of Mr. Léon Daudet with Mr. Georges Hugo as a provocation, and since I have been asked for my personal opinion, I must say that he [J-B. Charcot] was not in the wrong.'"*[70]

In conclusion, Gilles de la Tourette's personality comes through in the various letters Charcot addressed to him, some of which deal with more personal matters. Gilles de la Tourette was a loyal friend and endeavored to be useful to others, a task to which he applied his exceptional capacity for hard work.

Notes

1. Gilles de la Tourette G. Réponse au Dr Vibert. Etude médico-légale sur les blessures produites par les accidents de chemins de fer. Séance du 9 avril 1888. *Bulletin de la Société de Médecine Légale*. 1888-89;10:170–171.
2. Gilles de la Tourette G. Blessures produites par les accidents de chemins de fer. Réponse à Ch Vibert. *Archives de l'Anthropologie criminelle et des Sciences pénales*. 1888;3:296–297.

3. *Currente calamo* (Latin); literally, "with running pen"; i.e. rapidly and without attention to style.

4. Charcot JM. *Leçons de Mardi à La Salpêtrière, note de cours de MM. Blin, Charcot, et Colin.* Paris: Aux Bureaux du Progrès Médical et Librairie A. Delahaye et Emile Lecrosnier. 1887.

5. Elliott B, Joyce E, Shorvon S. Delusions, illusions and hallucinations in epilepsy: complex phenomena and psychosis. *Epilepsy Res.* 2009;85(2–3):172–186.

6. Goldstein J. The wandering Jew and the problem of psychiatric anti-semitism in fin-de-siècle France. *J Contemporary Hist* 1985;20(4):521–552

7. Foville A (fils). *Les aliénés voyageurs ou migrateurs. Etude clinique sur certains cas de lypémanie.* (Mémoire lu à la Société médico-psychologique le 26 avril 1875). Paris: JB. Baillière. 1875.

8. Beaune JC. *Le vagabond et la machine, essai sur l'automatisme ambulatoire, médecine, technique et société (1880–1910).* Seyssel: Champ Vallon. 1983.

9. Morel BA. *Traité des dégénérescences physiques, intellectuelles et morales de l'espèce humaine et des causes qui produisent ces variétés maladives.* Paris: JB. Baillière. 1857.

10. Dowbiggin I. Degeneration and hereditarianism in French mental medicine 1840–90: psychiatric theory as ideological adaption. In W Bynum, R Porter, M Shepherd (eds.), *Anatomy of Madness: Essays in the History of Psychiatry, People and Ideas.* London and New York: Tavistock Publications. 1985;1:188–232.

11. Gilles de la Tourette G. *Traité de l'hystérie. Tome I seconde partie. Hystérie paroxystique.* Paris: Plon-Nourrit. 1895.

12. Tissié P. *Les aliénés voyageurs. Essai médico-psychologique.* Thèse no. 29. Bordeaux: Vve Cadoret. 1887.

13. Dubourdieu VC. *Contribution à l'étude de l'automatisme ambulatoire. De la dromomanie des dégénérés.* Thèse no. 66. Bordeaux: Imprimerie du Midi, P. Cassignol. 1894.

14. Pitres A. *L'automatisme ambulatoire dans ses rapports avec l'épilepsie: le vagabondage pathologique. Congrès des médecins aliénistes et neurologistes de France et des pays de langue française.* Bordeaux: de G. Gounouilhou. 1895.

15. Meige H. *Etude sur certains névropathes voyageurs Le Juif errant à la Salpêtrière.* Thèse no. 315. Paris: Bataille. 1893.

16. Meige H. Le juif errant à La Salpêtrière. *La Nouvelle Iconographie de La Salpêtrière.* 1893;6:191–204, 277–291, 333–358.

17. Hacking I. Les aliénés voyageurs: how fugue became a medical entity. *Hist Psychiatry.* 1996;7(27):425–449.

18. Medford N. Dissociative symptoms and epilepsy. *Epilepsy Behav.* 2014;30:10–13.

19. van der Kruijs SJ, Jagannathan SR, Bodde NM, Besseling RM, Lazeron RH, Vonck KE, Boon PA, Cluitmans PJ, Hofman PA, Backes WH, Aldenkamp AP, Jansen JF. Resting-state networks and dissociation in psychogenic non-epileptic seizures. *J Psychiatric Res.* 2014;54:126–133.

20. Richer P. *Etudes cliniques sur l'hystéro-épilepsie ou grande hystérie.* Paris: A. Delahaye et E. Lecrosnier. 1881.

21. Gilles de la Tourette G. *L'hypnotisme et les états analogues au point de vue médico-légal.* Paris: Plon, Nourrit. 1887.

22. Tuke DH. *Sleep-Walking and Hypnotism.* London: J. & A. Churchill. 1884.

23. Charcot JM. *Leçons du Mardi à La Salpêtrière, Policlinique 1888–1889.* Notes de cours de MM. Blin, Charcot, Henri Colin. Paris: Aux Bureaux du Progrès Médical. 1889.

24. Charcot JM, Guinon G. Du somnambulisme hystérique, phase passionnelle de l'attaque, attaque délirante, attaque de somnambulisme. *Le Progrès Médical.* 1891;19(2ᵉ TXIV)(29):41–49, 136–141.

25. Charcot JM, Guinon G. Du dédoublement de la personnalité d'origine hystérique (vigilambulisme hystérique). *Le Progrès Médical.* 1892;20(2ès tXV):193–196, 236–238, 361–364, 401–40; (tXVI):17–21/73–76/131–134./

26. Joffroy A, Dupouy R. *Fugues et vagabondages. Etude clinique et psychologique.* Paris: F. Alcan. 1909.

27. Bourneville DM, Regnard P. *Iconographie Photographique de La Salpêtrière.* Paris: Aux Bureaux du Progrès Médical. 1879–1880.

28. Gilles de la Tourette G. Des attaques de sommeil hystérique. *Archives de Neurologie.* 1888;15(43):92–107.

29. Charcot JM. *Leçons de Mardi à La Salpêtrière. Policlinique 1888–1889.* Notes de cours de MM Blin, JB Charcot, H. Colin. Paris: Aux Bureaux du Progrès Médical. 1889.

30. *Il Morgagni; Istituto di anatomia e istologia patologica dell'università di Milano.*

31. Gilles de la Tourette G. Dell'influenza di una intossicazione o di una malattia anteriore sulla localizzazione e sulla forma dei fenomeni isterici (Clinica delle malattie nervose alla salpetriere, prof. M. Charcot). Il Morgagni. Dott. Leonardo Vallardi Edit., Napoli-Milano, 1888. The Italian translation of the title of the article published in *Le Progrès Médical* of December 17, 1887: "Hystérie et syphilis: de l'influence d'une maladie ou d'une intoxication antérieure sur le mode de localisation et sur la forme des accidents hystériques."

32. Charcot JM. Hystérie et syphilis: de l'influence d'une maladie ou d'une intoxication antérieure sur le mode de localisation et sur la forme des accidents hystériques. Leçon recueillie par Gilles de la Tourette. *Le Progrès Médical.* 1887;15(51):511–512.

33. Marie P. Eloge de JM Charcot. *La Revue Neurologique.* 1925–1;32(6):731–745.

34. Electrotyping is a printing process used at the time to reproduce relief or intaglio plates.

35. Gilles de la Tourette G. *L'hypnotisme et les états analogues au point de vue médico-légal.* Paris: Plon-Nourrit. 1887.

36. Goetz CG. The prefaces by Charcot: leitmotifs of an international career. *Neurology.* 2003;60(8):1333–1340.

37. Gilles de la Tourette G. *Der Hypnotismus und die verwandten Zustände vom Standpunkte der gerichtlichen Medicin.* Hamburg: FF. Richter. 1889.

38. Gilles de la Tourette G. *L'hypnotisme et les états analogues au point de vue médico-légal.* Paris: Plon-Nourrit. 1887.

39. Lacassagne A. *L'affaire Gouffé, acte d'accusation; rapport de MM. les Drs Paul Bernard, Lacassagne, Brouardel, Mottet et Ballet.* Lyon: A Storck. 1891.

40. Lèbre G. *Revue des grands procès contemporains.* Paris: Chevalier-Maresq. 1891;9:19–107.

41. Bernheim H. *L'hypnotisme et la suggestion dans les rapports avec la médecine légale.* Nancy: A. Crépin-Leblond. 1887.

42. Meyer H, Fichot K. L'affaire Gouffé: la révélation, l'accomplissement du crime, le colis funèbre devant la maison rue Tronson-Ducoudray. *Le Petit Journal.* 2 février 1891;27(5):34–36.

43. Plas R. Hysteria, hypnosis, and moral sense in French 19th-century forensic psychiatry. The Eyraud-Bompard case. *Int J Law Psychiatry.* 1998;21(4):397–407.

44. Gilles de la Tourette G. L'épilogue d'un procès célèbre. *Le Progrès Médical.* 1891;19-1(5):89–96.

45. Brissaud E. Les suggestions hypnotiques au point de vue médico-légal. *La Nouvelle Rome.* 1889;11(56).

46. Bouchardon P. *La malle mystérieuse, affaire Eyraud-Bompard.* Paris: Albin Michel. 1933.

47. Gilles de la Tourette G. *Bibliographie. Liégeois J. De la suggestion et du somnambulisme dans leurs rapports avec la jurisprudence et la médecine légale.* Paris: O Doin. 1889; and *Archives de Neurologie.* 1889;17(49):156–161.

48. Liégeois J. *De la suggestion et du somnambulisme dans leurs rapports avec la jurisprudence et la médecine légale.* Paris: O Doin. 1889.

49. Bernheim H. Hypnotisme et suggestion, doctrine de La Salpêtrière et doctrine de Nancy. *Le Temps.* Supplément du jeudi 29 janvier 1891;31(10848):1–2.

50. Bernheim H. *Hypnotisme & suggestion, Hystérie, Psychonévrose, Neurasthénie, Psychothérapie.* Paris: O. Doin. 1910.

51. Bellanger AR. *Le magnétisme, vérités et chimères de cette science occulte.* Paris: Guilhermet. 1854.

52. Gilles de la Tourette G. *Exposé des titres et travaux scientifiques. Concours de l'Agrégation de 1892.* Paris: E. Plon-Nourrit. 1892.

53. His first name was indeed Amand and not Armand, as it is too often written.

54. Chastenet AM, dit Marquis de Puységur. *Mémoires pour servir à l'histoire et à l'établissement du magnétisme animal.* A Londres, 1786.

55. Bernheim H. *Valeur relative des divers procédés destinés à provoquer l'hypnose et à augmenter la suggestibilité au point de vue thérapeutique. Comptes-Rendus du Premier Congrès International de l'hypnotisme expérimental et thérapeutique.* Paris: Doin. 1890:79–98. Ibid., 99–101; discussion par Gilles de la Tourette G.

56. Liégeois J. *Rapports de la suggestion et du somnambulisme avec la jurisprudence et la médecine légale. La responsabilité des hypnotiques. Comptes-Rendus du Premier Congrès International de l'hypnotisme expérimental et thérapeutique.* Paris: Doin. 1890:244–264; discussion par Gilles de la Tourette G, 264–268.

57. Voisin A. *Suggestions criminelles ou délictueuses et responsabilité pénale. Actes du Troisième Congrès International d'Anthropologie Criminelle.* Bruxelles: Henri Lamertin. 1893.

58. Ottolenghi S. *Suggestion et crime. Section de Médecine Légale. Comptes Rendus XIIIe Congrès International de Médecine Paris 1900.* Paris: Masson. 1900.

59. Harris R. Murder under hypnosis. *Psychol Med.* 1985;15(3):477–505.

60. Henry D. *Arsène Lupin, gentleman-cambrioleur: un nouveau type de personnage?* Université Sorbonne nouvelle-Paris 3. UFR Littérature et Linguistique françaises et latines. Thèse 2007PA030160. 2007.

61. Beaujoint J (de Grandpré). *La malle sanglante: assassinat de l'huissier Gouffé, affaire Eyraud et Gabrielle Bompard.* Paris: Fayard. 1890.

62. Laurent E. *Les suggestions criminelles: viols, faux et captations, faux témoignages, viols moraux, les suggestions en amour, Gabrielle Fenayrou et Gabrielle Bompard.* Lyon: Strock. 1891.

63. Locard E. *La Malle sanglante de Millery.* Paris: Gallimard. 1934.

64. Bouchardon P. *La malle mystérieuse, affaire Eryaud-Bompard.* Paris: Albin Michel. 1933.

65. Babiński J. Grand et petit hypnotisme. *Archives de Neurologie.* 1889;17(49):92–108.

66. Liégeois J. *De la suggestion hypnotique dans ses rapports avec le droit civil et le droit criminel. Mémoire lu à l'Académie des sciences morales et politiques (séances des 5, 19, 26 avril, 3 et 10 mai 1884).* Nancy: Imprimerie de Berger-Levrault. 1885.

67. Robert H. Plaidoirie. In G Lèbre (ed.), *Revue des grands procès contemporains.* Paris: Chevalier-Maresq. 1891;9:75–107.

68. Bernard J, Najean Y, Alby N, Rain JD. Les anémies hypochromes dues à des hémorragies volontairement provoquées. Syndrome de Lasthénie de Ferjol. *Presse Médicale.* 1967;75(42):2087–2090.

69. Barbey d'Aurevilly J. *Une histoire sans nom.* Paris: A. Lemerre, 1882.

70. Bataille A. Gazette des tribunaux. *Le Figaro.* 1898;11(181):3–4.

4

The Assassination Attempt

1893, *Annus Horribilis*

The year 1893 got off to a promising start. Gilles de la Tourette had finished the second part of his treatise on hysteria, *Hystérie pathologique*, which he gave to his teacher, Charcot, to revise. On June 3, 1893, he was pronounced "Chevalier de la Légion d'honneur" on behalf of the French Ministry of the Interior for the decisive role he had played in the erection of a statue to honor Théophraste Renaudot (1586–1653), inaugurated on June 4, 1893. But everything shifted dramatically when summer arrived. His eldest son, Jean, aged five, died on July 11, 1893, of meningitis. Gilles de la Tourette wrote to the journalist Georges Montorgueil (1857–1933), his close friend, on the twentieth of that same month:

Dear Sir and Friend, I have returned from my painful pilgrimage to Loudun very tired. I find on my desk this brochure that we are publishing in L'Iconographie de la Salpêtrière, No. 4. It is new, unpublished material for everyone. Granted, it was the subject of a friend's thesis, but this thesis will not be in circulation before the Iconographie is released.[1] I think you will find material in it for an amusing book. Life is not a happy affair when your hopes are dashed; good friendships are the only consolation. Most sincerely yours.[2]

Having just returned from his son's funeral in Loudun, Gilles de la Tourette turned to his friend, Montorgueil, for support. Six weeks later, on August 16, 1893, Jean-Martin Charcot (1825–1893) died during a journey to the Morvan region of Burgundy, where he had intended to rest. The cause of death was pulmonary edema associated with angina, from which Charcot had suffered for two years. A few weeks earlier, on July 29, 1893, Henri Lamy (1864–1909), Charcot's *interne* in 1892, had defended his thesis on syphilitic meningomyelitis.[3] The defense of Pierre Janet (1859–1947) took place the same day. Theirs were the last two juries Charcot would preside over. It is likely that Gilles de la Tourette was referring to Lamy's work in his letter to Montorgueil.

The year 1893 also ended dramatically.

The Assassination Attempt

On Wednesday, December 6, 1893, a woman by the name of Rose Kamper, born Laurence-Rose Lecoq (1864–1955), made a fateful visit to Gilles de la Tourette's home at 39 Rue de l'Université (Figure 4.1). Georges Guinon (1859–1932) recounted the events: *"That day, at around seven-fifteen in the evening, a young, respectable-looking woman presented herself, asking to speak with Gilles de la Tourette. As he was away and she insisted, she was shown to a waiting room where she remained for about a quarter of an hour. Upon his return, Gilles de la Tourette took her into his office. She then asked him: 'Are you Doctor Gilles de la Tourette? The one who has written books on hypnotism?' After our friend's response, the young woman explained that various practitioners had already hypnotized her, that she was currently destitute and needed 50 francs. Gilles de la Tourette could not recall meeting her, or only vaguely remembered her lucubrations about hypnotism; in any case, he asked her for her name and address, promising to help her obtain assistance if her situation merited it. As the woman's only reply was to ask for money again, Gilles de la Tourette walked toward the door as if to escort her out, turning his back to her as he put his hand as he did so. At that moment, he heard a shot and felt a violent impact in his neck. Before he had the time to move, he heard two more shots. He then hastened to leave the room. Once out of range, he touched his neck, which was covered in blood. He could also feel the presence of a hard body between the bone and the skin, which he supposed was a bullet. During this time, the woman was arrested, not resisting in any way. Fortunately, the bullet had touched the occipital bone at an angle, then flattened, and after traveling around 5 cm between bone and skin, had stopped. It was immediately removed by Doctor Delbet,[4] hospital surgeon, and today we are relieved to know that our friend is out of danger."[5]*

In his report, the police commissioner stated that he had found two bullets in the office, one in the bookshelf and the other in a leg of the desk. Taken by Marie Gilles de la Tourette to her husband's room, he found Gilles de la Tourette lying in bed, *"his head stabilized in a brace."* When the commissioner

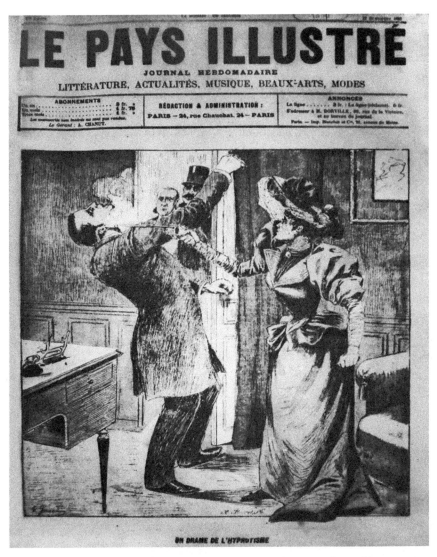

FIGURE 4.1 *"Hynotism Drama,"* the assassination attempt on the cover of a weekly newspaper. Private collection of the author.

asked Kamper why she had attempted to murder Gilles de la Tourette, she repeated *"that she lived in poverty and had long ago, either voluntarily or without her knowledge, agreed to be a subject for hypnotism experiments at La Salpêtrière."* The commissioner's report continues: *"She had lost her will to such an extent that she found it impossible to continue working, and consequently, asking money of those who had taken away her livelihood appeared logical to her. Continuing with the dream that seemed to obsess her, she vehemently insisted she had within her a duality. One part was physical, the other part was moral and not herself. She said that she had acted under the influence of the person who controlled her will, but that in fact, she had willfully attempted to shoot Mr. Gilles de la Tourette because she was destitute. She mentioned the name of Mr. de Rochas d'Aiglun, Director of the Ecole Polytechnique,[6] with whom she shared certain ideas, as evidenced by three real letters addressed to her by this individual. Her attitude was that of a person who acts with cold determination, dominated by an idée fixe. She had left her home at 52 Rue de Cléry on Sunday, the third of this month, without any money. Incidentally, no one had ever made any particular remarks about her at this address. She does not know the whereabouts of her husband, who left her some time ago and was apparently a hairdresser's assistant. Her father lives in Poissy (Seine-et-Oise) where he is the head road worker. Civil status: Lecoq Laurence Rose, aged thirty, born in Poissy on May 12, 1863, to François Lecoq and Quettier Antoinette, married in Paris (7th arrondissement) to Jean Kamper on September 28, 1886, no children. I have submitted my report today to the State's Council. Police Commissioner Chilot, Saint-Thomas d'Aquin district. December 7, 1893."[7]*

Upon shooting Gilles de la Tourette, Kamper sat down on a bench in the anteroom, her revolver still in her hand. To the servant instructed to watch her until the police arrived, she declared: *"I know that what I've done is wrong, but I had to do it and now I'm satisfied."*[8] In 1892, Kamper had been a patient at La Salpêtrière, under the care of Jules Séglas (1856–1939), a young physician filling in for Jules Falret (1824–1899) at the time. More recently she had been released from Hôpital Sainte-Anne, where she had been committed for delusions of persecution. Published in *L'Eclair*, her hospitalization papers indicate that her condition was complicated by *"insomnia, disturbances of cutaneous sensation, sensorial illusions, and delusional interpretations. She says that she has been hypnotized, that she is in contact by means of hypnotism with Colonel Rochas. . . . She is fascinated by Sâr Péladan."*

On the evening of the murder attempt, Gilles de la Tourette wrote to Montorgueil in an unsteady hand (Figure 4.2): *"I shall be happy to see you today. The bullet has been taken out. I am better, better. Sincerely, Gilles de la Tourette. What a strange story!"*.

Played up by the Press

This event sparked considerable media coverage, occurring a few months after the public courtroom dispute between the Nancy and Salpêtrière Schools. Certain newspapers went so far as to insinuate a publicity stunt orchestrated by Gilles de la Tourette himself. One tabloid article was reportedly entitled "Injury as Advertising." Many years later, in 1911, Dr. Felix Regnault (1863–1938), a

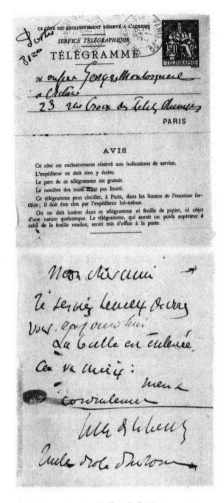

FIGURE 4.2 After the assassination attempt, Gilles de la Tourette wrote to his friend Montorgueil in an unsteady hand.
Copyright Musée Charbonneau-Lassay, Ville de Loudun, with kind permission.

French physician, anthropologist, and prehistorian, would relate in *Le Journal* his difficulties establishing a clientele at the start of his career, and, among his many anecdotes, was this one: *"Some take advantage of a simple accident. Gilles de la Tourette told those close to him that after struggling to have a regular clientele, the problem resolved itself rapidly after a drama that nearly cost him his life, a drama that all of the newspapers covered, printing his name and address in their stories; a woman had entered his office and tried to shoot him to death with a revolver."*[9]

On Friday, December 8, 1893, Guy Tomel (1855–1898) reported in *Le Figaro*, under a headline in the form of a question: "Laboratory crime?"

"According to the first reports, Kamper, taken to see the district's police commissioner, said she had attempted the murder under the influence of suggestion. There are always well-informed newsmongers in such cases, and this time they went so far as to suggest they knew the name of the hypnotizer and were keeping it 'provisionally quiet.' Despite the unlikelihood of the rumor, is it possible that a rival physician pushed his love of experimentation to the point of becoming an accomplice to a crime? If this were true, is the crime a bloody demonstration of the errors of Charcot's disciples? A rapid but meticulous investigation has clearly shown that the Nancy School will not have to defend itself against accusations of an extravagant experiment; nor will it have any reason to triumph over the Salpêtrière skepticism. Kamper is simply a woman with hallucinations and delusions of persecution who was released prematurely from the department of Dr. Falret."[10]

On Saturday, December 9, 1893, Montorgueil, with information from Gilles de la Tourette himself, devoted more than half of the first page of *L'Eclair* to the story under the title: "A madwoman, the attempted murder of Gilles de la Tourette, the criminal's motives, a dispute amongst physicians, and criminal suggestion."[11] He began this way:

"On Wednesday night, as we know, Dr. Gilles de la Tourette was the victim of an assassination attempt that owes its peculiar nature ('mysterious' would be going too far) to the physician's personality, his work, and the mental state of the would-be murderer. Another circumstance adds to the strangeness of this crime. A few days before it occurred, L'Eclair published an article on the views of two opposing camps, represented on one side by Mr. Dumontpalier[12] *and Mr. Mesnet, who defended the possibility of criminal suggestion, versus Mr. Gilles de la Tourette and Mr. Guinon, who denied it."*

Montorgueil's account is complete in every detail: *"She had spoken to Gilles de la Tourette and the commissioner about her double personality. One of these personalities was in contact with Dr. Luys or Dr. de Rochas. The names of these two physicians were written on a list before that of Mr. Gilles de la Tourette. In particular, she claimed to have been at Mr. Luys's home the day before. We found out that she had in fact gone to this address. Her plan, her* idée fixe, *was to seek out these three men and to kill the first one she met."* Montorgueil's tone is ironic when it comes to the prognosis of the alienist who authorized her release from Sainte-Anne: *"She was much improved after her stay in the hospital, according to the physician who signed her release certificate, which the subsequent events quickly made absurd: 'Is calmer than at admittance, and since she came of her own will, she does not appear to be a danger to herself or others. We feel she can be released on a trial basis.' Trial there was, and it was a disaster. Dr. Gilles de la Tourette, who greeted us with his head in bandages, would no doubt concur!"*

Montorgueil also explored Kamper's motives: *"In the end, her impoverished condition took control of her delusions, and she decided to kill those she deemed responsible for her material and spiritual distress. She was obsessed, and her delusions were chronic. She conceived of her plan, which was to kill one of the men who, she believed, was hypnotizing her, inventing any necessary pretext. She came up with a list of three names: Dr. Luys, Dr. Gilles de la Tourette, and Mr. de Rochas."*

As Jules Luys (1828–1897) was not in Paris at the time, and de Rochas had given orders to send her away, Kamper's victim was Gilles de la Tourette. Montorgueil quoted Guinon in his conclusion: *"This lamentable accident, which almost cost the life of one of our most distinguished physicians from the early days of the School, might be seen as having no practical moral. Georges Guinon, who treated Mr. Gilles de la Tourette, does not hold this view. 'What is going to happen?' he asks. 'There can be no doubt; this woman is a lunatic. The incompetent judge will call on her physician to testify. Deemed sick, she will be put away and considered as just another patient. If one day she appears to be cured, as has already happened once before, she could be released. Can we be certain that she will not attempt to take other lives? Do we once again not feel the need to protect innocent human beings from the delusions of the criminally insane? No, we do not feel the need to create asylums where judges could send those criminals unfit for prison due to their mental condition. Prison, which is a punishment, would be an unfair sentence, but asylums from which they can be released so easily are hardly reassuring for us. There is an imperative need to create a place of both treatment and detention where those criminals not fully aware of the gravity of their actions, are nonetheless unable to cause harm."*

Guinon also testified to the nature of the press campaign at the time: *"The newspapers use this as a means for building up a fiction around the possibility of crimes by hypnotic suggestion. As reported in* Le Figaro *yesterday, some well-informed newsmongers went so far as to hint at knowing the name of the person responsible for the criminal suggestion, which they were keeping 'provisionally quiet'. . . . Criminal suggestion is impossible in this case, since the alleged hypnotization only existed inside the delirious brain of this woman. It is no less true that, if hypnotism were not so carelessly popularized, the mentally weak wouldn't seize upon it for their delusions of persecution."*

On Monday, December 18, 1893, Gilles de la Tourette, the *"miraculous survivor,"* sent out an invitation to celebrate his prompt recovery:

My dear friend, On Saturday 23, at 7.30, my internes are coming over to drink to my "resurrection" with Boudin[13] and a few friends. We are counting on you for dinner, 7.30 without fail, I shall remind you.

Montorgueil later stated: *"This accident taught him to distrust the hysterics who came to see him and to be more circumspect in his communications, so as not to designate himself in their schemes; but he in no way slowed his frenetic activity."*[14] A note confirming the precautions Gilles de la Tourette began taking can be found in the National Archives. Most likely for some role he was playing in a trial, Gilles de la Tourette gave these instructions to Montorgueil on May 22, 1894:

My dear friend, My wife is scared silly of bombs, and my landlord, who is a friend, continues to worry. . . .

So please use the following in the text if possible: "One of our venerable alienist physicians whose authoritative words have often rung out in the courts, whereby we are obliged to withhold his respected identity, gave us the following interview, of evident importance." At my age, you are not yet venerable unless you are in a Masonic lodge, where incidentally I never got beyond the level of apprentice.[15]

Also, if Guinon gave you an interview, put it as far away as possible and, of course, do not mention either Charcot or La Salpêtrière. Excuse me for this request. . . And grant it. Affectionately.

P.S.: It goes without saying that the same applies to your *L'Eclair* collections; the interview must remain anonymous.

The tone is directive. Gilles de la Tourette did not want to be attacked again. He gave interviews to the press, but more anonymously than before. We learn in passing that he was initiated by the Freemasons, but apparently put little time or energy into their organization. The unspoken rivalry with his friend Guinon, dating from the publication of *La maladie des tics convulsifs,* also comes through in his words.

And Rose Kamper?

After Ballet's expert assessment, the judge declared Rose Kamper immune from liability. She was committed on March 13, 1894. Le Gendre wrote: *"Committed for the third time, she almost injured a nurse by hitting her with a fork. After staying at Sainte-Anne for some time, she was sent to Villejuif, but space was limited and she was eventually sent to a small asylum in the Charente region. She quickly escaped. The prefect of police, who knew how dangerous she was, sent one of his officers to warn our colleague and encourage him to be careful. He even offered to assign him a permanent officer for his consultations, a very effective means for attracting clients! Gilles de la Tourette preferred to have private detective work done and discovered his persecutor's hideout just when she was about to return to Paris with the avowed aim of repeating her crime against the physician whom she had only seen once, the day of the murder attempt."*

In *Gil Blas* on February 7, 1902, the columnist Jean Bernard (1858–1936) wrote again of the affair. He was strolling the boulevards with an unnamed physician when *"suddenly, the doctor took me by the arm and pointed out a woman passing by. . . . 'It's that hysteric who tried to assassinate Dr. Gilles de la Tourette. She was put under observation and, based on the physicians' reports, declared immune from liability, committed for a time to an asylum, and finally released. There she is, moving freely about Paris while her victim, suffering the effects of overwork, has been committed to a rest home; unfortunately, there is every reason to fear he will never be released. So this wretch kills a man, or tries to murder him with a revolver, and she escapes justice. She's mad, it's an established fact. Or is it really madness? Isn't she only half-mad? What motive drove her? So many questions. What's certain is that Mrs. K. . . . who injured Dr. Gilles de la Tourette, was placed in an insane asylum; the physicians declared her cured and let her out among the mentally sound. Were they mistaken? The curious thing about it all is that the victim, Dr. Gilles de la Tourette, published a brochure when the assassins of the bailiff Gouffé were on trial. It was in response to my deposition of the Nancy doctor. Called as a defense witness, he had said that Gabriel Bompard's involvement in the bailiff's murder was under Eyraud's suggestive impulsion. Gilles de la Tourette argued to the contrary in a paper that did not go unnoticed. In any case, opinions of that crime aside, we can state that scientifically, it is possible that Mrs. K. shot Dr. Gilles de la Tourette under the suggestive influence of a third party."*[16]

Hospitalized once again, Kamper escaped in 1910. Police identified her several years later, at which point she was working as a seamstress under her maiden name. Since her mental health had improved, she was not rehospitalized. But she relapsed during World War II. She spent the last twelve years of her life in Hôpital Sainte-Anne, where she died in 1955 at the age of ninety-two. Finally, we should note that the day Montorgueil used the murder attempt as his headline—December 9, 1893—the anarchist Auguste Vaillant (1861–1894), seeking vengeance for the death of Ravachol,[17] threw a nail bomb into the benches of the National Assembly and injured some fifty people.

Surprisingly enough, this drama remains a source of novelistic inspiration to this day. An American novelist, predestined by her name, Aileen La Tourette, constructed a plot bringing together Charcot, Freud, Colette, and Gilles de la Tourette, in which the victim is Rose Kamper, a woman suffering from delusional obsessions.[18]

Notes

1. Lamy H. De la méningo-myélite syphilitique, étude clinique et anatomo-pathologique. *Nouvelle Iconographie de La Salpêtrière.* 1893;6(2):86–101; 1893;6(3):153–176; 1893;6(4):205–237; 1893;6(5):251–276.

2. Archives Nationales 428AP/2 Correspondance Montorgueil-Gilles de la Tourette.

3. Lamy H. *De la méningo-myélite syphilitique*. Thèse no. 433. Paris: Battaille. 1893.

4. Pierre Delbet (1861–1957).

5. Guinon G. Attentat contre le Dr Gilles de la Tourette. *Le Progrès Médical*. 1893;18(49):446.

6. Eugene Auguste Albert de Rochas (1837–1914) was a French soldier and administrator and an author of historical studies and books on paranormal phenomena.

7. Dossier G. Gilles de la Tourette. Archives de la Préfecture de Police de Paris. 25–27, rue Baudin 93310 Le Pré Saint-Gervais.

8. Anonyme. Attentat contre Gilles de la Tourette. *La Patrie: journal quotidien, politique, commercial et littéraire*. 8 décembre 1893. BNF Notice FRBNF32833792.

9. Regnault F. L'art de se faire une clientèle. *Le Journal*. Jeudi 10 août 1911;19(6892):6.

10. Tomel G. Crime de Laboratoire? *Le Figaro*. Vendredi 8 décembre 1893;39(342):1.

11. Montorgueil G. Une folle, la tentative d'assassinat contre M. Gilles de la Tourette. *L'Éclair*. 9 décembre 1893;6(1889):1.

12. Prof. Victor Dumontpallier (1826–1899), Dr. Ernest Mesnet (1825–1898).

13. Name difficult to make out; identification impossible (Baudouin of *Le Progrès Médical*?).

14. Montorgueil G. Georges Gilles de la Tourette. *L'Éclair*. 24 mai 1904.

15. A congratulatory letter sent by Charles Beaumont in May 1884 to Gilles de la Tourette when his book on Théophraste Renaudot was published confirms this involvement with the Freemasons.

16. Bernard J. Courrier de Paris. *Gil Blas*. 7 février 1902;21(8117):1.

17. François Claudius Koënigstein known as "Ravachol" (1859–1892); see Chapter 16 on *La Revue Hebdomadaire*.

18. La Tourette A. *Late connections*. Melbourne: Ilura Press. 2008.

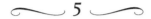

Glimpses of Gilles de la Tourette's Personality

Hospital Life and the Driout Scandal

S TARTING IN 1893, Georges Gilles de la Tourette's behavior gradually changed, a sign of syphilitic general paralysis. His manic tendencies, his irascibility, and his arrogance led to disputes that were not always legitimate. We present the previously unpublished letters he sent to the administrators of his hospital, where he was in charge of a department, and we describe his reaction to a slanderous press campaign. In addition to Gilles de la Tourette's condition, the new documents elucidate the state of Parisian hospitals and the challenges of hospital physicians at the end of the nineteenth century.

Accounts of Hospital Life

On March 2, 1895, Gilles de la Tourette wrote to the Director General of the Paris public hospital system. Visitors had invaded his department at Hôpital Cochin, where he was replacing a *chef de service*.[1]

March 2, 1895, Dear Sir, It is my duty to inform you of the condition of the sheds at Hôpital Cochin that have been assigned to me. The patients cannot rest due to the bugs and other vermin that have infested the bedding and the walls. These pests are so numerous that they nearly prevent the physicians and students from auscultating the patients; we often have to undress in the department to rid ourselves of their presence. I do hope, sir, that in the interest of the patients and the medical personnel, you will order a disinfection of the premises as soon as possible.

Gilles de la Tourette took his duties as chef de service seriously and tried to improve conditions for his patients. His letter also testifies to how dilapidated certain Parisian hospitals were at the time. As for the response he received, it reveals the impotence and resignation of hospital administrators:

This situation, inherent to the wooden construction of the sheds, can only be attenuated by measures that the personnel take at all times: steam sterilization of the sheets and cleaning of the beds, bed bases, walls, and floors with antiseptic solutions. As often as possible, the Hospital Director will proceed with various disinfections which, while they cannot totally eradicate the vermin, should attenuate to the greatest degree possible the difficulties that you report.

The director of Hôpital Cochin, after conducting his own investigation, wrote:

March 7, 1895. The question of bugs in our sheds is not new and I have not waited until today to address it. . . . Doctor Gilles de la Tourette also claims that the students are often obliged to undress in the department to rid themselves of bugs. The head nurse could only recall one person who had to undress, and that was Doctor Gilles de la Tourette himself, on the same Saturday, March 2. It is possible that the disagreeable fact of finding a bug on his person led Doctor Gilles de la Tourette to write his letter and to draw general conclusions from this particular event."

In another letter written shortly after he was transferred to Hôpital Hérold in May 1896, Gilles de la Tourette sought to improve conditions in his department. Basing his argument on a complaint lodged by a patient's family for lack of appropriate treatment, he requested that the director of the hospital authorize the installation of a shower for hydrotherapy treatments, in common use at that time.[2] Gilles de la Tourette's tone was courteous but firm. His request was, however, refused for lack of funds.

All of these letters were written with the same pugnacity that Gilles de la Tourette used elsewhere to impose his will. Other contentions between Gilles de la Tourette and the hospital administration, while of a different sort, would arise later.

The Driout Scandal

The chapter on Gilles de la Tourette's correspondence with journalist Georges Montorgueil (1857–1933) shows how he often succeeded in disseminating ideas and opinions to a broad audience, using the "mainstream press" as his intermediary. In 1901, the press focused its attention on him again, in a story meant to uncover scandalous practices in the hospitals. Against his wishes this time, Gilles de la Tourette found himself at the center of a controversy.

On February 1, 1901, the newspaper *Petit Soir* featured an article headlined "A Macabre Story" which developed as follows: *"This past July, a policeman named Driout (Emile) was the victim of a carriage accident on the Pont Mirabeau. He passed away a few months later and the State Council's Office, to determine whether he had died of his injuries, appointed Doctor Socquet, a forensic medical examiner, to perform the autopsy on the cadaver. . . . The body was then transported to the morgue and laid out on a slab. Dr. Socquet was shocked to discover that any serious examination of the cadaver was impossible: the brain had been replaced by copies of the paper* La Gaudriole *and the sheet music of Bruant; the intestines had disappeared and the spinal cord had been completely removed. As for the thorax, it contained two livers instead of one. The honorable medical examiner immediately sent a report to the State's Council, who in turn opened an investigation into the odious mutilations to which this cadaver had been subjected, and which undoubtedly took place in the lecture hall of Hôpital Necker where the unfortunate officer had been taken."*

This led journalists first to Hôpital Necker, then Hôpital Boucicaut, and finally Hôpital Saint-Antoine where the ill-fated police officer had died. The newspapers played up the suspense with day-by-day accounts, complete with commentaries on the hospitals and their personnel. At Boucicaut, considered the most modern hospital in Paris, the director was adamant: *'The internes of Hôpital Boucicaut are incapable of such an odious act!' "* Driout had indeed been hospitalized briefly at Boucicaut, starting on October 15, 1900. *"The diagnosis, signed by Doctor Letut, was neuropathy."* To satisfy the journalists, the director of Hôpital Boucicaut called in the head nurse, who *"stated that Doctor Clément must have sent Driout to his colleague, Doctor Gilles de la Tourette."*

On February 2, 1901, a few more details emerged: *"Doctor Gilles de la Tourette, who specializes in nervous diseases, did indeed treat Sergeant Driout in his department at Hôpital Saint-Antoine. . . . The patient died on January 18, 1901, and the autopsy, performed immediately, was aimed at examining and studying the nervous centers: brain, cerebellum, and spinal cord. But this in no way explains or excuses the mutilation of the body, or sheds any light on why these indecencies were committed after the autopsy! The internes of Hôpital Saint-Antoine have a very peculiar way of treating the mortal coil. [signed] Mayer-Lévy."*

Gilles de la Tourette had to respond to these allegations. On February 16, 1901, he wrote to the Director General of the Paris hospital system (Figure 5.1):

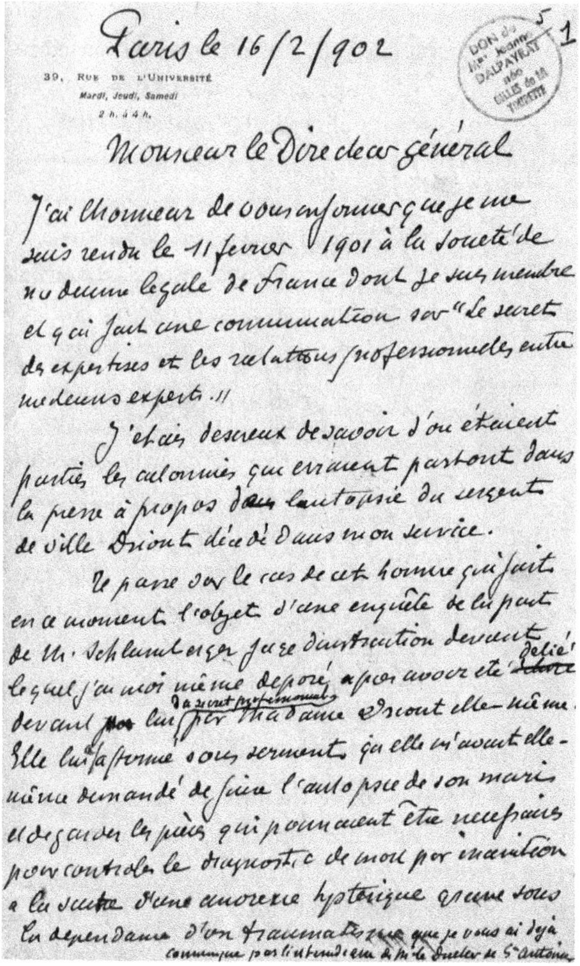

FIGURE 5.1   On February 16, 1901, Gilles de la Tourette wrote to the Director General of the Paris hospital system.
Copyright Musée Charbonneau-Lassay, Ville de Loudun, with kind permission.

"Paris, February 16, 1902, I have the honor of informing you that on February 11, 1901, I attended a meeting of the Société de Médecine Légale de France, of which I am a member, and I presented a paper on the confidentiality of medical examinations and the professional relations between medical examiners. I wished to uncover the source of the slander spread by the press regarding the autopsy of Sergeant Driout, who died in my department. I shall not go into further details about this case, currently the subject of an investigation ordered by the examining magistrate, Mr. Schlumberger, before whom I myself testified after Mrs. Driout granted her permission that I speak of confidential matters regarding her husband's health. She confirmed under oath that she had asked me to autopsy her husband and keep the parts necessary to verify the diagnosis of death by starvation, following hysterical anorexia secondary to trauma. . . . Mr. Socquet performed a new autopsy and this is the key point to which I draw your attention. The press said that the cadaver was mutilated and defiled at Saint-Antoine, that organs were found that did not belong to Driout, along with bits of cigar and trash, and that sheets of a humorous newspaper had been stuffed inside the skull. The brain and spinal cord were absent, but Mr. Socquet made a formal declaration before the Société de Médecine Légale that the facts had been distorted. . . . As to the newspaper stuffed into the skull, it was placed there by a janitor at Saint-Antoine, who filled the empty space left by the brain to ensure the head's stability. This is standard practice in such a case. It so happened that he did not have any other material on hand, and had to take the only paper he could find. By an ironic twist of fate, the newspaper he used was none other than *La Gaudriole*, with its humor columns and romantic stories. This has occasioned sarcasm and ironic remarks . . . even insults aimed at both the janitor and myself, and in some cases targeting your administration. . . . He might have added that from now on, the lecture halls where the autopsies are carried out should be provided with better material for maintaining the condition of the cadavers, such as: clean paper without humorous commentary, wooden packing material, kelp or other substances that are, in reality, very inexpensive. . . . This memorandum was not forthcoming, I do not know why; I can only make the observation without asking for the reason. What I have suffered will be quickly forgotten; I have the clean conscience of one who has done his duty. In short, I believe that everyone at Saint-Antoine has done their duty and nothing but their duty, whereas the administration has not entirely done its duty. I have heard the janitor is going to be reprimanded.

Apart from attesting to Gilles de la Tourette's position and his aggressive way of defending himself, this letter reveals symptoms of the disease that was slowly destroying his health. He misstates the name of the hospital where he worked, referring at times to Saint-Louis, instead of Saint-Antoine. He also dated his letter "1902," whereas the controversy took place at the beginning of 1901. While only extracts are presented here, the style of the long original text is pompous and repetitive.

Dr. Henry Napias (1842–1901), at the time Director General of the Paris hospital system, had published a memorandum one year earlier, on January 20, 1900: *"The regulatory order of December 3, 1834, and that of April 23, 1872, strictly prohibit any dissection work in the hospitals. These two orders only authorize autopsies; that is, the observation of scientific facts, which must never go beyond observation or lead to mutilation by the removal of organs or anatomical parts, regardless of any benefit."* Not all of the letters exchanged have been kept, but the Loudun archives do contain a reply from the administration, sent to Gilles de la Tourette on February 1, 1901, undoubtedly in response to a letter from him:

Dear Sir, You thought it necessary to write to me in protest against the memorandum in which I reminded the Hospital Directors of the regulations concerning the lecture halls and morgue. The Administration has never meant to hamper the Chefs de Service in their scientific research on the bodies of deceased patients in the hospitals, or to hinder autopsies to which the families give their consent; nor does the Administration have the intention to prohibit in all cases the removal of organs or anatomical parts that could facilitate this research. But it is obligated to respect the wishes of the families, with regard to whom it is the sole responsible party. . . . The Director General of the Assistance Publique.

Gilles de la Tourette wasted no time in replying:

Paris, February 17, 1901.

Dear Sir, Yesterday I received a letter from you, reminding me of the "general rules," in response to an objection which I thought it necessary to submit to you and which I maintain regarding your regulations on autopsies in the hospitals. It is my duty to respond and I hope this time to convince you. . . . My objective was to uncover the origin of the slander that has inundated both the political and the medical press in recent days—you may judge for yourself in reading the enclosed article from a certain *Journal de Médecine* which targets myself and my students, the management of Hôpital Saint-Antoine, and also your Administration.

Clearly, Gilles de la Tourette's indignation was intense.

Support from the Press

Gilles de la Tourette likely discussed this dispute with his friends Marcel Baudouin (1860–1941) and Paul Le Gendre (1854–1936), especially in view of what Baudouin wrote in La Gazette Médicale de Paris on February 16, 1901: "A recent incident at the morgue calls attention to the matter of hospital autopsies, highly relevant to Medical Science. We are aware of the details. . . . This produced a great stir in the mainstream press, which is always admirably well informed when it comes to police affairs of no interest to the public! There is really nothing here to make a fuss about, as they say. . . . Of course, it would be preferable that Medical Science come to us from the heavens, all questions resolved! But at present this is not the case. It is from cadavers, and not gods, that we must painstakingly extract the secrets of the human machine.

"Autopsies are utterly indispensable, not only to the progress of medicine, but also to medical practice itself. Since they currently cannot be performed anywhere but in the hospital, and since very few are carried out, relative to the needs of Science, it is not *surprising that an* interne *should autopsy a subject who may one day become, and this nearly by chance, an article of forensic evidence."³*

On February 5, 1901, the newspaper *Le Temps* published an open letter from Le Gendre, at that time *chef de service* at Hôpital Tenon, in support of his friend. Entitled "Autopsies in the hospitals," it picked up the same theme:⁴

To the Director of Le Temps,

. . . If the instructions contained in the above-mentioned memorandum were strictly applied, then autopsies would no longer be possible in our hospitals. Indeed, the memorandum's terms are such that autopsies should entail no more than opening the body's cavities, examining the viscera with the naked eye and returning them immediately to the body. . . . All of us, after reading this memorandum, scratched our heads and wondered if Doctor Napias, a member of the Académie de Médecine, had in fact written it.

In this day and age, what would be the value of an autopsy in which the physician could do no more than verify the relationships and appearance of the viscera with the naked eye? Who would dispute the fact that examining tissues under the microscope, after various procedures of hardening, cutting, and coloring, is the only means of diagnosing most lesions? These procedures require several days, several weeks in some cases. The laboratory work is possible only if certain viscera have been removed, in whole or in part, when the autopsy is performed. If this removal can only be performed once the Director General has granted his authorization, it must be abandoned forthwith, since the short period before the funeral would not allow sufficient time. This means that we must abandon here in Paris any autopsies that might further medical progress. . . . What the public should know is that autopsies, which are indispensable for scientific progress, are performed by physicians of the Paris hospital system with the utmost respect for the deceased and their families. But the public must also realize that an incomplete autopsy is useless and that the public interest does not lie in unduly restricting these procedures, if medicine is to continue to progress in our country as in other civilized nations.

Dr. P. Le Gendre

To sum up, a sensational newspaper story led Gilles de la Tourette and his friends Baudouin and Le Gendre to confront the hospital administration in an exchange mediated by the press, on an issue with implications for scientific research. Julien Noir (1866–1948) participated in the discussion in *Le Progrès Médical* after reproducing Le Gendre's article published in *Le Temps*: *"Accidents like the one at Saint-Antoine are rare and exceptional, and it is only too regrettable that the press is given free rein to interpret and generalize them in such a way as to galvanize public opinion. In the interests of medical science, which coincide with the* interests of patients, it would be useful to refute the commonly held idea that autopsies are a profanation. We should insist on the advantages to the family of the deceased. We should point out that illustrious men, monarchs, and even popes undergo autopsies, which are in no way degrading for common mortals. Rather than hindering these procedures, we should encourage chefs de service to perform them and to teach these practices to their students."[5]

These controversies forced the Société de Médecine Légale to take up the issue, to appoint a commission, and to debate the report issued on May 13, 1901. Emile Leredde (1866–1926) wrote: *"The commission set up to examine this question maintains that the administration should organize autopsy rooms to prevent errors from occurring when the autopsied organs are handled. The administration should take every measure so that the autopsy personnel perform their duties with attention and decency."*[6]

Notes

1. Archives de l'AP-HP. Hôpital Cochin. Hygiène et salubrité. 9L71. Service des archives de l'Assistance publique-Hôpitaux de Paris, 7 rue des Minimes, 75003 Paris.
2. Archives de l'AP-HP. Hôpital Hérold. Services hospitaliers. 9L97. Service des archives de l'Assistance publique-Hôpitaux de Paris, 7 rue des Minimes, 75003 Paris.
3. Baudouin M. Les autopsies dans les hôpitaux. *Gazette Médicale de Paris.* 1901;72–1(7):51.
4. Le Gendre P. Les autopsies dans les hôpitaux. *Le Temps.* Mardi 5 février 1901;41(14484):3.
5. Noir J. Les autopsies dans les hôpitaux. *Le Progrès Médical.* 1901;30-1(6):91–92.
6. Leredde E. Société de Médecine Légale. Séance du 13 mai 1901. *Annales d'hygiène publique et de médecine légale.* 1901;65(série 3 no. 45):539.

6

Chief Physician for the 1900 World's Fair in Paris

WORLD'S FAIRS DEVELOPED from the French tradition of national exhibitions, a tradition that culminated with the French Industrial Exposition of 1844, held in Paris. This fair was followed by other national exhibitions in Europe. For example, the "Great Exhibition of the Works of Industry of All Nations" was held in London in 1851 and is usually considered the first international exhibition of manufactured products. These fairs influenced various societal trends, including art-and-design education, international trade and relations, and tourism. World expositions were the platforms where state-of-the-art innovations in science and technology from around the world were brought together. After the world expositions in London (1851), New York (1853), London (1862), Philadelphia (1876), Paris (1889), Chicago (1893), and Brussels (1897), Paris hosted the exposition in 1900.

1900 World's Fair in Paris

An excerpt from the preliminary material for the 1900 World's Fair is enough to convey the excitement that this grand event aroused: *"As the 1889 World's Fair reached its apotheosis and came to a close, the participants and visitors were already making plans for the 1900 event in Paris. Still impressed by the imposing spectacle they had just seen and partaken in, they asked themselves what genius France and its guests could marshal to, if not outshine the 1889 gathering, at least bring the nineteenth century to a fitting close and mark the new milestone in the forward march of contemporary civilization.*"[1]

The 1889 fair would be a hard act to follow, given its showpiece was the Eiffel Tower. Momentum gathered in 1892 after Germany showed interest in organizing a world's fair in Berlin. Deputy François Deloncle (1856–1922) quickly brought a resolution before the French National Assembly, on July 2, 1892, inviting the government to decree that a world's fair would take place in Paris in 1900. On July 13, 1892, the President of the French Republic, Sadi Carnot (1837–1894), issued a decree whereby *"a world's fair of artwork as well as industrial and agricultural products would open in Paris on May 5, 1900, and close the following October 31."* The terms used by the press and in official reports were pompous, grandiloquent, and not without a spirit of revenge, albeit understated: *"France, aware of her grandeur, sure of herself, will deploy the treasures of her industrial and agricultural production amidst those of other nations."* Or this example: *"Peaceful celebrations to which will be invited all of the workers of the world"*; or, *"Man emerges comforted, full of valor and with a profound faith in the future . . . and this is the general religion of modern times, a fruitful rite where the universal expositions figure as majestic and useful solemnities, as the manifestations necessary to the existence of an industrious nation driven by an irresistible need for expansion."*[2] The Paris Metro would be one outcome of the fair in 1900.

Alfred Picard (1844–1913) (Figure 6.1), a graduate of the prestigious Ecole Polytechnique and part of the Bridges and Roads Engineering Corps of the French State, penned the preceding citation. A rapporteur for the 1889 fair, he was named the 1900 Commissioner General.

1900 World's Fair: The Nomination

The clauses concerning the fair entrepreneurs called for a medical department, run by the administration, for workers suffering injury or illness during the preparatory work and then for participants and visitors during the fair itself. A commission was set up in 1896 to propose an organization for the fair's health department. Paul Brouardel (1837–1906), at the time Dean of the Faculté de Médecine, was appointed President. Among others, he brought together Louis-Ernest Peyron (1836–1908), Director of the Assistance Publique; Adrien Proust (1834–1903), Professor of Hygiene; and Auguste Le Dentu (1841–1926), Professor of Surgery. *"This commission first examined and unanimously set aside a privately sponsored project with passionate supporters that entailed building, on the fair's premises, a central hospital for the*

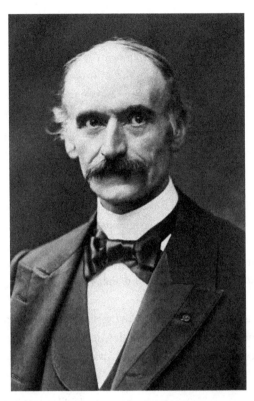

FIGURE 6.1 Alfred Picard (1844–1913), the 1900 Paris World's Fair Commissioner General.
Private collection of the author.

injured and sick." Three separate care centers were instead planned: at the Champ de Mars, at the Esplanade des Invalides, and on the right bank of the Seine River. For the first time, auditory warnings and telephone technology made it possible to alert the crowds and communicate with the hospitals where the injured would be transferred. *"A primordial step was naming a Chief Physician, responsible for the entire department and for making proposals in the planning stages. The commission voted by secret ballot and unanimously appointed Dr. Gilles de la Tourette, Hospital Physician and Professor at the Faculté de Médecine. This appointment was officially confirmed in an order dated September 10, 1896."*[2] Despite the method of appointment, rumors spread that Gilles de la Tourette *"had managed to get himself designated as the fair's Chief Physician by his powerful relations."*[3] It is true that Brouardel had been his teacher and Deloncle was a deputy who, like his friend Bourneville, belonged to the extreme left in the French Parliament, led by Alexandre Millerand (1859–1943). While their support may have allowed him to present his candidacy, he was chosen in a fair election by secret ballot.

Emile Berr (1855–1923), explaining the organization of the fair's medical department in *Le Figaro* on February 11, 1900, advanced arguments in favor of his nomination: *"Dr. Gilles de la Tourette was selected on account of his scientific merits; he is Professor at the Faculté de Médecine and a Hospital Physician, and he lectured for ten years on hygiene in the city's nursing schools. Moreover, he is a sensitive, erudite writer and a polyglot, into whose care the foreign commissioners will feel reassured placing their injured nationals. The fair's Chief Physician can consult in French, German, Spanish, English, Portuguese, and Italian, a consideration that can only confirm the excellent choice of Mr. Brouardel and his committee."*[4]

Gilles de la Tourette's friend, Paul Le Gendre (1854–1933) wrote: *"This desire to create, this intense activity found an outlet in the task of medical department organizer for the 1900 World's Fair. The nomination of a 40-year-old doctor to such a sought-after position, which would affirm and augment his fame by conferring distinction along with material and moral advantages, such as the opportunity to be useful to his confreres and students, would also cause him great fatigue and generate a number of jealous enemies."*

In the National Archives, there is a hand-written note on plain white paper without a letterhead. Composed by Gilles de la Tourette himself, it suggests he distributed some sort of curriculum vitae to journalists to publicize his nomination:

> Mr. Boucher,[5] Minister of Commerce, has named Gilles de la Tourette as Chief Physician of the 1900 Fair and associated works, after his unanimous election by a technical commission organized by the minister. This nomination will be met by approval on all sides. Mr. Gilles de la Tourette is one of our most eminent scientific personalities. He was a favorite student of both Charcot and Brouardel, and his publications on nervous and mental diseases lead the field. Through his initiative and efforts, the statue of Théophraste Renaudot, founder of journalism and charitable consultations, was finally erected. As a professor of hygiene for ten years at the municipal nursing school, he is entirely prepared for the organization of this important department. The Press as well as the scientific world can only welcome his nomination. Mr. Gilles de la Tourette is a Professor at the Faculté de Médecine, a Hospital Physician, and Chevalier de la Légion d'honneur.

On August 24, 1896, in *Le Figaro*, the journalist Jean de Malonne described what was in store: *"Doctor Gilles de la Tourette, recently appointed Chief Physician for the 1900 World's Fair, will return on August 25 from his holiday in Saint-Vaaste la Hougue to oversee the organization and installation of the medical department during the construction period, which is already underway. Directing such a vast and complex department is certainly no sinecure. On the immense worksites soon to fill* with thousands of workers, there will be accidents and illness requiring immediate, high-quality medical care. Upon his return, Mr. Gilles de la Tourette will have to co-ordinate several physicians and set up his offices, an ambulance service with nurses, and a pharmacy. The daily consultations and house visits will start immediately." Malonne noted the medical department statistics from the 1889 fair: 21,000 consultations, several dozen cases of typhoid fever, and thirty-three deaths, twenty-seven of which were accidental.[6] In *Gil Blas*, Charles Bardin asked Gilles de la Tourette about the malicious gossip: "*I found Mr. Gilles de la Tourette very affected by the two or three objections regarding his nomination. 'I honestly cannot say who initiated these attacks. Imagine, they even criticized me for giving interviews too easily, further claiming that I sought out the interviews myself. You will understand why I have decided to keep quiet from now on. . . . There can be no doubt that certain people are envious of my nomination, and this is how they express it.'* "[7]

Julien Besançon (1852–1952) distilled venom in his memoir: "*Gilles de la Tourette made influential friendships. At the Café Flory, a café of France's youth, I drank beers with him and two of his friends, a big boy with a pince-nez named Alexandre Millerand. . . . The other man's name was Stephen Pichon.*[8] *Both were clerks in the offices of La Justice, Clemenceau's paper. The boss got Millerand elected in the 12th arrondissement, as a revolutionary socialist. Some may recall that he was driven out of the Elysée as a horrible reactionary. As for Stephen Pichon, appointed Ambassador of France in Peking, he embarrassed the few Frenchmen living there by hiding in his cellar during the Boxer Rebellion. He was later named Minister of Foreign Affairs under Clemenceau, as "the Tiger" liked his orders obeyed promptly and precisely. So to see my old friend, the whore, lording over the 1900 World's Fair as the Chief Physician came as no surprise. The red rosette in his buttonhole is as big as the butt of an artichoke.*"[9]

Le Gendre wrote: "*He explained that the hostile ones must be fought with as much ardor, that he enjoyed striking them down. His combativeness inspired enmity in some, and led certain writers to tarnish his legacy. When appointed, he was criticized for being a physician and not a surgeon. However, rigorous statistics suggest that the medical obligations far exceed, in such circumstances, the surgical eventualities. In spite of everything, Gilles de la Tourette proved himself a skillful organizer and over-came the difficulties of the fair's immense scope. From a surgical point of view, the emergency units were well equipped, and the instruments and sterilization systems were impeccable thanks to his appointment of hospital surgeon Louis Beurnier.*[10] *The complex hierarchy, the perfect order, and the care Gilles de la Tourette devoted to this project over several years proved that the selection committee had not made their choice in error. The Commissioner General, Mr. Alfred Picard, expressed his sat-isfaction with Gilles de la Tourette in the most flattering terms. Since he is a good judge with a basis for comparison, his support must have been precious to Gilles de la*

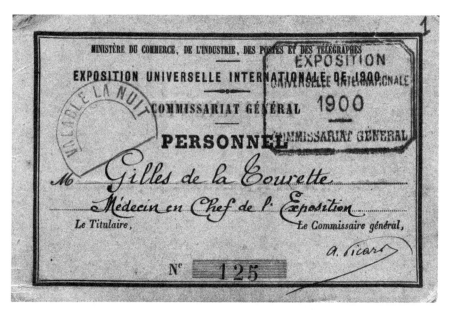

FIGURE 6.2 Gilles de la Tourette's personnel entry card for the Fair.
Copyright Musée Charbonneau-Lassay, Ville de Loudun, with kind permission.

Tourette—*more precious than the Officer's rosette that replaced his Knight's ribbon* [Legion d'Honneur] *at an age when such a promotion is unheard of in the civil or even the military medical corps, and more flattering than the foreign decorations he wore during official ceremonies"* (Figure 6.2).

Gilles de la Tourette wrote to Montorgueil on December 1, 1897. He wanted to introduce his friend to the fair's Commissioner, undoubtedly hoping for an article in Montorgueil's newspaper, *L'Éclair,* that would highlight the fair and his own initiatives.

My dear friend, Please find enclosed my invitation. I would be very pleased if you were to accept, as this will be a dinner amongst friends with Risler, Bouvard, and also Mr. Picard, the Commissioner General for the fair, who promised me he would attend. . . . And I shall stop by to see you the first day of the fair. I saw Mr. Barthou about Miss Bottard and gave him your article; he was very nice indeed. Saturday, I am seeing the Prefect of the Seine. But will the Minister come to my dinner? . . . Yours truly.

In passing, he mentioned seeing the Minister of the Interior, Louis Barthou (1862–1934), to promote Charcot's head nurse as a candidate for the Légion d'honneur. Was he worried about the meeting between the minister and the journalist?

1900 **World's Fair: Hard Work and Its Rewards**

Gilles de la Tourette wrote to Claretie on April 5, 1900: *"This month—and just between us, of course—we had 1,300 patients; fortunately, none of them with serious conditions. It's a real battlefield, because they are working so fast, and because alcohol flows much too freely, despite my efforts, as you can imagine. But that is the way things are."*

Another letter, dated September 12, 1900, barely conceals Gilles de la Tourette's vanity: *"Upon returning to Paris I found your* Vie à Paris de 1899 *on my table, which I naturally read straightaway. I was eager to see my name in something you had written; that may be why I enjoyed my reading so thoroughly."*

The title of the book's twenty-sixth chapter translates as "The battlefield, October 4, 1899," an expression borrowed from Gilles de la Tourette. In it, Claretie described a visit to the worksite during a rainstorm: *"In the mud at Champs-de-Mars after a meeting with the fair's Commissioner General, with my felt hat, my pants rolled up, and my umbrella open, I braved the October weather and visited the construction sites where work is accelerating. To learn more about the emergency units for the workers, we spent several hours with the Chief Physician of the medical department, our friend Dr. Gilles de la Tourette. Returning from the esplanade, we met the General in charge of his army of workers. . . . The main rule, of prime importance, is that all injured workers must report to the nearest emergency unit immediately, even for minor injuries, to prevent infection. The penalty for breaking this rule is a loss of pay. . . . The result is that workers report to the medical unit with the slightest scratch. During the three years of worksite operation, there have been no serious abscesses, and no epidemics. As for the Chief Physician's excellent hygienic beverage, though some find it amusing, ten to twelve thousand liters of spring water are delivered every day in the summer to keep the workers refreshed. All forms of alcohol are prohibited, but it is still consumed and some construction companies even provide absinthe for difficult tasks."*

After describing a fall from a scaffold, Claretie continues: *"Every day claims at least one of the men. The victims are taken away as their companions say 'Adieu' with a sideways glance. Like soldiers, they have their ambulances, and they have their surgeons, also deserving of our appreciation. The* internes *and physicians have been caring for injured workers since December 15, 1896. The medical staff is always present; the physicians replace each other every three hours. . . . With intelligent zeal, Mr. Gilles de la Tourette pays close attention to cleanliness, as do his colleagues, who are devoted to their chief."* Needless to say, Claretie was not stingy with his compliments!

One of Gilles de la Tourette's duties was to manage the medical personnel. On May 30, 1899, he wrote to Brouardel, the dean of the medical school and his former teacher:

My Dear Master, You mentioned that students wishing to perfect their skills sometimes inquire at the Faculté. Since I have an open *interne* position for the fair, I went to see Mr. Pupin[11] so as not to disturb you. I then received a visit on your behalf from Mrs. Béclard.[12] But it is impossible to arrange things for various reasons, mainly because the department is too demanding for an *internat* candidate. . . . The position is paid with a small part of the Chief Physician funds. I remain yours in devotion and gratitude. P.S.: Full-time duty every other day, including at night. 150 francs per month plus 300 francs of in-kind compensation per year: housing, heating, lighting, and a few other benefits. If possible, a commitment of 2.5 to 3 years, to cover the rest of the fair as well as the demolition period that will follow.[13]

There must have been no shortage of eager candidates. The archives in Loudun contain a handwritten note on paper with a French parliamentary letterhead. It was sent by Charles Dupuy (1851–1923), Président du Conseil when Captain Dreyfus was condemned. Dupuy was an ardent partisan of the refusal to grant Dreyfus a retrial and thus very far from Gilles de la Tourette's political opinions:

July 6, 1896, Dear Sir, I have been told you are in charge of recruiting medical personnel for the 1900 World's Fair medical department. If I may, Sir, I would like to highly recommend a family member by marriage. Dr. Laborde (Fortuné) resides in Paris, 70 Rue Condorcet, and has recently set up his medical practice. I remain yours sincerely, Ch. Dupuy.

One of the most serious accidents of the fair took place on April 29, 1900. A walkway collapsed, killing nine people and injuring nine others: *"Gilles de la Tourette, Chief Physician for the fair, arrived immediately and took charge of the situation."*[14]

Prior to that event, on May 4, 1897, the fair's medical department had been called upon when a fire broke out in the Bazar de la Charité: *"Bystanders were witness to a horrifying spectacle in the bazaar's immense framework, where everything was burning at once: boutiques, walls, flooring, and facades. Men, women, and children writhed in pain, screaming like the damned, vainly trying to find a way out, before catching fire themselves and falling onto the ever-growing mound of burnt cadavers."* On May 14, 1897, *Le Figaro* reported: *"We have noted the courageous conduct of the* interne *Roussel, employed by the fair's medical department and who, from the first alert, ran to the Bazar de la Charité where he saved several ladies, before returning to his unit to care for the wounded. Mr. Picard, the fair's Commissioner*

General wrote: 'Sir, Mr. Gilles de la Tourette, Chief Physician for the 1900 fair, told
me of the great energy and conviction with which you cared for the victims of the ca-
tastrophe on Rue Jean Goujon. I would like to congratulate you for carrying out your
duties so thoroughly in these tragic circumstances, and I shall inform the Police Chief
of your dedication. Commissioner General Picard.'. . . However, what Dr. Gilles de
la Tourette did not say in his report is that the fair's Chief Physician, as soon as he
received word of the catastrophe, ran to his unit and hardly left until the Saint-Jean
ward closed around midnight. He came back and took up his duties the following day,
and the day after that, whenever he was not needed by his patients at the hospitals.

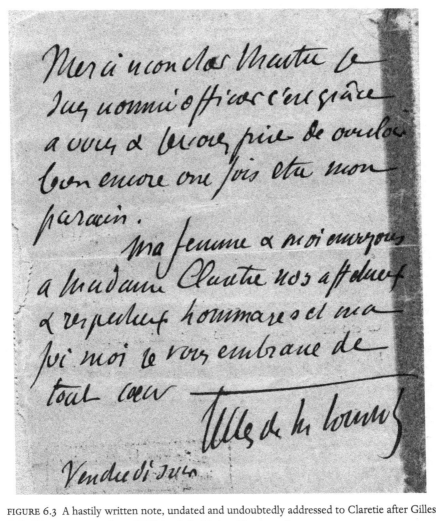

FIGURE 6.3 A hastily written note, undated and undoubtedly addressed to Claretie after Gilles
de la Tourette was made an "Officier de la Légion d'honneur."
Copyright Musée Charbonneau-Lassay, Ville de Loudun, with kind permission.

Dr. Gilles de la Tourette impressed everyone with the heroic accomplishment of his duties."[15]

Gilles de la Tourette's service during the fair earned him the rank of Officier de la Légion d'honneur. A hastily written note, undated and probably addressed to Claretie, reads as follows (Figure 6.3): *"Friday evening, Thank you my dear Master. If I have been named an officer, I owe it to you, and I thank you for being my sponsor."* The surprising familiarity in the beginning of the message suggests that Gilles de la Tourette was showing signs of his insidious disease.

In his April 5, 1900 letter to Claretie, Gilles de la Tourette mentioned his officership in these terms: *"As for the other redness, the blush that rises to my forehead before the red medal is pinned to my chest, there is nothing new to report. I do not dare speak of it to our excellent chief, who will be lucky if he manages to avoid neurasthenia. As for me, I am up to my neck and would like this period of feverish activity to be over."*

He is probably referring to Alfred Picard, the fair's commissioner with whom Gilles de la Tourette was often in contact. He must have recognized a state of exhaustion or depression in Picard, making him fear that Picard would refuse to participate in the Légion d'honneur ceremony. In any case, Gilles de la Tourette also expressed his own fatigue and his desire to be free of his responsibilities. Not long thereafter, the May 12, 1900 edition of *Le Progrès Médical* announced a banquet: *"The medical department of the fair, along with the students and friends of Dr. Gilles de la Tourette, will hold a banquet on May 25 at 7.30, at the Hôtel Continental, to celebrate Gilles de la Tourette's promotion to the rank of Officier de la Légion d'honneur. Professor Brouardel will preside over the event. Dr. Deschamps, 76 Rue de la Victoire, will be accepting subscriptions."*[16] In Gilles de la Tourette's letters to Claretie, we discover that he organized this banquet himself. As early as April 26, 1900, he wrote the following: *"I hoped that with Mr. Brouardel, you would agree to preside over a banquet that my friends and students are putting on to celebrate the rosette medal I owe to you. Mr. Brouardel has accepted for Friday, May 25 at the Hôtel Continental. . . . I am so grateful to you and this would be the perfect occasion to express my gratitude with everyone present!"* The fair's Commissioner General, Alfred Picard, did indeed attend, along with all of the public figures who had made it possible for Gilles de la Tourette to direct the medical department.[17]

In Conclusion

Gilles de la Tourette's nomination inevitably made him the object of intense jealousy. He responded in the best way possible, by devoting himself to his duties. The fair's medical department was perfectly organized and fulfilled all of its missions throughout the five years the event lasted, including its set-up and dismantling. The initial criticism was forgotten once Gilles de la Tourette set to work, leaving no room for further censure. As usual, he managed to bring his success to the media's attention. His disease apparently did not hinder his work, although his condition must have worsened, as he was hospitalized a few months after the fair ended. During his time as Chief Physician, he probably remained focused on his reputation, by that time firmly established, in the hope of entering the Académie de Médecine, for example, or obtaining an academic promotion.

Notes

1. Picard A. *Préambule. Exposition Universelle Internationale de 1900 à Paris. Rapport général administratif et technique.* Paris: Imprimerie Nationale. 1892, tome 1.
2. Picard A. *Services divers de l'Exposition Universelle Internationale de 1900 à Paris. Rapport général administratif et technique.* Paris: Imprimerie Nationale. 1892, tome 7.
3. de Lavarenne E. Gilles de la Tourette. *La Presse Médicale.* 1904;1(45):1–2.
4. Berr E. L'Exposition de 1900, le service médical. *Le Figaro.* Dimanche 11 février 1900;46(42):1–2.
5. Henry Boucher (1847–1927).
6. de Malonne J. Le Médecin chef de l'Exposition. *Le Figaro.* 24 août 1896;42(234):2–3.
7. Bardin Ch. Le Médecin en chef de l'Exposition. *Gil Blas.* Jeudi 27 août 1896;18(6128):2.
8. Stéphen Pichon (1857–1933), a diplomat and minister of foreign affairs in the government headed by Clémenceau in 1906.
9. Besançon J. *La pie borgne.* Paris: La Clé d'Or. 1948.
10. Charles Louis Edmond Beurnier (1860–1917), who began his *internat* the same year as Gilles de la Tourette.
11. Dr. Charles Pupin (1875–1964), secretary general of the Faculté de Médecine.
12. Mother of Henri Béclard (1877–?).
13. La Faculté de Médecine de Paris, personnel de la faculté: dossiers, fiches, gestion 1750–1953. Académie de Paris. Archives Nationales AJ/16/6509 Gaillard-Gilles de la Tourette.
14. Anonyme. L'accident d'hier. *Le Figaro.* Lundi 30 avril 1900;45(120):1–2.
15. Anonyme. Les victimes de l'incendie. *Le Figaro.* 14 mai 1897;43(134):3.
16. Anonyme. Announcement. *Le Progrès Médical.* 12 mai 1900;29(19):319.
17. Picard A. *Exposition universelle internationale de 1900 à Paris. Le bilan d'un siècle (1801–1900). France, Ministère du commerce, de l'industrie et du travail.* Paris: Imprimerie nationale. 1906.

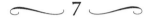

A Sad End

Eclipse, Twilight, and Death

G EORGES GILLES DE la Tourette died an agonizing death from general paralysis when he was only forty-seven. We report on several episodes, from his professional life as well as his social and public life, that reveal his slow psychic decline, especially from 1893 onward. In response to his erratic behavior, several articles were published by the press that were either ill-intentioned or downright slanderous. His reputation and his legacy were undeniably tarnished. We begin with the history of a pathology that is now largely forgotten due to the 1943 discovery that penicillin is an effective treatment.

A Brief Historical Account: Neurosyphilis
or "General Paralysis"

Neurosyphilis is the third stage of syphilis, a disease that was inevitably fatal before the era of penicillin. Although the illness was first documented by the Italian Vicenzio Chiarugi (1759–1820) in 1793, followed by the Englishman John Haslam (1764–1844) in 1798, the first description is classically attributed to Antoine Laurent Jessé Bayle (1799–1858), who wrote in his 1822 thesis: *"The symptoms of chronic arachnitis may all be reduced to general and incomplete paralysis and derangement of the intellectual faculties. . . . The delirium is generally maniacal, frequently accompanied by dominant ideas. The patient speaks in an agitated manner and moves about continuously, to the point of the most violent and uncontrollable furor."*[1] In 1825, he completed his description, noting: *"Some patients speak much more articulately than usual, throwing in witticisms and making associations that are ingenious, bizarre, and amusing."*[2]

Working regularly with Alfred Fournier (1832–1914), who maintained that general paralysis was caused by syphilis in 1876, Gilles de la Tourette eventually came to accept the syphilitic origin of tabes and of conditions affecting the spine (myelitis), medulla, and pons. But this was not until 1893, after the death of his master, Jean-Martin Charcot (1825–1893), who had always contested the syphilitic origin of nervous system diseases. Progressive locomotor ataxia (for which Charcot did not yet use the German expression "tabes") was, to his mind, due to *"nervous heredity."* Did this view conceal anti-German ideology? Charcot clearly expressed his thoughts in commenting on the Civrieux prize that one of his students, Isaac Seeligmann, was awarded in 1882 for his research on the causes of locomotor ataxia: *"As nervous heredity has proven superior to the other etiological conditions, the author considers nervous heredity to be the major cause of tabes. The other conditions which certain authors describe as leading directly to tabes, for instance syphilis, appear with varied frequency, as adjunct and occasional causes."*[3] Although a friend of Pasteur and Fournier, Charcot did not realize the importance or the implications of Pasteur's bacteriological discoveries, unlike Alfred Vulpian (1826–1887).

The syphilitic origin of the psychic and cognitive problems in general paralysis would begin to gain acceptance in France at the end of the 1890s. Fournier used an elegant metaphor for syphilis: *"This indiscreet person capable of the most illegitimate trespassing."* In 1893, Jean Nageotte (1866–1948) categorically concluded in his thesis: *"Syphilis is indeed the primary efficient cause of general paralysis and tabes."*[4]

As he had for the theories of hysteria, Gilles de la Tourette saw himself as the guardian of the intangible dogmas laid down by Charcot, and he remained attached to the notion of multiple causes for tabes and general paralysis. Charcot, in his correspondence with Freud concerning the translation of his Lessons, had adopted a peremptory tone worthy of his status as a professor and had clearly explained that there could be no doubt that *"syphilis is nothing but an inducing agent"* in a hereditary context predisposing patients to tabes and general paralysis.[5] It is unlikely that Gilles de la Tourette ever realized he was suffering from general paralysis.

First Faux Pas in Public

In early 1901, Gilles de la Tourette made a public appearance that put his health problems on display. We have reconstructed the events based on unpublished letters Gilles de la Tourette wrote after the fact to explain his behavior. The result is an honest account, unlike the narratives in previous biographies that rely on fragments and attempt to discredit Gilles de la Tourette.

In its "Theater" section, *Le Temps* ran the following announcement on February 4, 1901: *"At the Odéon: Monday,* Le Cid et les Plaideurs; *Tuesday, Wednesday, Thursday, Friday, and Saturday:* Château historique. *Saturday, five o'clock, talk by Gilles de la Tourette, followed by the premiere of* La Dormeuse, *a dramatic play consisting of two tableaus, by Mr. André de Lorde."*[6]

This play, staged by Paul Ginisty (1855–1932), premiered on February 9, 1901. Ginisty, a chronicler and journalist who wrote for *Gil Blas*, was the director of the Odéon Theater from 1896 to 1906. He was an acquaintance of Gilles de la Tourette and had already written about *Traité clinique de l'hystérie* in his periodical.[7] The text of the play *La Dormeuse* appeared in the book *Théatre d'épouvante*, published by Lorde in 1909.[8] Two short scenes portray a woman in a *"lethargic state,"* who has been a *"zombie"* for six years following a *"terrible fright."* She is visited in her home by physicians, curious friends, and magnetizers. One day she awakens, learns that her two sons are dead and—immediately dies herself.

On January 10, 1901, Gilles de la Tourette wrote to Jules Claretie (1840–1913), a well-known writer who was also the administrator of the Comédie Française from 1885 to 1913. In his letter, Gilles de la Tourette explained to his friend why he had agreed to give an introductory lecture for the play's premiere.

My Dear Master. . . , Yesterday I saw Mr. Géo Dupuy, your illustrator. I gave him every possible recommendation for La Salpêtrière, where I hope he will be welcomed, though I would prefer to be there myself. I, or rather we, have the honor of inviting Mrs. Claretie, yourself, and Georges to attend a lecture that I shall give at a date to be set, on a Saturday, five o'clock, at the Odéon. It is a long story that begins with Ginisty. We are on excellent terms and he recently sent a young man by the name of Mr. de Lorde to see me. Lorde, who had sent Ginisty a pathological play called *La Dormeuse*, is the son of Mounet-Sully. As a favor to Mounet-Sully, Ginisty asked me to read the play and invited me to give an introductory talk before its performance at the Odéon. Well, I accepted, as a favor to Mounet-Sully, Paul Mounet, and Ginisty, and I think the performance will take place early in February. I shall see to it that you have a nice box. And of course, you will not be forgotten because I shall speak at length of La Salpêtrière. As soon as I know the exact date I shall let you know; a few friends will be in attendance.

In a word, I am planning on covering pathological sleep in the entire animal series and finishing at the summit, with human sleep, accompanied by the projection of figures, diagrams, and so forth. This should be relevant for madness in the contemporary world.

Here is a rapid summary of the protagonists mentioned in Gilles de la Tourette's letter. Géo Dupuis (and not Dupuy; 1875–1932) was a painter and engraver. He illustrated books by Honoré de Balzac, Guy de Maupassant, Maurice Barrès, and Arthur Conan Doyle. In 1902, Paul Ollendorff (1851–1920) published a deluxe edition of Claretie's book, *Les amours d'un interne*, in which the evocative illustrations of Dupuis, consisting of tableaus of La Salpêtrière patients, were engraved by Georges Lemoine. Gilles de la Tourette apparently helped the artist gain access to the hospital wards (Figure 7.1). Jean-Sully Mounet, known as Mounet-Sully (1841–1916), was a famous actor who mainly worked with the Comédie Française. Jean-Paul Mounet, known as Paul, was Mounet-Sully's younger brother. Also an actor, first at the Odéon then at the Comédie Française, he was known for his portrayal of Balthazar in *L'Arlésienne*, written by Alphonse Daudet (1840–1897). As for André de Lorde (André de Latour, Count de Lorde, 1869–1942), whom Gilles de la Tourette did not yet know, he would become famous for his Grand Guignol plays written with Alfred Binet (1857–1911) and for his horror plays, between 1900 and 1935. Gilles de la Tourette's letter reveals that, in addition to his close friendship with Claretie, he had other ties to the theater and took a passionate interest in dramatic works. We should also note that, in 1883, a case of abnormal sleep had fascinated the press and its readers. It undoubtedly inspired Lorde. Marguerite Bouyenval (1861–1903), who became known as *"la dormeuse de Thenelles,"* gave

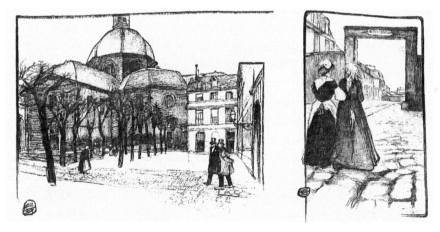

FIGURE 7.1 *La Salpêtrière* by Géo Dupuis (1875–1932) for *Les amours d'un interne* by Jules Claretie (P. Ollendorff, 1902).
Private collection of the author.

birth out of wedlock in 1883 to a stillborn child.[9,10] During the police investigation that followed the birth, Bouyenval had *"several hystero-epileptic attacks,"* then fell into a *"cataleptic sleep"* that lasted twenty years. She died soon after *"her awakening."*[11]

In the days following this play and Gilles de la Tourette's lecture, no mention of either appeared in *L'Eclair*. The *Gil Blas* account was slightly mocking: *"Gilles de la Tourette may have gratified us with an erudite lecture, but the spectators, mainly there for the play, found it rather long, and were at one point ready to riot. In which case Gilles de la Tourette would have ended up as the Sleeping Doctor."*[12] The tone in *L'Aurore* was also gently ironic: *"Dr. Gilles de la Tourette gave a lecture-lesson from a thick manuscript but had to shorten his presentation due to the fierce, noisy complaints in the audience. His medicine seemed to go down with some difficulty and the doctor, who had set out to show that sleep could last for six years, was unable to prove that he himself could last longer than an hour."*[13]

It was only in the Sunday, July 14, 1901 edition of *L'Eclair*, five months later, that Montorgueil headlined the "Current Events" section with "The disease of Dr. Gilles de la Tourette/The 'Dormeuse' incident": *"The last time he appeared in public was at the Odéon, for a matinee. He gave a lecture on 'La Dormeuse.' With his usual rigor, he presented his subject meticulously. The audience, accustomed to less solid fare, showed a few vague signs of impatience. Dr. Gilles de la Tourette, instead of hastening to conclude, defied the unhappy spectators. He had the support of his friends, but the incident suggested he was overworked and needed to curb his activities. He received even more specific warnings, which made the rounds and point to the fact that the desire to work is not always reduced by pain. But now he is following a regimen of rest, which should help to ease his temporary over-exertion. He is feeling better, much better. We initially saw no reason to mention this catastrophe, given our certainty that Gilles de la Tourette would quickly recover and write some wonderful new book. But with the rumors that have been circulating, we could not abide by our discretion. The truth of the matter is just as we have reported it, though it saddens Gilles de la Tourette's confreres and friends, whom the physician has always treated with such loyal, courteous generosity, and will do so once again."*

In a letter to Claretie a week after his talk, Gilles de la Tourette reflected on what had happened that day and how it had affected him. Although clearly disappointed with his performance and the poor impression he had made on the audience, he was quick to excuse himself on account of overwork:

February 11, 1901. My Dear Master, Thank you for your words, so full of affection and good will. I was overworked when I gave that lecture and I was unable to prepare it as I would have liked; I simply did not have the time. I plan to revise the material, which matters so much to me because it is the bulk of what I did with my dear illustrious

Charcot. Its length, which I was criticized for, and rightfully so in those unpleasant circumstances, is also important to me, in spite of everything, because I hope it will bring me closer to you. The book in which it will be included is, in fact, not very long; adding this pathological sleep material will considerably increase the length. Then will come the denouement of Froufrou, I think, for which you have given me the best elements. That is how *La folie au théâtre* will take shape, with a preface by Jules Claretie, of the Académie Française, who I know will give the best of himself and his considerable talents.

Gilles de la Tourette was aware that his long lecture was poorly organized. His letter also reveals that he intended to publish a new book. Some of Charcot's lessons, which Gilles de la Tourette had prepared, dealt with *"la dormeuse."* They aimed to elucidate hysterical sleep and lethargy.[14] Inspired by Charcot, Gilles de la Tourette probably wanted to make his findings on hysteria accessible to the general public. He had already written about *L'état mental de Froufrou* in *La Revue Hebdomadaire* in 1892. This play was staged by Henri Meilhac (1831–1897) and Ludovic Halévy (1834–1908) in 1869. As other letters to Claretie also attest, Gilles de la Tourette intended to write a book on madness in dramatic works (*La Folie au Théâtre*). He planned to use the material from his talk for one of the chapters, in which he would address pathological sleep. As it turned out, the book was never published, and there is no trace of the manuscript in the Loudun archives. It remains a mystery how Gilles de la Tourette would have approached this subject, though he mentioned it several times in his *Revue Hebdomadaire* articles. When Gilles de la Tourette invited Claretie to the banquet for his decoration, Claretie responded: *"What a preface I shall write for your wonderful book!"*

In 1913, Lorde would publish a book with this same title, *La Folie au Théâtre*, prefaced by Gilbert Ballet (Chair of Mental Illnesses and the Brain at Hôpital Sainte-Anne) and dedicated to Binet. The book consists of text from three plays illustrating mental pathologies: one deals with sexual obsession (*La Petite Roque*), the second with delusions of persecution (*L'Homme Mystérieux*), and the third with a ward in an asylum (*Les Invisibles*).[15] In 1921, like Gilles de la Tourette during his lecture, Lorde had to face a discontented audience after staging an execution at the Grand-Guignol Theater. He defended this choice in *Le Journal*: *"Illness, madness, and death are my favorite subjects. I try to tell the truth, relying on brutal facts. I am like a surgeon who plunges his scalpel into an abscess. The masters of science, such as Gilles de la Tourette, Alfred Binet, and Gilbert Ballet, encouraged me in my approach when I began long ago."*[16]

Severe Disorders

Not long after his talk, Gilles de la Tourette mentioned his difficulties walking. The letter he sent his friend Montorgueil on April 14, 1901, is nothing short of a clinical picture, including both cognitive and physical symptoms:

I really thought I was done for, my dear friend, my legs were leaden, a frightening sluggishness took over my entire body, and my mind refused to focus on anything in a sustained way . . . but I am feeling better now, in control once again.

Edouard de Lavarenne (1855?–1907) described Gilles de la Tourette's downfall this way: *"Priding himself on his knowledge of aesthetics and literature, he had many acquaintances in the artistic world and zealously sought out their company. He absorbed the ideas he heard expressed and took part in conversations on literature and other matters. With charismatic vivacity and ease, he introduced his listeners to the psychological mysteries that the science of Charcot elucidated, and he was well known in certain literary circles, as one member of the Académie Française, Jules Claretie, recently noted in one of his* Le Temps *chronicles of Parisian life. In this intellectual milieu Gilles de la Tourette became a sought-after speaker, with something of a following, and soon he began to give public lectures. It was during one such lecture at the Odéon Theater, directed by a friend of his, that his mental breakdown became apparent, surprising even those closest to him."*[17]

Gilles de la Tourette's behavior became increasingly erratic. In *Paris Vécu*, although this text dates from 1930, Léon Daudet gives his view of how Gilles de la Tourette's general paralysis came to light: *"[His] delirium, due to a neglected treponemal infection, revealed itself publicly in the most comical way. While conducting an exam he asked the candidate: 'Who, Sir, are the three greatest French physicians of the nineteenth century?' The student thought for a moment and answered: 'Laennec, Duchenne de Boulogne, and Charcot,' because he knew that Gilles de la Tourette had been Charcot's student. 'No, Sir, you're wrong. The correct answer is my grand-father, my father, and me, Mate. That is why'—at this moment, the examiner put his own professor's cap on the head of the speechless young man— 'that is why a potassium bromide statue will be erected for me!' "*[18]

Already in 1915, Daudet had written in his "medical memoir": *"Contrary to the views expressed by Professor Fournier, who saw clearly in spite of everything—and with an eagle's eye!—Gilles de la Tourette argued that general paralysis bore no relation to syphilis. He would prance and skip and dance when people drew his attention to certain coincidences. He would repeat, 'This is my firm conviction.' Alas! His own ideas, poor boy, were becoming less and less firm, such that one day, during an exam, having asked a candidate, 'What disease initially causes bleeding from the left nostril,' and having received the answer, 'Typhoid fever, Sir,' he shook his head and, after a five-minute silence, solemnly declared, 'It's typhoid fever, Sir, you're worthless and I shan't admit you.'*

Some time before his death, as I was leaving my home on Rue de l'Université, Gilles de la Tourette, whom I had not seen for several years, caught sight of me, rushed over and threw his arms around my neck. I was taken aback by this excessive affection that nothing in our previous relations could justify. He said in a halting voice: 'My dear Daudet, I feel such affection for you. I have hoped for this formal reconciliation for so long.' Then, taking a step back, he repeated: 'Formal reconciliation. . . .' He was red in the face, with big tears in his eyes. I knew immediately what the problem was. The diagnosis was not difficult to make. . . . Gilles de la Tourette, poor devil! Only for that brief moment had he ever been nice to me. He nearly wrecked everything by insisting on accompanying me, wherever I was headed. I could not get away from his panting expressions of tenderness and devotion."[19]

Not long after Gilles de la Tourette died, a certain "Michaud" exposed the rumors to which Montorgueil had made veiled references: *"For several long months, he had already presented the clinical picture for pre-paralytic megalomania and, since no learned assembly of alienists oversees our medical schools, this insane man continued to interrogate candidates at doctoral examinations. His questions were so bizarre and his behavior so mad and clownish that he might have been a character in a comedy play. This famous neuropathologist continued with his consultations until the day his family found him completely naked, flailing about in front of a terrified patient, who was hiding behind a commode from the doctor he had come to consult . . . about his health. The comedy play was something of a vaudeville act as well. A few days before he was taken away, the brilliant professor shocked the lycée students and the young ladies who attend the Odéon matinees with a baffling lecture. The critics understood not a word, and with good reason; the lecturer had entirely lost his wits."*[20]

A Record of Megalomaniacal Delirium

In 1901, despite his failing health, Gilles de la Tourette decided to submit his candidacy for the Chair of Medical History, which Edouard Brissaud (1852–1909) had recently vacated for the Chair of Medical Pathology. To this end, he began writing the required dissertation, which he entitled: *"Chair of Medical History, The Scientific Titles and Works of Gilles de la Tourette."* The dissertation was never submitted and remained nothing more than a draft; Dejerine was named to this chair from 1901 to 1907. The manuscript reveals a sincere and passionate man, but one who was clearly disturbed. There are thirty-eight handwritten, unbound pages, in different formats, written in different orientations, with numerous cross-outs. The text is at times illegible, with significant changes in letter size and shape from one page to the next. Gilles de la Tourette most likely wrote it at intervals spanning several days, as indicated by the multiple versions of certain chapters. The page numbering is complex, often crossed out and corrected. Different pages have the same number, and the overall impression is one of extreme confusion. The beginning appears to have a structure, which by the end has been totally lost. The publication dates for his own works are often wrong. There are few spelling mistakes, but grammar and punctuation become increasingly erratic: *"Based on these facts and others that I have also drawn attention to for 25 years plus 12 more for the Iconographie, I have in all sincerity served the good cause of the Chair of Medical History so that I now have the right to ask you for distinction through words, for me, for my work (which has for too long remained 'barren' in the words of Montaigne) and for my applied photographic work. I thereby align myself with the moral principles that I have adhered to for many years in medicine without compromise."*

At several points, megalomania is obvious, with flight of ideas and loss of critical self-appraisal: *"We have published more than 100 articles exclusively dedicated to the History of Medicine. As a result we have almost made this subject popular among our colleagues who have rushed to join our enterprise, an enterprise so unusual that it has become the only one of its kind in the world. We think it a magnificent service we have rendered to the History of Medicine by bringing attention to these old treasures in our museums and also by making them appealing. These documents are so specific and so accurate in their representation, and were almost completely ignored until now and unknown to most of the public as well as those physicians most specialized in the posthumous objects of medicine."*

An example of flight of ideas: *"The impostor Urbain Grandier could be seen with a rope around his neck, his shirt dirty, his pants crumpled about his feet, making amends on the steps of Saint Pierre du Marché, his church and where I married with my witnesses Brouardel and my poor beloved Damaschino looking on, before the Collégiale de la Croix, where he had offended Richelieu who had him killed after imprisoning him for a rather stupid question of precedence."*

An example of loss of critical judgment (Figure 7.2): *"But let us return to our meditations which have perhaps frolicked too long in the tender grasses, for spring has just sprung, winter retreated and the green grasses make our thoughts heady with their liquorous succulence. We are all familiar with the chemical reactions that transform sweet substances into alcohol, a slightly aromatic alcohol that is all the more heady and the result is that all of the tissues of the economy are broadly inhibited for a long spell, reproducing in the poor languishing [illegible word] . . . and the sleepyheads all bundled up who drowse at the ringing of the little Savoyard's bell which I applauded*

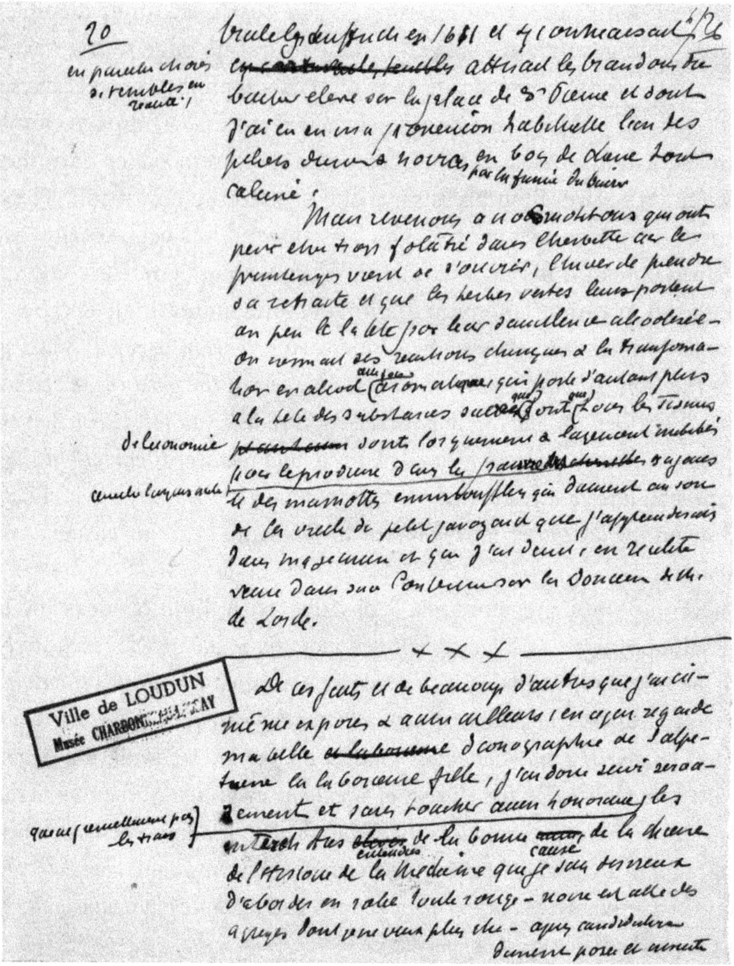

FIGURE 7.2 Dissertation for the Chair of Medical History. Never submitted, it remained nothing more than a draft.
Copyright Musée Charbonneau-Lassay, Ville de Loudun, with kind permission.

in my youth and which I described in actual reality in a lecture on the charming works of A. de Lorde."

These haphazard musings seem totally out of place in a university document. Gilles de la Tourette also mentions Charcot's article on faith-healing, *"La foi qui guérit,"* published in *La Revue Hebdomadaire* and the *New Review* in London. Not only does he confuse the journal titles; in his mythomaniac élan he claims authorship of the text: *"The article requested by The North American Review from my dear and lamented Master was written entirely by my own hand under his illustrious direction."* While Gilles de la Tourette does not appear to have authored this article, it is true that he worked with Emile Zola (1840–1902): *"For* Lourdes, *Zola consulted one of Charcot's students, Gilles de la Tourette, sending him a questionnaire."*[21]

Gilles de la Tourette refers to *La folie au théâtre* as if it were in press, whereas he had probably only started to write it, as noted earlier. *"The book is in press and the articles will be published at the same time in* La Revue Hebdomadaire. *The manuscript is completed and readily available to my judges."*

The passages in which Gilles de la Tourette explains his interest in the Chair are just as pathological: *"I ask only to be allowed to continue our work and my research and publications which I have been pursuing for so long. I would be most grateful to my judges if they would provide me with the desired means to disclose and further disseminate my work by according me the Chair of Medical History which would encourage me even more to develop my efforts. This position has been the aim of my industrious ambition since I began my studies and if I am appointed I will loyally commit to fulfilling my duties and never leaving the Chair."*

Self-satisfaction shows through in several passages: *"I have thus published, taught, and made the history of medicine known to a wider public for more than twenty years. As such I am worthy of those who have preceded me in occupying the Chair."* He doesn't hesitate to predict the fame he hopes to achieve, which seems to have eluded him in his teaching of legal medicine: *"If you wish to teach and have numerous students, become famous, and achieve success in the high position conferred by your Chair, this requires solid preparation and you must not think of moving as fast as possible to another Chair where success will not come either."*

The same symptoms were already perceptible in the preparatory note he sent to Fulgence Raymond in late October 1900, concerning the speech for Marguerite Bottard's retirement ceremony. The beginning of 1901 must have been particularly difficult. As noted, he requested a leave from April 7 to 14, which was *"rescinded."* Why? There is no surviving explanation. He was absent without interruption starting May 26, 1901. The Secretary of the Assistance Publique wrote to him on June 4, 1901: *"Dear Sir, I have the honor of informing you that the three months leave you requested has been granted, starting June 4. Based on his availability, I have appointed Dr. Boulloche, hospital physician, to replace you during your absence."*[22]

Dean Brouardel, on behalf of the Faculté de Médecine, sent his letter later, on November 19, 1901: *"Sir, Attached please find a copy of the order dated November 14, 1901, granting you three months of leave as per your request, for health reasons."* This leave was renewed every three months, then every six months, and in October 1903, for a year[23] (Figure 7.3).

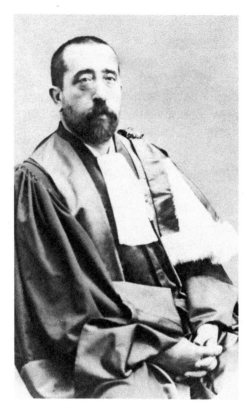

FIGURE 7.3 Gilles de la Tourette dressed in his university professor gown. Notice the signs of his disease on his face.
Private collection of the author.

Keeping Things Quiet

Marie Gilles de la Tourette wanted her husband to be treated with as much discretion as possible. In early June 1901, his old friend Jean-Baptiste Charcot (1867–1936) (Figure 7.4) managed to persuade him to go to Lucerne, Switzerland, to rest. Once he arrived at the Hôtel Schweizerhof, Gilles de la Tourette received a dispatch from Dr. Albert Mahaim (1867–1925), a Belgian psychiatrist in charge of the Bois-de-Cery asylum and a friend of J-B. Charcot. Dr. Mahaim asked Gilles de la Tourette to come to his clinic, supposedly for a consultation with a famous patient.[24] Gilles de la Tourette fell into the trap and was himself interned. He, of course, resisted violently. On June 25, 1901, J-B. Charcot wrote to Marie Gilles de la Tourette, as her friend and neighbor (he lived at 80 Rue de l'Université):

Dear Madam, there is no point in telling you how sorry I am I could not write sooner. With great emotion, I have been following the events since your return to Prilly.[25] You

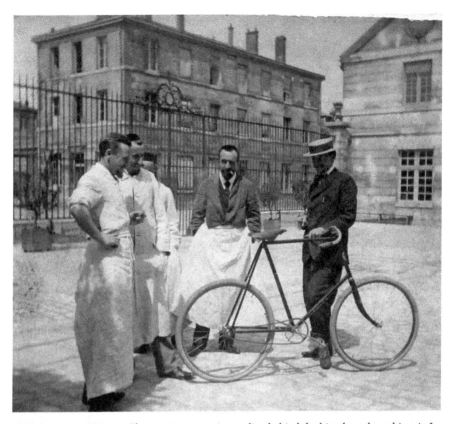

FIGURE 7.4 Jean-Baptiste Charcot (1867–1936), standing behind the bicycle and smoking, in La Salpêtrière courtyard.
Private collection of the author.

must be experiencing some very difficult moments, my dear lady, and unfortunately your life will be a trial for some time to come. One cannot imagine a more dreadful convalescence! . . . I saw your servant, Pierre, twice; he is trying to find work at the Hôtel de Ville. . . . The Faeroe Islands will rapidly cure all of that for me."

This letter and those that follow bear witness to J-B. Charcot's personal involvement with the entire Gilles de la Tourette family, including the management of their assets. The servant who had worked at the Rue de l'Université home must have been dismissed, and Charcot was helping him find employment. And his mention of the Faeroe Islands reminds us of his passion for navigation.

There are multiple signs of the Charcot family's affection; for example, the following card, one of several from Jeanne Charcot (1869–1941), dated Thursday, December 26, 1901: *"Thank you, my dear lady, for remembering us so affectionately. We think often of you and of what a difficult time you are having at present. I always tell you the same thing and yet cannot bring about what I so wish. It would make me so happy to be at your side, especially now, and to be able to surround you with our affection. Please know that I hold you and your dear little ones in my heart. My husband joins me in sending you his respectful regards."*

A letter from JB. Charcot, one year later, dated June 2, 1902, recalls his arrival in Switzerland: *"Alas! A year has already passed since we made that sad voyage, which I will always remember, but I beg you, do not thank me, for I was only performing my duty for a master whom I admire, for a friend whom I love as he loves me. Your sole consolation is knowing that you have done, and continue to do what few French people could have done in your place. Dear lady, I think of you once again and of your poor husband, and I remain, and will always remain yours, most affectionately, Charcot."*

Marie also received this letter from her father-in-law, Théodore Édouard Gilles de la Tourette (1827–1902), dated June 30, 1901:

My dear Marie, I received your letter in good time. I write to tell you how deeply affected we are by the misfortunes of our poor Georges. We think of him night and day; in spite of everything, we must not despair but on the contrary, continue to hope that with the good care he is receiving, he will recover his health. He is still young. This is an important point. There can be no doubt that overwork led to his predicament. He gave good advice to others while utterly neglecting himself. Here no one knows of his situation and when we are asked for news, we simply reply that he is doing a little better. Please, my dear Marie, keep us informed of what happens and above all, hide nothing from us.

I understand all too well how cruel this state of affairs is for you. You were obligated to leave Paris with your children, who for the time being cannot know what is going on, although you must still see to their education. You will need courage, and a great deal of it, to get through this critical moment, but I have every reason to hope that you will rise to your task and provide our dear sufferer with the consolation he so needs. I bid you adieu. Berthe and Marie join me in sending our most affectionate regards, to you and your children. Your loving father-in-law, E. Gilles de la Tourette."

Marie in Lausanne

Gilles de la Tourette was fortunate that his wife could accompany him to Switzerland and attend to him throughout his long hospitalization. Marie's correspondence gives some idea of her daily life, which in turn reflects the progression of her husband's disease. Staying in Lausanne, she had to request a resident's permit, granted on November 18, 1901 (on the "profession" line of the form she noted "person of independent means"). It was renewed on December 18, 1902, then again on December 24, 1904. During the first weeks of her stay, she received letters in care of Madame Perrin, 1 Rue Beauséjour, and so must have taken lodgings with a private individual. She was not very happy there, as attested by a brief message from J-B. Charcot on October 30, 1901: *"I hope, my dear lady, that in your new lodgings you will no longer be tormented by an irritable old Huguenot and that you will spend this winter as peacefully as possible."*

The Loudun archives contain her accounting, which she kept on one of her husband's prescription pads. Her budget was around 1,000 Swiss francs per month, including 250 f for rent at the Villa Gai Coteau, Avenue des Alpes, 100 f for a servant, 15 f for "maintenance," and so forth. This record also indicates where she moved during the rest of her stay in Lausanne.

On July 13, 1901, J-B. Charcot wrote a letter on the letterhead of his famous boat, the *Yacht Pourquoi Pas* (Figure 7.5): *"Dear Madam, I arrived in Gosport to find your letter. . . ."* On July 30, 1901, JB. Charcot tried to ease Marie's worries and give her hope: *"Dear Madam, I have finally been in touch with Brissaud, and have spoken to him of your poor husband. He responded that nothing Mahaim said would modify his opinion, which remains unchanged, and he added that he could only repeat what he has already told us. In any case, he noted, there is no way our poor patient could be receiving better or more intelligent care."*

Edouard Brissaud must have already sent this undated letter to Marie Gilles de la Tourette (Figure 7.6):

Dear Madam, I do hope that you will excuse my delay in writing to you. . . . I believe Dr. Mahaim must have communicated my response to you. What you have told me about the health of my poor friend does not differ much from what Mr. Mahaim has said. I do not know how to advise you about your husband's return. I am well aware of how difficult it must be for you when your dear husband reproves you so lamentably, and I deeply regret that you suffer so from the silence with which you must answer his perpetual pleas for freedom. Would it nonetheless be wise to compromise the modest benefit so painfully gained by a premature release? And then, is his improvement going to last? Truly, the wisest course of action is to follow the advice of Mr. Mahaim. He alone is in a position to assist you with regard to any decisions you are called on to make. I do not believe that a change of residence would improve the situation. . . . I remain yours in devotion and respect. Brissaud.

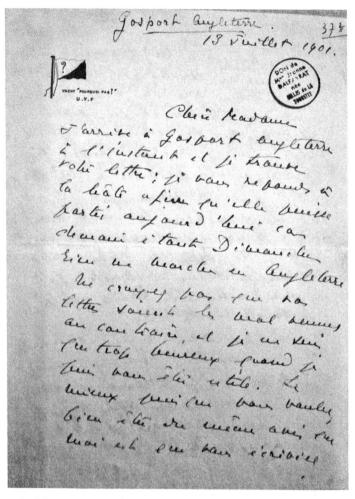

FIGURE 7.5 On July 13, 1901, J-B. Charcot wrote a letter on the letterhead of his boat, the yacht *Pourquoi Pas.*
Copyright Musée Charbonneau-Lassay, Ville de Loudun, with kind permission.

Response from Friends and Colleagues

Marie Gilles de la Tourette received more messages of sympathy than can be included here. The following example is representative. Using letterhead from the Faculté de Medecine, Dean Paul Brouardel (1837–1906) sent a brief undated message, most likely upon learning his disciple had been hospitalized: *"Dear Madam, I cannot tell you how saddened we were to learn of the illness of poor Gilles. We stand by you whole-heartedly and will do anything within our power for your husband, you, and your children. I sent a note to Gilles and told him what matters most is his health. I assured him that his department is taken care of until he is cured and can return to it. Brouardel."*

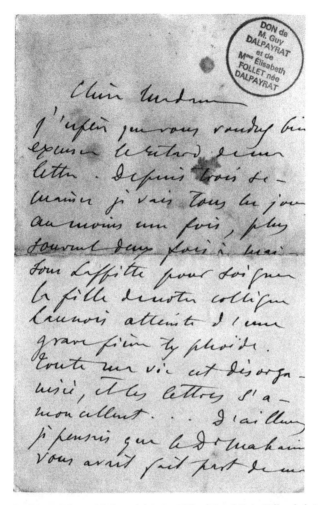

FIGURE 7.6 In this letter, Edouard Brissaud (1852–1909) advises Marie Gilles de la Tourette.
Copyright Musée Charbonneau-Lassay, Ville de Loudun, with kind permission.

Nearing the End

The exact nature of Gilles de la Tourette's illness and where he was being treated were carefully kept secret, as attested by this letter sent to Marie at her address in Paris. It was written on July 17, 1901, by Alphonse–Rémi Mauté (1873–1940) (Figure 7.7), an *interne* at Hôpital Saint-Antoine, worried about his teacher, who had been absent for more than a month.

Madam, All of us here are impatiently awaiting news of our Master, Mr. Gilles de la Tourette. I have gone several times to Rue de l'Université but no one there can reassure me. News from you, Madam, would be invaluable and might even give us a bit of hope. Please pardon me, Madam, for taking this liberty. My excuse is the great sympathy I feel for your suffering and my ardent wish that you should find happiness again, with the return of our venerated Master. I remain yours most respectfully.

Managing her family's affairs must have been complicated for Marie Gilles de la Tourette. Based on the Family Council's deliberations, the decision was made to legally seek a guardianship. On December 10, 1902, a civil court in the Seine handed down this decision:

> Interdiction upon Gilles de la Tourette. Jurisdiction states non-appearance of Gilles de la Tourette,
>
> Failure by him to appoint an attorney although he was served due process on December fourteenth, nineteen hundred and one
>
> Whereas according to the documents for the cause, while on a journey to Switzerland, Doctor Gilles de la Tourette suffered from mental disorders

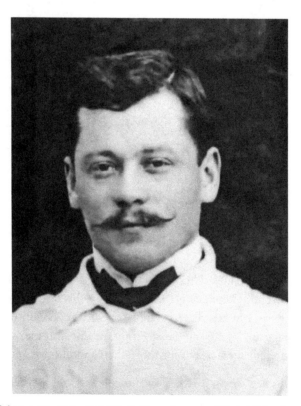

FIGURE 7.7 Alphonse-Rémi Mauté (1873–1940), an *interne* at Hôpital Saint-Antoine, was worried by the lack of news concerning his teacher.
Private collection of the author.

of such violence that he had to be committed to the asylum in Cery, near Lausanne,

Whereas his health condition has not improved and it is currently impossible for him to care for himself and to manage his estate,

Whereas the anamnesis that has been ordered cannot take place due to his state of extreme agitation

Whereas it is fitting, in these conditions and in compliance with the unanimous opinion from the Family Council, to accede to the conclusions in the petition:

On these grounds:

declare that Doctor Gilles de la Tourette is legally restrained from managing his affairs and himself, orders that a Family Council be held for the purpose of appointing a supervising guardian in compliance with the law. Furthermore sentences him to all costs, provisionally liquidated at the amount of 50 francs to the benefit of Deschamps, attorney

appoints Guillé bailiff-at-law to serve this ruling upon the defaulting defendant. Deschamps

For Madame Gilles de la Tourette, address 39 Rue de l'Université in Paris.

Undoubtedly for financial reasons, Marie Gilles de la Tourette terminated the lease for the apartment on Rue de l'Université and moved to Avenue Mozart. In the letter that the owner, the banker Charles Risler (1848–1923), sent on January 20, 1902, with the termination papers, he wrote: *"You may stay in the apartment until the end of April. And now, my dear lady, how to express our bitter sadness at ending this lease that was to keep you many more long years under our roof! Not a day goes by that we don't think of you and your poor dear husband to whom we are so grateful. How we wish we could do something to help him! You have not spoken to me of his condition and this silence troubles us as we fear his progress has not been substantial enough to reassure your friends. Please do not forget us. Especially during this cruel ordeal, please be assured of the sincere and profound sympathy of your faithful friends."*

The real diagnosis was never mentioned in these letters or in the articles of Montorgueil or other journalists. For example, in *Le Journal*: *"Mr. Gilles de la Tourette has died, struck down at the peak of his talents by the excessive demands that he relentlessly placed on himself to excel as a physician and dominate in his fields of research and teaching. Despite the absolute rest and perfect calm imposed on him for more than four years already, he succumbed the day before yesterday to the final attack of his illness."*[26]

Exhaustion due to overwork was the only cause ever mentioned. Was this because people truly did not know what his diagnosis was? Or, by leaving significant matters unsaid and misusing language in a catachrestic way, did they choose to ignore the facts for cultural reasons?

The Hidden Truth

Despite the treatment he received, Gilles de la Tourette died on May 22, 1904, following status epilepticus (Figure 7.8). Whereas in Paris every effort was made to ensure discretion on what caused Gilles de la Tourette's death, in Switzerland, this little obituary appeared in *La Feuille d'avis de Lausanne* on Tuesday, May 24, 1904: *"On Sunday morning, at the Cery Asylum, Dr. Gilles de la Tourette passed away after being treated there for two years for general paralysis. . . . His body will be returned to France for burial."*[27]

Marie Gilles de la Tourette wrote immediately to Montorgueil. This letter provides some explanation as to why the diagnosis was kept secret:

Lausanne, Sunday, May 22, 1904, Dear Sir, I did not want you to learn from some stranger that my poor husband passed away this morning. My telegram to you was brief, but because of the faithful friendship that always bound you to my husband, I wanted to ask you a favor. This sad and unfair ending to his life is something I would like to keep quiet. But if you foresee this to be impossible, please say that following a long illness due to overwork and fatigue, which led him to move with his family to Switzerland where the climate is more amenable, my poor husband succumbed to an attack of apoplexy that lasted 26 hours. This, in any case, is the exact truth. Thank you, I am very tired, especially from grief. I send you all of my best regards. Marie Gilles de la Tourette.[28]

Gilles de la Tourette was buried in Loudun.

Tracing a Commitment to Medicine and to Medical History

Writing with elegance, Montorgueil penned Gilles de la Tourette's portrait in *L'Eclair* on May 24, 1904. Although his eulogy included several new biographical details, it began with a dissimulation of the cause of death:

We learn with deep regret of the death in Lausanne of Dr. Gilles de la Tourette. He succumbed to an attack of apoplexy. Exhausted by exceptional professional demands, the eminent specialist and historian of nervous diseases had sought

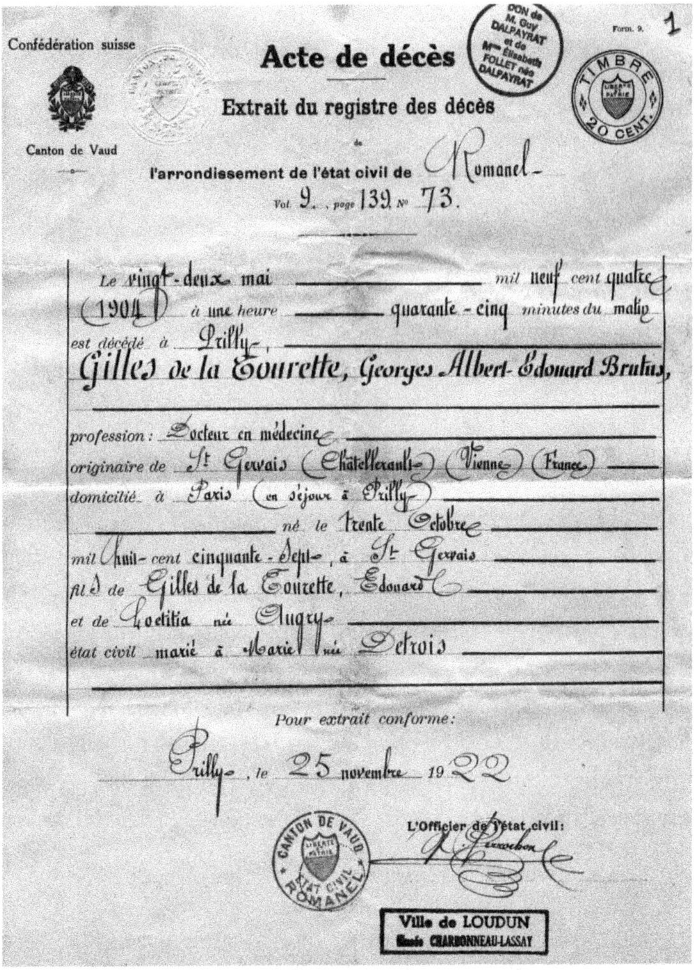

FIGURE 7.8 Georges Gilles de la Tourette's death certificate.
Copyright Musée Charbonneau-Lassay. Ville de Loudun, with kind permission.

out a better climate and calmer surroundings in which to recover his health, though ultimately it eluded him. His family remained at his side, departing with him very soon after the 1900 World's Fair, for which he directed the medical department. If the deepest affection and most faithful devotion could have accomplished the miracles vainly asked of science, he would have regained the clairvoyant energy for which he was so admired.

This learned man, having made a name for himself at such an early age, was taken from us at the peak of his maturity. As Charcot's disciple, it was as if he inherited his popularity. He had entered the Salpêtrière School when the Master's brilliant teachings had such a powerful effect that the extra-medical public grew fascinated with this new, or cleverly renewed science of hypnotism, which revealed to us the mysteries and ills of our nervous centers. . . .

Dr. Gilles de la Tourette, combative by nature, moved out ahead of the phalanx of Charcot's disciples, most of them now famous, and besieged the traffickers. . . . He was an erudite as well as a practitioner. . . . The proof that a reputation is established lies in its influence on public opinion. During Charcot's lifetime, and even more so after his death, every time one of these phenomena concerned our poor human condition, reporters ran to Gilles de la Tourette. We found a warm and welcoming man, in his magnificent offices on Rue de l'Université. As an artist, he had surrounded himself with paintings and valuable curios, his most prized being those he had discovered himself. Ferreting around the stalls, along with hunting, were his favorite ways of spending what little leisure time he allowed himself. In his own surroundings, when he was questioned, he would examine the question briefly and clearly, without pedantry, skilled at honing in on what would impress and educate those with the least knowledge. . . . He wrote, taught, diagnosed patients, and gave lectures, always springing to the defense of his causes, in a continual need for movement and combat. The force of his solicitude was keenly felt by his entourage—he astutely warned us to avoid the shortcuts we are wont to take, he indicated the dangerous curves and fatal drop-offs along the way—but all the while, his ambition to be another Charcot drove him onward at full speed. He never realized that in the prime of his life, worn down by overwork, he would die of this pursuit.[29]

Celebrating a Friend and a Man of Science

In *Le Temps* of May 27, 1904, Claretie wrote a very different eulogy in terms of form, but the substance was much the same:

Every era is bound to have its faults, just as it has its strengths—and its diseases. I was told as much by Doctor Gilles de la Tourette, who knew and studied our neuroses, our neurasthenias, our fatigues, and who guided me, as Doctor Gilbert Ballet had done, through the hell of La Salpêtrière, a hell that for many sufferers, is a paradise, or at least a resting place, an asylum. This man whom science has just lost, I can still see him as a young *interne*, gay and charming. . . . He was a talented writer, and he roused his audience when he spoke. I listened to more than one of his lessons. His diction was picturesque and elegant, giving wings to his ideas. . . . This literary work, which Gilles de la Tourette enjoyed, was a respite from his scientific labors. This learned man left us with books unlike any others. . . . He did a lot of good for those around him, and his charming wife, so admirable in recent years, helped him with this task. He made great efforts for the welfare of others. And now he has died at the age of 47. But at least the author of so many enduring works leaves an honored name and a glorious *oeuvre*. . . . I regret the loss of my dear friend from La Salpêtrière who could have spoken about this matter, when he was at his most eloquent, with so much charm and intelligence![30]

"He Died in the Prime of His Life"

Mrs. Dejerine-Klumpke paid homage with this very brief eulogy at the Société de Neurologie on June 4, 1904:

> Sirs, the Société de Neurologie recently lost one of its members. Dr. Gilles de la Tourette, a professor at the medical school and physician at Hôpital Saint-Antoine, died on May 24. Our colleague was a founding member of our Society and participated assiduously in its activities. A student of Charcot, Gilles de la Tourette published important works, including his studies on the tic disease and on gait in nervous system diseases. Together with his Traité de l'Hystérie, these works made him well known as a neuropathologist. He died in the prime of his life, at a time when he was starting to savor the fruits of his labors, struck down by a condition that had kept him far away from us for some time. On behalf of the Society, I bid our late lamented colleague a final farewell.[31]

Gilles de la Tourette's grave, in the middle of the Loudun cemetery (aisle K, No. 127) is in a state of neglect, overrun with moss and lichen (Figure 7.9). It is inscribed with a cross, whereas he was an atheist; there were no religious signs on either his death announcement or that of his son, Jean. Erosion of the tufa stone has erased all written inscriptions, making the grave entirely anonymous. And there is no indication at the cemetery's entrance to compensate for the guard's lack of knowledge. Not only has Gilles de la Tourette's grave been forgotten; most inhabitants of Loudun know little or nothing about one of their most famous adopted sons. Although a property management company registered in Poitiers is named after him, no streets or buildings in Loudun honor his memory. On the Loudun Wikipedia page, Gilles de la Tourette is not featured as one of the city's celebrities.[32] While Gilles de la Tourette syndrome is known throughout the world by physicians and by patients who have the disease, the man himself is mostly unknown.

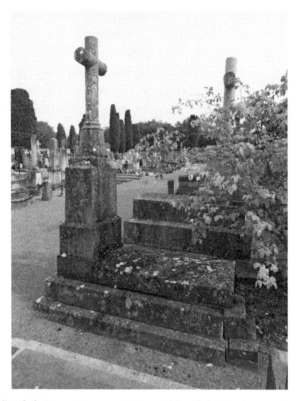

FIGURE 7.9 Gilles de la Tourette's grave, in the middle of the Loudun cemetery (aisle K, No. 127), is in a state of neglect, overrun with moss and lichen.
Photographed by the author in 2015.

Notes

1. Bayle ALJ. *Recherches sur les maladies mentales*. Thèse no. 247. Paris: Imprimerie Didot le Jeune. 1822.
2. Bayle ALJ. Nouvelle doctrine des maladies mentales. *Revue médicale*. 1825;1(2):169–216.
3. Charcot JM. Rapport sur le concours du Prix Civrieux de 1882. *Bulletin de l'Académie de Médecine*. 1883;47:977–979.
4. Nageotte J. *Tabes et paralysie générale*. Thèse no. 93. Paris: G. Steinheil. 1893.
5. Gelfand T. "Mon cher Docteur Freud": Charcot's unpublished correspondance to Freud, 1888–1893. *Bull Hist Med*. 1988;62:563–588.
6. *Le Temps*, Lundi 4 fevrier 1901;41(14483):3.
7. Ginisty P. Causerie littéraire, un chapitre du Traité clinique de l'hystérie. *Gil Blas*. vendredi 13 novembre 1891;13(4378):3.
8. de Lorde A. *Théâtre d'épouvante*. Paris: E. Fasquelle. 1909.
9. Bérillon E. La léthargique de Thenelles. *Revue de l'hypnotisme exéprimental et thérapeutique*. 1887;1:289–296.
10. Lancereaux E. *La dormeuse de Thenelles. Un sommeil pathologique de vingt années consécutives*. *Bulletin de l'Académie de Médecine*. Paris: Masson. 1904.

11. Ganteaire. Les mystères de la nature. La Belle au bois dormant. *Gil Blas*. Jeudi 22 octobre 1896;18(6484):2.

12. ROM Propos de coulisses. Odéon, La dormeuse de M. André de Lorde. *Gil Blas*. Lundi 11 février 1891;23(7756):3.

13. Md Ch. Théâtres. *L'Aurore*. Dimanche 10 février 1901;5(1210):3.

14. Hysterical sleep differs from normal sleep by the absence of muscular hypotonia, often replaced by a hypertonia similar to catalepsy.

15. de Lorde A. *La folie au théâtre, l'homme mystérieux, la petite Roque, les invisibles*. Paris: Fontemoing et Cie. 1913.

16. de Lorde. Après la manifestation du Grand-Guignol. *Le Journal*. Samedi 10 décembre 1921;29(10646):4.

17. de Lavarenne E. Gilles de la Tourette. *La Presse Médicale*. 1904;1(45):1–2.

18. Daudet L. *Paris Vécu*. Paris: Gallimard. 1930.

19. Daudet L. *Devant la douleur. Souvenirs des milieux littéraires, politiques, artistiques et médicaux de 1880 à 1905*. Paris: Nouvelle Librairie Nationale. 1915.

20. Michaut. Varia, nécrologie. *La Vie Médicale*. 1904;13(516):333.

21. Lancelot A. Lourdes d'Émile Zola. *Revue scientifique*. Lundi 20 octobre 1902;6(1827):3.

22. Pierre Boulloche (1864–1923).

23. La Faculté de Médecine de Paris, personnel de la faculté: dossiers, fiches, gestion 1750–1953. Académie de Paris. Archives Nationales AJ/16/6509 Gaillard-Gilles de la Tourette.

24. Müller C. Rapports entre la psychiatrie suisse et la psychiatrie francaise. *Annales de Thérapeutique Psychiatrique*. 1969;4:59–65.

25. Swiss town west of Lausanne, in the canton of Vaud. Where the Bois-de-Cery asylum was located.

26. Deuil. Le docteur Gilles de la Tourette. *Le Journal*. Mercredi 25 mai 1904;13(4255):2.

27. Nécrologie. G. Gilles de la Tourette. *Feuille d'Avis de Lausanne et Résumé des Nouvelles*. 1904;143(120):15.

28. Archives Nationales 428AP/2 Correspondance Montorgueil-Gilles de la Tourette.

29. Montorgueil G. La mort du Docteur Gilles de la Tourette. *L'Éclair*. 24 mai 1904.

30. Clarétie J. La Vie à Paris. *Le Temps*. 1904;44(15 885):2–3.

31. Dejerine A. Nécrologie: M. Gilles de la Tourette. *Revue Neurologique*. 1904;12(12):614.

32. http://www.ville-loudun.fr/decouvrir-loudun-1/personnage-celebre-loudun-vienne

~~ Part II ~~

Medical Writings, Fame

~ 8 ~

Doctoral Thesis

GILLES DE LA Tourette defended his thesis on Monday, December 28, 1885: *Etudes cliniques et physiologiques sur la marche; la marche dans les maladies du système nerveux étudiée par la méthode des empreintes* (Clinical and physiological studies of gait; walking in patients with nervous system diseases, studied by the footprint tracing method.) The jury was presided over by Jean-Martin Charcot (1825–1893) and was composed of François Damaschino (1840–1889), Louis Landouzy (1845–1917) (Figure 8.1), and Alix Joffroy (1844–1908) (Figure 8.2). Only Joffroy did not have Gilles de la Tourette as an *interne* (house officer or resident). The subject was suggested by Charcot in 1884, when Gilles de la Tourette was an *interne* in his department. Gilles de la Tourette collected the necessary data under Paul Brouardel (1837–1906) during 1885.

In Competition with Augusta Klumpke

Borrowing from the practices of the Académie Impériale de Médecine, the Société de Biologie in Paris, founded in 1848, awarded prizes annually to distinguish theses in specific domains, as determined by the benefactors who bequeathed the necessary sums, for whom these prizes were named. For example, the anatomist and anthropologist Ernest Godard (1827-1862) left instructions in his will that 5000 francs be donated for the prize that would bear his name and eventually become much sought after.

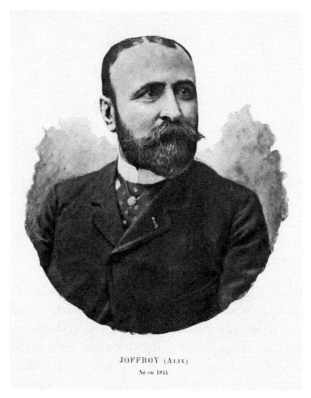

JOFFROY (Alix)
Né en 1844

FIGURE 8.1   Alix Joffroy (1844–1908).
Private collection of the author.

The commission set up by the Société de Biologie to judge the dissertations submitted for this prestigious Prix Godard for 1886 was composed of Auguste Chauveau (1827–1917), president; Charles Féré (1852–1907); Victor Hanot (1844–1896); Isidore Straus (1845–1896); and Jules Dejerine (1849–1917), acting as rapporteur. In its session on October 23, 1885, the commission examined five dissertations, including those of Benjamin Lœvenberg (1836–?), Georges Assaky (1855–?), Augusta Klumpke (1859–1927) *"interne,"* and Georges Gilles de la Tourette (*Etudes cliniques et physiologiques sur la marche*).

Only the last two dissertations were selected for presentation. Dejerine, a favorite pupil of Alfred Vulpian (1826–1887), made an in-depth report of these presentations in which he highly praised the work of Klumpke, carried out in the laboratory of Vulpian (Figure 8.3), and in which Dejerine himself most likely participated: *Contribution à l'étude des paralysies radiculaires du plexus brachial* (Contribution to the study of the brachial plexus palsy). In fact, she was a temporary *interne*; the examination jury did not actually name a woman

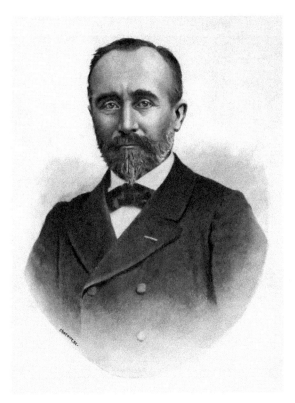

FIGURE 8.2 Louis Landouzy (1845–1917).
Copyright BIUSanté Paris, with kind permission.

interne, even though she had obtained the best grades on the written test: 29/30 on the question of *"signs and causes of organic hemiplegia."* She would later write: *"One of the examination judges, expressing the general opinion of his colleagues, remarked: 'If your oral results are as good as your written results, we will name you at the top of the list; otherwise, you will fail.' Another said: 'We are receiving injurious letters about your written grade; if we can get a letter from Vulpian to cover us, you will be named an interne.' I had too much respect and veneration for the great Vulpian to ask for a recommendation; I wouldn't have even wanted him to hear about the matter. So, I was only named a temporary interne. During the following examination, without my saying anything to Vulpian, he spontaneously recommended me. And then I became a regular interne."*[1] Klumpke was the first woman *interne* in the Paris hospitals, in 1886. Knowing that they were getting married a later in 1888, we will never know whether personal or professional scruples led Dejerine to orient the commission toward Gilles de la Tourette's dissertation.[2] At the time, Augusta Klumpke (Figure 8.4) was spending an enormous amount of energy helping Dejerine prepare for his *agrégation* exam: *"She was*

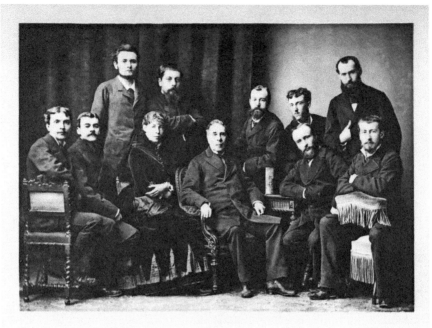

LA CLINIQUE DE LA CHARITÉ — 1881

Prof. A. Hardy ; L. Landouzy, agrégé, Médecin du Bureau Central ; J. Dejerine, Chef de Clinique ; A. Josias, Chef de Clinique Adjoint ;
A. Malherbe, Chef de Laboratoire ; L. Queyrat, R. Semelaigue, Grisel, Gomet, Delahaye, externes, Mlle A. Klumpke, stagiaire.

FIGURE 8.3 In 1881, Augusta Klumpke-Dejerine (1859–1927) worked under the young *chef de clinique,* Jules Dejerine (1849–1917), and the *agrégé,* Louis Landouzy (1845–1917), in the department of Professor Alfred Hardy (1811–1893) at Hôpital la Charité (1849–1917).
Copyright BIUSanté Paris, with kind permission.

cool and calm, supporting with all the strength of her love and her ingenious activity the man who would triumph and, eventually, become her husband."[33]

Honored with a Prize

Gilles de la Tourette was the official laureate of the Prix Godard in 1886 for his dissertation, which he would use for the physiological gait chapter in his thesis. André Thomas (1867–1961), in his 1927 homage to Augusta Klumpke-Dejerine, said that the 1886 Prix Godard went to her, undoubtedly an honest mistake. But it is also an indication that, at the time, Gilles de la Tourette was in a sort of purgatory (because of the bad reputation linked to his demented death) before his work was rediscovered in the 1960s.[4]

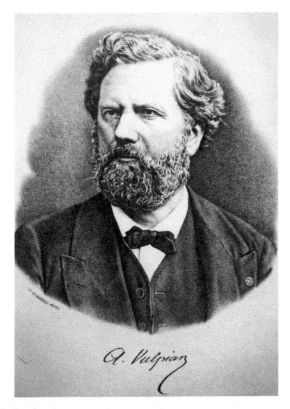

FIGURE 8.4 Alfred Vulpian (1826–1887).
Private collection of the author.

Work Method

Gilles de la Tourette explained how he carried out his work: *"Over the two years we were involved in this project, our excellent friend, Albert Londe, head of the chemistry and photography laboratory at La Salpêtrière, was a constant and invaluable help to us. Without his aid, we would not have been able to publish the footstep traces that are the fundamental basis of the study. This work will be published jointly, since we both presented the general results to the Société de Biologie at the October 23, 1885 session."*[5] In 1882, Albert Londe (1858–1917) (Figure 8.5), a non-physician photographer, took over the photographic laboratory that Charcot had asked Désiré-Magloire Bourneville (1840–1909) and Paul Regnard (1850–1927) (Figure 8.6) to create in 1878 in his own department. The joint presentation given by Gilles de la Tourette and Londe to the Société de Biologie probably also influenced the attribution of the Prix Godard.[6]

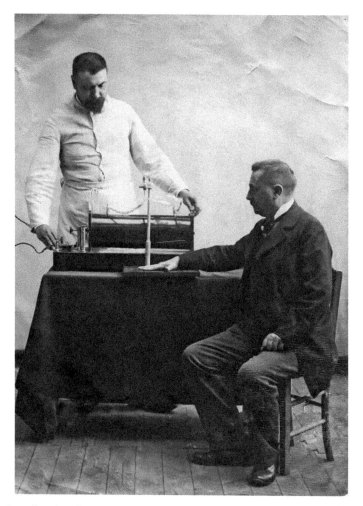

FIGURE 8.5 Albert Londe (1858–1917) radiographing a hand.
Private collection of the author.

Gilles de la Tourette was pleased that his study provided *"some interesting results based on the extensive research and experiments we conducted between 1884 and 1885, both on patients and the healthy personnel at the La Salpêtrière and La Pitié hospitals, and on the patients at the Hospice Vieillesse-Femmes and at the Nervous Diseases Clinic."* At Hôpital de la Pitié, in addition to the patients hospitalized in Brouardel's department, Gilles de la Tourette examined patients in the department of Victor Dumontpallier (1826–1899).

His thesis is divided in two parts. The first provides data on physiological gait, while the second provides data for gait dysfunction in nervous system diseases. His aim was to obtain an easily applicable method that could be used for comparative analysis of the results, then to compare his results to those of

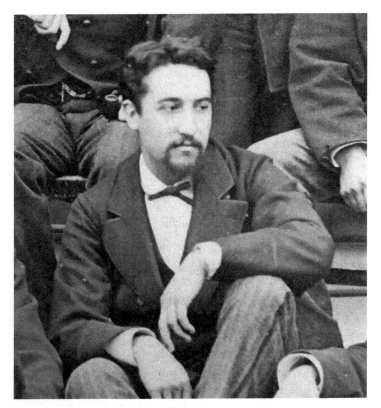

FIGURE 8.6 Paul Regnard (1850–1927) in 1878.
Private collection of the author.

authors using more complicated equipment. His larger project was to develop a simple, reproducible method that could be applied in daily clinical use.

His Predecessors

Gilles de la Tourette did not fail to acknowledge the debt he owed to certain predecessors. First of all, he mentioned the brothers Wilhelm Weber (1804–1891), a German physicist and his brother Eduard Weber (1806–1871), an anatomist and physiologist in Göttingen, who *"introduced calculations and step measurements during walking in their study."* That is, they built a mathematical theory of human modes of locomotion, which was supposed to determine the human body's center of gravity and introduce the action of weight in the movement of stepping.[7] Gilles de la Tourette omitted to mention Guillaume Duchenne de Boulogne (1806–1875), who demonstrated the inaccuracy of the Weber brothers' theory in 1855: *"They would have never formulated this theory had they applied pathological observation as a control for their experiments.*"[8] In 1867, Duchenne repeated the entire study of the action of each muscle group of the thigh, lower leg, and foot involved in walking for his famous book *Physiologie des mouvements*: *"Using muscular electro-physiology and clinical observation as mutual controls gives the results of this sort of research the highest degree of certainty."*[9] Charles Lasègue (1816–1883) and Straus qualified this work as *"a veritable masterpiece, in which Duchenne's genius for observation is even more apparent than in his other publications."*[10]

Gilles de la Tourette chose to focus on the 1872 study of Gaston Carlet (1845–1892), a student of Etienne-Jules Marey (1830–1904). Carlet recorded himself walking around a circular track while pushing a recording cylinder: *"On his feet were shoes in which the sole had two little balls of compressible rubber in two compartments: one at the heel, the other at the forefoot. Protruding from this ball was a rubber tube that transmitted the footsteps to Marey's recording device."*[11] Following his study, Carlet developed *"a theory of gait,"* which breaks down the kinetics of human steps with remarkable accuracy and which Marey confirmed the following year using chronophotography.[12] Carlet only examined normal gait; the modifications of pathological gaits had not yet been studied. Almost ten years later, in 1881, it was Hermann Vierordt (1853–1944) in Germany who would implement a method of ink jets projected under the foot, based on a particularly complex device known as the kymograph. This enabled him to compare normal gait with abnormal gait, mainly from deformations secondary to orthopedic dysfunction.[13] Gilles de la Tourette concluded that *"this method will certainly give results less scientifically rigorous than Carlet's method."*[14]

Was Gilles de la Tourette aware of the work of Eadweard Muybridge (1830–1904)? He did not mention the innovations Muybridge developed and used to break down a horse's run (*The Horse in Motion*) in 1878. Muybridge set up twelve photographic devices in a series along the track where the horse ran. In 1879, he developed his *"zoopraxiscope,"* a projector that simulates movement through rapid and successive viewing of photographs taken in series, giving the illusion of movement phases. This invention made him a forerunner to modern cinema.[15] The American Francis Xavier Dercum (1856–1931), an "instructor in nervous diseases" at the University of Pennsylvania, is known for the eponymous disease. In 1888, three years after Gilles de la Tourette's thesis, Dercum obtained *"zoopraxiscopic"* images of pathological modifications to gait with the help of Muybridge.[16] He made several collotype prints of his patients.[17] Some of these prints are included in volume 8 (of 11) of Muybridge's monumental 1887 work, which was an expanded edition of the 1881 original publication.[18,19,20]

Data Acquisition

Here is how Gilles de la Tourette recorded normal or pathological gait: *"We take a roll of ordinary wallpaper, the kind used by building painters, gray to blue-gray and affordable, though of high quality. Each roll is around 7 or 8 meters long and 0.50 meters wide."* He drew a continuous line down the middle of this sheet, and then nailed it to the floor. *"The experimental subject sits at one end of the paper. An assistant rubs the ball of his feet and his toes with iron sesquioxide[21] reduced to a very fine powder. This inexpensive substance, which produces very strong coloration, seemed better than the powdered carmine used by our friend Neugebauer. Initially, the subject's two feet are placed in the position they will take during normal standing, with the axis line passing between them. The individual then walks straight ahead, as usual. The sheet of footprints made from the coloration material is removed for photography purposes, and reduced as needed for reproduction."* Gilles de la Tourette did not invent this process. Joseph Rohmer (1856–1921) in Nancy, for his 1880 thesis on the plantar arch, coated the ball of the foot with lampblack.[22] Franciszek Ludwik Neugebauer (1856–1914) was an obstetrician in Warsaw interested in the deformations in the position and shape of the pelvis in pathologies affecting spinal alignment (especially spondylolisthesis) that could lead to dystocia.[23] Gilles de la Tourette appears to have known him well, attributing his use of the dye to Neugebauer, and described *"the indisputable advantage"* of his improvement on Neugebauer's process this way: *"It obfuscates the shoe and allows a direct print of the ball of the foot in healthy subjects and in patients."*

Interpretation of Results

Gilles de la Tourette compiled statistical tables of his results. Men's steps measure 0.63 cm on average, women's measure 0.50 cm; the step that sends the right foot forward is longer than the left step, and so forth. He corroborated his results with anatomy and was able to distinguish normal steps from steps where the subject had neuromuscular deficits.

In the second part, he differentiated what he called *"bilateral rectilinear gait"* and *"unilateral gait."* He described several degrees of *"spasmodic gait."* *"Locomotion is of the same type (although there are varying degrees), whether the pyramidal system is entirely affected, as in the amyotrophic lateral sclerosis discovered by Charcot, or is only affected relatively locally, as in spinal compression or transverse myelitis."* Discussing the different explanations for these dysfunctions, he focused on *"spinal tremor"* and the different locations of contraction that lead to a reduction in step length, a reduction of foot pressure applying exclusively to the forefoot, and so on.

In his description of gait during "paralysis agitans," he observed that the *"body is rigid, bent forward to find the center of gravity,"* and *"the patient is subject to antepulsions after a short walk,"* but he did not explicitly describe festination. He also noted that *"the step is very small, 20 to 22 cm,"* curiously omitting to mention patients' difficulty with lifting their feet from the ground.

During locomotor ataxia, *"the patient throws his legs out while walking; the foot, with the tip turned out, falls strongly on the heel, with the revolution of the sole's surface occurring in two separate phases (the first of which is always more accentuated than the second) rather than the regular rolling succession of foot phenomena. . . . The muscular energy of the lower limb is wasted by the exaggerated projection of the foot forward and outward, rather than accomplishing the phenomena of progression."*

Gilles de la Tourette had much more difficulty explaining *"staggering bilateral or zigzagging gait,"* the etiology of which, he claimed, was simple chorea or hysterical chorea, Ménière's disease, or multiple sclerosis. *"The two main factors of a zigzagging gait are trembling of the lower limbs, in the largest sense, and vertigo. . . . It is obviously difficult, in the staggering gait, to assign special characteristics to the various actions that comprise the step."* His conclusions were vague and of little interest in 1885 and are even more so today.

In the introduction to the *"unilateral gait"* observations, Gilles de la Tourette cited several possible etiologies: infantile paralysis[24] or cerebral or brainstem hemorrhage or softening, which can be due to syphilis as well as tuberculosis, *"by compression of the transmitting pathway."* He focused on hemiplegia, regardless of etiology, in the flaccid or spastic phase. *"Among nervous gaits, the hemiplegic gait is indeed that found in the oldest descriptions and is the most frequently described. The result is that today, no further description is considered necessary, other than to say that the hemiplegic drags his leg, with circumduction. As we hope to demonstrate, this type of locomotion, however, deserves more precision."* Studying the evolution of several hemiplegics from onset of *"apoplexy"* to the *"fixed"* paralysis stage, he identified a first period where *"the affected leg, when it is the walking leg, does not overstep the healthy, weight-bearing foot. It thus never forms the step and only aids progression by providing support, albeit insufficient, to the healthy, oscillating limb."* Gilles de la Tourette accurately described the action of each muscle, at every level, indicating the effect on the step of still-functional patients as well as hypotonic patients and those with secondary contraction. After analyzing and providing the drawings of footprint traces of hemiplegics walking with circumduction, he discussed the final stage: *"The contracted foot remains almost constantly in clubfoot position, resulting in a characteristic print. The patient does not exhibit circumduction; the leg, entirely rigid, is carried forward in one piece; the space it covers is so short that the oscillation curve is perfectly negligible."*

As Dejerine noted in his report, Gilles de la Tourette's conclusions *"seem unexpected at first, but the author justifies them in this way: 'The pathological step, if not to say the gait, is always more regular in itself, than the normal step or gait, as a result of the length, lateral gap, and angle of opening of the feet.' This, according to Gilles de la Tourette, is easy to understand, because in the normal case, it is the individual who walks and who may modify or vary his gait; in the second case, it is the disease itself that walks and not the patient, and if the patient has some control, he will use it in an attempt to normalize the locomotion created by the disease. The results obtained by the author seem well-founded, at least in certain respects, because he has substantiated them with comparisons and calculations for several similar cases, which has allowed him to establish comparative averages. As one of the first of its type, this study is original. The numerous footprint traces taken over the course of the study, and shown in a summary table, make it possible to visually understand the various types of gait described by the author."*

Peer Analysis

Gilles de la Tourette must have been pleased to see that an analysis of his thesis, written by the alienist Jules Séglas (1856–1939), deputy physician to Jules Falret, head of a division for the insane at La Salpêtrière, was published in *Le Progrès Médical* on June 12, 1886.[25] While it is surprising that an alienist took an interest in a thesis far from his area of specialization, Séglas had himself defended his thesis before Charcot in 1880.[26] Séglas wrote regularly for *Le Progrès Médical* from 1885 to 1930, touching on all medical fields, and he seemed to have been assigned many of the reports on publications in Italian. It was in *Le Progrès Médical* that he first wrote on the *"delusion of negation,"* his precise description ensuring him the posthumous fame that continues to this day.[27] It is highly possible that Gilles de la Tourette and Séglas met at La Salpêtrière, and Séglas may have seen him recording patients' footsteps. He speaks highly of the study: *"The results Mr. Gilles de la Tourette obtained are the fruit of prolonged research over nearly two years on numerous healthy and affected individuals. These results are thus highly valuable. Several figures add to the clarity and relevance of this work. What makes these figures all the more interesting is that they are not simple diagrams, but actual photographic reductions of the footprint traces the author obtained, measuring seven to eight meters in length. . . . Mr. Gilles de la Tourette has not limited himself to the simple observation of facts; he also provides anatomical as well as physiological explanations. . . . Needless to say, his work is one of the most important documents available today on the controversial question of gait characteristics in healthy and affected individuals."*[28]

While Simon Duplay (1836–1924) mentioned this thesis in a few purely descriptive lines, without commentary, in *Les Archives Générales de Médecine*,[29] Gilles de la Tourette's friend Paul Le Gendre (1854–1936) wrote a detailed, point-by-point analysis. He concluded with this favorable remark: *"The intelligence of the text on this rather arid subject is greatly enhanced by the many graphics. Gilles de la Tourette has neglected nothing to make his work as complete as possible. Hence this new publication by our colleague, who has already distinguished himself through his successes in a wide range of genres, will undoubtedly open the way for him to the Société de Biologie. We cordially congratulate him."*[30] Le Gendre's prediction turned out to be false. Despite several attempts from 1886 to 1892, Gilles de la Tourette was never admitted to the Société de Biologie.

Commercial Version

Doctoral theses in medicine were printed at the expense of the applicants and were often costly. The luckiest applicants, whose work won recognition, as in Gilles de la Tourette's case with the Prix Godart, could then hope that a Paris publisher like J.-B. Baillière, Félix Alcan, or Gustave Steinheil would put out a commercial version of their work to be sold in bookstores. This was the case for Gilles de la Tourette; the commercial version of his thesis indicates the publisher as: *"Paris, Aux Bureaux du Progrès (14 rue des Carmes) et A. Delahaye et Lecrosnier (Place de l'Ecole de Médecine)."* Because of a quarto sheet (30 × 49 cm) at the end of the volume showing reproductions of the walking anomalies described in each chapter, the publication costs were probably high and required the support of a publisher.

Gilles de la Tourette never returned to gait dysfunction during his career, nor did he pursue the research undertaken for his thesis. There are no citations of his study in the most well-known treatises of nervous system diseases published over the subsequent thirty years, notably those of Grasset and Rauzier (1894)[31] and Pierre Marie (1911),[32] and also Dejerine's monumental *Sémiologie des affections du système nerveux* (1914).[33] Octave Crouzon (1874–1938) cited a number of names in his excellent chapter on motility in *La Pratique Médico-Chirugicale* of Brissaud, Pinard, and Reclus (1907) but omitted Gilles de la Tourette.[34] Only Paul Blocq (1860–1896) mentioned the results obtained by Gilles de la Tourette in the initial part of his 1892 book on gait dysfunction in nervous system disorders,[35] in which he indicated all of the exploration techniques used up to that point. Blocq was Charcot's *interne* in 1887 and remains known for his seminal publication on psychogenic astasia-abasia in 1888.[36]

Nevertheless, the subject of Gilles de la Tourette's thesis, proposed by Charcot, is still of interest today. Sophisticated instrumentation based on modern technology is now used for recording step prints in both rheumatology and neurology.[37] The pathophysiology of gait dysfunction and its exploration in neurology remain the focus of numerous publications.[38,39] "Posturology" has become a "super-specialty" that is covered in journals on functional rehabilitation, among others. The titles of scientific journals published over the past two decades or more recently are a clear indication that the relevant techniques have moved far beyond those of Gilles de la Tourette's day. While not the case for *Human Movement Science*, there are journals named for recording technologies, such as *Sensors* or *IEEE Transactions on Neural Systems and Rehabilitation Engineering*, as well as *Frontiers in Computational Neuroscience*.

Brief biographies of Gilles de la Tourette regularly appear in neurological journals, but rarely do they mention his thesis.[40,41]

Notes

1. Dejerine A. Discours au nom des anciens élèves de Vulpian. In *Centenaire de la naissance de Vulpian (1826–1887)*. Paris: Masson. 1927:30–40.
2. Rapport fait au nom de la commission instituée par La Société de Biologie pour examiner les Mémoires présentés pour le Prix Godard de 1886. *Comptes rendus hebdomadaires des Séances et Mémoires de La Société de Biologie*. 1887;39(1):1–6.
3. Letulle M. Madame Dejerine 1859-1927. *La Presse Médicale*. 1927;35(96):1468.
4. Thomas A. Augusta Klumpke-Dejerine (1859–1927). In *Madame Dejerine 1859–1927*. Paris: Masson. 1929.
5. Gilles de la Tourette G. *Etudes cliniques et physiologiques sur la marche, la marche dans les maladies du système nerveux étudiée par la méthode des empreintes*. Thèse no. 84. Paris: Imprimerie de la Société de typographie. 1885.
6. Gilles de la Tourette G, Londe A. La marche dans les maladies du système nerveux étudiée par la méthode des empreintes. *Comptes Rendus hebdomadaires des Séances et Mémoires de la Société de Biologie*. 1885;37(35):606–609.
7. Weber W, Weber E. *Die Mechanik der menschlichen Gehwerkzeuge. Eine anatomisch-physiologische Untersuchung*. Göttingen in der Dietrichschen Buchandlung. 1836.
8. Duchenne GB. *Du Second temps de la marche, suivi de quelques déductions pratiques, mémoire présenté à l'Académie des Sciences. Extrait de l'Union médicale. 13 et 15 septembre 1855*. Paris: F. Malteste, 1855.
9. Duchenne GB. *Physiologie des mouvements démontrée à l'aide de l'expérimentation électrique et de l'observation clinique, et applicable à l'étude des paralysies et des déformations*. Paris: JB. Baillière. 1867.

10. Lasègue Ch, Straus I. Duchenne (de Boulogne) sa vie scientifique et ses œuvres. *Archives Générales de Médecine.* 1875;52(26 série 6):687–715.

11. Carlet G. *Essai expérimental sur la locomotion humaine. Etude de la marche.* Paris: E. Martinet. 1872.

12. Marey EJ. *La machine animale, locomotion terrestre et aérienne.* Paris: Germer Baillière. 1873.

13. Vierordt H. Das *Gehen des Menschen in gesunden und kranken Zuständen: nach selbstregistrirenden Methoden.* Tübingen: Laupp. 1881.

14. Le Dœuff-Calin S. *Les techniques d'analyse de la marche des origines à 1950.* Thèse Nancy 1, NAN11149. 1999.

15. Muybridge E. "The Horse in Motion 'Sallie Gardner,'" (Leland Stanford ©) running at a 1:40 gait over the Palo Alto track, June 19, 1878. See the film: http://en.wikipedia.org/wiki/Eadweard_Muybridge

16. Dercum FX. The walk and some of its phases in diseases, together with other studies based on the Muybridge investigation. *The Transactions of the College of Physicians. Philadelphia.* 1888;3(10):308–338.

17. Lanska DJ. The Dercum-Muybridge collaboration and the study of pathologic gaits using sequential photography. *J Hist Neurosci.* 2016;25(1):23–38.

18. Muybridge E. *Attitudes of Animals in Motion: A Series of Photographs Illustrating the Consecutive Positions Assumed by Animals Performing Various Movements Executed at Palo Alto, California in 1878 and 1879.* San Francisco. 1881.

19. Muybridge E. *Animal Locomotion: An Electrophotographic Investigation of Consecutive Phases of Animal Movement.* Philadelphia: University of Pennsylvania. 1887.

20. Medved V. *Measurement of Human Locomotion.* Boca Raton, FL: CRC Press. 2000.

21. Iron(III) oxide or Fe_2O_3 or red iron oxide.

22. Rohmer J. *Les variations de forme normales et pathologiques de la plante du pied étudiées par la méthode graphique.* Thèse no. 101. Nancy: Imprimerie N. Collin. 1879.

23. Neugebauer FL. *Zur Entwickelungsgeschichte des spondylolisthetischen Beckens und seiner Diagnose: mit Berücksichtigung von Körperhaltung und Gangspur, casuistisch-kritische Monographie.* Halle: Niemeyer. 1882.

24. At the time, this referred to both the sequela of poliomyelitis and Little's syndrome.

25. Haustgen T, Bourgeois ML. Le dr Jules Séglas (1856–1939), président de la Société Médico-Psychologique, sa vie et son œuvre. *Annales Médico-psychologiques.* 2002;160:701–712.

26. Séglas J. *De l'influence des maladies intercurrentes sur la marche de l'épilepsie.* Thèse no. 17. Paris: Goupy et Jourdan. 1881.

27. Séglas J. Mélancolie anxieuse avec délire des négations. *Le Progrès Médical.* 1887;15(46):417–419.

28. Séglas J. Etudes cliniques et physiologique sur la marche. La marche dans les maladies du système nerveux, par Gilles de la Tourette. *Le Progrès Médical.* 1886;14-1(24):505–506.

29. Duplay S. Index Bibliographique: Etudes Cliniques et Physiologiques sur la marche par le Dr Gilles de la Tourette. *Archives Générales de Médecine.* 1886;18.7ᵉ série(2):512.

30. Le Gendre P. Bibliothèque: Etudes Cliniques et Physiologiques sur la marche par le Dr Gilles de la Tourette. *L'Union Médicale.* 1886;42-3ᵉ série:510–513.

31. Grasset J, Rauzier G. *Traité pratique des maladies du système nerveux.* Montpellier: Camille Coulet and Paris: G. Masson. 1894.

32. Marie P. *La pratique neurologique.* Paris: Masson. 1911.

33. Dejerine J. *Sémiologie des affections du système nerveux.* Paris: Masson. 1914.

34. Crouzon O. Motilité In Brissaud E, Pinard A, Reclus P. *Pratique Médico-Chirurgicale.* Paris: Masson. 1907.

35. Blocq P. *Les Troubles de la Marche dans les Maladies du Système Nerveux. Bibliothèque Charcot-Debove.* Paris: Rueff et Cie. 1892.

36. Blocq P. Sur une affection caractérisée par de l'astasie et de l'abasie. *Arch Neurol (Paris)*. 1888;15:24–51,187–211.
37. Falconer J, Hayes KW. A simple method to measure gait for use in arthritis clinical research. *Arthritis Care Res*. 1991;4(1):52–57.
38. Nolan KJ, Yarossi M, Ramanujam A. Measuring ambulation in adults with central neurologic disorders. *Phys Med Rehabil Clin N Am*. 2013;24(2):247–263.
39. Vachranukunkiet T, Esquenazi A. Pathophysiology of gait disturbance in neurologic disorders and clinical presentations. *Phys Med Rehabil Clin N Am*. 2013;24(2):233–246.
40. André JM, Paysant J, Martinet N, Beis JM, Beyaert C. Georges Gilles de la Tourette, initiateur de l'enregistrement de la marche dans les maladies du système nerveux. *Revue Neurologique (Paris)*. 2001;157(3):293–296.
41. Acharya HJ, Camicioli R. The forgotten thesis of Gilles de la Tourette. *University of Alberta Health Science*. 2005;2(2):32–33.

~ 9 ~

Gilles de la Tourette Syndrome

Phenomenology

Gilles de la Tourette syndrome currently refers to an association of motor and phonic tics with variable but frequent psychiatric comorbidity. Prevalence in children is estimated at 0.3–0.9%.[1] In addition to their well-characterized phenomenology, tics display a peculiar variability over time, which is strongly influenced by a variety of contextual factors. Motor tics may be simple (eye blinking, eye movements, grimacing, sniffing, lip movements, head nodding, head flicks, shoulder shrugs, rapid arm or leg movements, sniffing, or throat clearing) or complex (touching or handling an object, squatting-rising, jumping, bending or twisting the torso or limbs, abdominal muscle tensing, complex head movements, or pronouncing syllables, words, or phrases) with the appearance of orchestrated sequences lacking a specific purpose or appearing out of context. The tics usually start in the face—eye blinking is the most frequent form—before generalizing to the entire body after several months of progression. Simple vocalizations may accompany sniffing and throat clearing. Complex phonic tics include barking and various animal noises but can also involve clearly articulated chains of words.[2] Other signs may be present but not invariably: echolalia (repeating words pronounced by others) and palilalia (repeating one's own utterances), echopraxia (reproducing the movements of others), coprolalia (pronouncing scatological expressions involuntarily or the uncontrollable expression of socially unacceptable words), which the patient often masks by deforming or shortening the words or by coughing, and copropraxia (uncontrollable gestures often involving vulgar, sexually obscene touching).

Suppressibility by volitional control, for a few minutes and in rare cases a few hours, is one of the cardinal features of tics; however, a rebound of greater intensity may follow this period. The premonitory urges, which correspond to unpleasant somatic sensations typically building up immediately beforehand, can be momentarily relieved by tics. Thus, tics may be differentiated from other nonvoluntary movements (e.g., chorea, dystonia, dyskinesias, and myoclonus) based on their association with preceding sensory phenomena and by their partial voluntary suppressibility.

Tic characteristics and frequency fluctuate over time. Successive periods of waxing and waning symptoms mark the first twenty years of life.[3] An improvement is observed at the end of the second decade for most patients, but symptoms may persist into adulthood in around one-third of them.[4] Changes in frequency and intensity of tics may also depend on environmental context. Exposure to strong emotions (positive as well as negative) may worsen tic severity in the short term. On the other hand, tics may improve when subjects are engaged in activities requiring high levels of attention (e.g., sustained intellectual concentration or when patients play music, drive a vehicle, or practice a sport), general physical exercise, or relaxation.

Comorbid psychopathological conditions are frequent (about 90% of cases)[5] including attention-deficit hyperactivity disorder, obsessive-compulsive disorder, and self-injury disorder, along with affective disorders involving anxiety and depression or dysphoria. The presence of comorbid attention-deficit hyperactivity disorder is the main determinant of cognitive dysfunction in patients and heavily influences the risk of developing disruptive behaviors. There is no increased risk of developing dementia with age.

Functional Neuroanatomy and Pathophysiology

The therapeutic success of haloperidol in the treatment of Tourette syndrome put an end to the discussion about a "hysteric" or "neurotic" origin of the disease. The cortico-striato-thalamo-cortical circuit has been identified as an underlying neurobiological correlate. Nevertheless, the cause of Gilles de la Tourette syndrome remains unknown.[6] While family studies have clearly indicated a major genetic component, the search for genes is complicated by the likely involvement of a multitude of genetic variants, both common and rare,[7,8] interaction with environmental factors (among the latter, repeated infections with group A beta-hemolytic streptococcus and psychosocial stressors encountered during development), and a genetically heterogeneous background across involved families.[9] In addition to immune dysfunction,[10] neuroendocrine mechanisms mainly involving sex (testosterone) and stress steroid hormones participate in the pathophysiology of Gilles de la Tourette syndrome, with a severity peak in the period around puberty and a male to female gender distribution of 3:4 to 1.[11] There is evidence of dysfunction in the dopaminergic, serotoninergic, and gamma aminobutyric acid (GABA)ergic systems present in the neural networks of the motor, associative, and limbic territories of the basal ganglia (depending on the symptomatology) and in the neural networks of the frontal and prefrontal cortex. These dysfunctions may be linked to an abnormal migration of GABAergic and cholinergic interneurons during development.[12]

Although tics can often be managed by psychoeducation, a more proactive approach is often required depending on the psychosocial and functional handicap induced. First-line treatment includes cognitive-behavioral therapy, oral pharmacotherapy, and botulinum toxin injections. In case of refractory, severe, or injurious tics, deep brain stimulation represents an emerging option.

A conceptual redefinition is evident in the *Diagnostic and Statistical Manual of Mental Disorders* (DSM-5), which classifies Gilles de la Tourette syndrome along neurodevelopmental rather than neuropsychiatric disorders.[13] This in turn gives some indication of the ground covered since 1885.

Clinical Description by Gilles de la Tourette in 1899

The description by Gilles de la Tourette during a lesson in 1899[14] is *"not given very much consideration in the current literature,"* but *"should be re-examined, in its original version, since all of the characteristics of the disease are set forth in a masterful way."*[15]

> Around the age of 7 or 8, often a little earlier, and sometimes later, a child, boy or girl—both sexes appear to be equally susceptible—whose nervous heredity is nearly always complex, presents involuntary muscular jerking, or tics, which are quickly noticed by his or her parents, but in most cases, they see no reason for serious alarm. The jerking is almost always limited, at least in the beginning; it mostly concerns the muscles of the face and involves eye blinking, mouth twisting, and sudden, rapid movements of the lips. During this period, there are sometimes also expiratory laryngeal noises that may later take on particular characteristics.

The jerking may, for some time, remain localized in the muscles of the face, but under the influence of causes which are difficult to precisely determine, as are those accounting for the first tics, the movements generalize, for example to the muscles of the shoulders and upper limbs. The child lifts alternately one then the other shoulder, leans the trunk right or left, as a single unit, moving arms or hands. As the motions become more complex and involve more parts of the body, the child bends forward or back, jumps in place, striking with the foot, bending alternately one then the other knee. . . .

The tics are limited and/or infrequent in benign cases and at the beginning of the condition, and occur at intervals of varying length, while ceasing during sleep; however, they always intensify during waking hours, under the influence of moral emotions. The patients, who are always highly impressionable, feel very strongly those emotions caused by pleasure or pain; at such moments, excitation and spasmodic movements increase in intensity and frequency; their amplitude is exaggerated, and they may generalize.

It is then that the relative calm, interrupted by only the small jerks in the face or limbs that I have described, may give way to fits of muscular agitation, paroxysms during which the subjects, under the influence of the spasms that torment them, have difficulty eating and going about their usual occupations. These fits are variable in length; however, some persist over weeks and months, with slight intervening lulls. They include a period of augmentation, decline, and stability and may thus be considered true paroxysms. But I would like to underscore the importance of the fact that at the height of the fit, unless it is exceptionally intense, the patients can, in response to an order, under the influence of will, reduce their agitation, abruptly stop their movements; this is only observed in the convulsive tic disease, at least as compared with Sydenham's chorea. In fact, this cessation lasts only an instant, is only momentary; the movements restart with as much intensity after the mental constraint self-imposed by the subjects, but this cessation is real and its observance is, I repeat, very important from a diagnostic point of view. . . .

When the fit is declining, the movements decrease in frequency, amplitude, and intensity, becoming more localized. . . . But while it seems that the patient has completely calmed down, there are still movements, jerking, particularly in the muscles of the face, indicating that the condition is dormant and only suspended. . . .

Many ticcers, co-incidentally most often those with a jerking in the trunk or limbs, make a rapid, expiratory noise: inarticulate hem's, oh's, and ah's. It may be that only such sounds are involved, but sometimes, especially as the subject advances in age, generally a few months or years after the beginning of jerks in the face or limbs, this inarticulate noise may take on a special form and become, as a result, pathognomonic to some extent. . . .

Under the influence of causes impossible to judge in most cases, the ticcer is one day heard to utter aloud and always briefly, a word, a short phrase belonging to language that can truly be qualified as filthy. In addition to coprolalia, there is another psychic stigma that is observed, but less frequently in ticcers: I have called it echolalia.

What Is a Tic?

But what is the origin of the word "tic," with its onomatopoeic click? The term comes from veterinary medicine. According to the lexicographer Emile Littré (1801–1881), *"in horses, a tic consists in a sudden contraction of the muscles of the neck and the walls of the barrel, accompanied by a particular noise, a sort of eructation to remove gas from the stomach."* The word *"tique"* was used for the first time in French by a physician, Jean Jourdin, in his 1647 book on horse diseases and remedies, *La Vraye cognoissance du cheval, ses maladies et remèdes* [16]: *"A tique, according to Ferrare, results from retractions of the nerves originating in the brain and is caused by excessive heat or cold, or by an immoderate flow of blood. The signs of this disturbance occur when the horse twists its head and its ears stand up, when its eyes roll and its mouth locks and its tail extends and its flanks are sunken, and when it presses its teeth into the feeding trough and damages the trough by arching its neck. . . ."* When a horse experiences discomfort, it may pull on its halter by arching its neck abruptly. In French, this is referred to as a *"tire-sec,"* a sharp pulling movement. Jourdin's reference to Giovanni Battista Ferraro (1528–1569) is most certainly an error because this author had described a spasm in a horse with tetanus,[17] said to be suffering from a *"tiro mortale."*[18] However, the origin of the word "tic" does appear to be Italian: *"tiro-secco,"* similar to the French *"tire-sec,"* became *"ticchio"* (caprice) by abbreviation; the French became *"tique,"* *"ticq,"* and finally *"tic."* The word is apt insofar as what defines the motor and phonic tics of Gilles de la Tourette syndrome—namely, the association of abrupt muscular movements accompanied by a noise—is similar to a horse's sudden movements and eructated sounds. As Edouard Brissaud (1852–1909) wrote: *"Here Greek and Latin are wrong. The acceptation of the word 'tic' is so precise that it would be difficult to imagine an idea better suited to a name, or a name better suited to an idea. It seems to carry within itself a specific definition, since it is used in all languages. . . . Coordinated movements, unjustified, and all the more untimely in that they repeat, could not really be regarded as simple morbid reflexes, as spasms. Rather, they are tics.*"[19]

Tics in Historical Medical Books

The first description of tics in a medical book probably dates from 1741. In his work on the prevention of skeletal deformities, or orthopedics,[20] a word he coined, Nicolas Andry de Boisregard (1658–1742), who worked on Diderot's *Encyclopédie*, explained how bad *"habits"* form and gave this advice: *"A child upon waking must never be exposed suddenly to broad daylight, which causes violent eye blinking; and if one cannot be bothered to accommodate the child in this way, his eye blinking, repeated over and over every day, becomes a habit, and the child then blinks throughout his life, as if a grain of sand or wisp of hay were stuck in his eye, which is very deformed.*"[21]

François Boissier Sauvages de Lacroix (1706–1767), a famous physician in Montpellier and author of the first medical nosography, which he wrote in 1763 in Latin, described what were *"spasms for the Greeks"* and *"convulsions for the Romans"* or *"better yet cacokinesis, depraved movements of the muscles for local movement. These movements affect only the upper & lower limbs, the head, the eyes, the tongue, and the jaw.*"[22] The sonorous word "cacokinesis," from the Greek *"kakos"* meaning bad and *"kinesis"* meaning movement, must have included different types of convulsions, notably those characteristic of Jacksonian epilepsy and dystonia. Tics appear in his classification among partial tonic spasms, along with strabismus, torticollis, contractions, cramps and priapism, tetanus, and other abnormal movements. Is a ticcer afflicted with *"depraved movements"*?[23]

In the famous Panckoucke dictionary published in 1821, the tic is first distinguished from trismus, a symptom of tetanus, and then is defined as follows: *"The name 'tic' is given to a neuralgia, either of the face, in general, or of certain parts of the face. Since this disease is often accompanied by intense pain, it is known especially as 'tic douloureux.' More often, the name 'tic' is applied to un- natural habits in the movement of body parts, strange attitudes, singular gestures, a vicious manner of speaking, etc., etc., whose rectification often requires a great deal of treatment as well as perseverance, which may not always suffice in obtaining a cure."* Armand Trousseau (1801–1867) gave the name of "epileptoid neuralgia" to trigeminal neuralgia, a condition also known as *tic douloureux*. *"In the tic, it is the muscular force (of Blumenbach)*[24,25] *or irritability (of Haller)*[26,27] *of the cor- responding organs that is exaggerated and pain is not present. Otherwise, it is the nervous power, or the organs of sensitivity, that are specially affected, in which case the pain is more or less considerable. In the same way that Galen recognized, correctly, a paralysis of movement and paralysis of sensitivity, we are authorized to recognize an exaggeration of the one and the other, and from there, the well-established distinction between the non-painful tic and the painful tic.* "[28] Classically attributed to John Fothergill (1712–1780) in 1773,[29] the description of trigeminal neuralgia[30] had already been proposed in 1671 by Johannes Laurentius Bausch (1605–1665)[31] in Germany and in 1756 by Nicolas André (1704–1780) in France.[32]

To gauge the state of knowledge on tics prior to the work of Gilles de la Tourette and Jean-Martin Charcot (1825–1893), the 1883 "tic" entry of Maurice Letulle (1853–1929) in the Jaccoud *Dictionnaire de Médecine*[33] is a useful source. It distinguished between convulsive tics, which we continue to consider tics, and coordinated tics, which encompassed banal movements automatically and subconsciously repeated (smoothing one's hair, licking one's lips, and so forth) and probably included dystonias. The entry stated that the pathophysiology of tics was completely unknown but noted with certainty the contagious nature of tics, along with the role of imitation and "bad habits" in their triggering.[34] A more recent review was proposed by Shapiro in 1982.[35]

Gilles de la Tourette's Interest in Movement Disorders and Chorea

Gilles de la Tourette spent his third year of *internat* in Charcot's department in 1884. He was twenty-seven years old. His biography of Théophraste Renaudot, written in 1883, was published at the beginning of 1884. Starting in mid-May of that year, he attended meetings of the Société de Biologie every week and of the Société de Thérapeutique every two weeks, and he wrote meeting reports that were published in *Le Progrès Médical*. As advised by his "eminent Professor Charcot," Gilles de la Tourette started to collect records on the gait of patients in the department, which would be the subject of his thesis. Prodigiously active, not only did he manage to meet all of these obligations successfully; at Charcot's request, he also delved into the clinical aspects of the pathology described in the article of George M. Beard (1839–1883), "Experiments with the 'Jumpers' of Maine," which Gilles de la Tourette had translated while still a medical student in 1881. Was this a form of chorea? At that time, chorea designated all conditions involving continual, irregular, or involuntary movements. The chorea identified by Thomas Sydenham (1624–1689) was well isolated, and its link with acute rheumatic fever and rheumatic heart had been established since the work of Jacques Pierre Botrel (1819–?)[36] and Germain Sée (1818–1896)[37] in 1850, and Henri Roger (1809–1891)[38] in 1868, and was confirmed in 1889 by William Osler (1849–1919).[39] In an exchange with Alix Joffroy (1844–1908) at a meeting of the Société de Neurologie on June 7, 1900, Gilles de la Tourette was still contesting the pathogenic link between these two conditions.[40]

Hereditary chorea (often called chronic chorea at the end of the nineteenth century) was recognized by George Huntington (1850–1916) in 1872[41] and its clinical picture was addressed in detail in various theses, such as that of Milan-Vladimir Vassitch (1856–?) in 1883.[42] But, in reality, for most physicians at the time, all abrupt, isolated, or repeated movements, whether psychological or organic in origin, were referred to as "chorea,"[43] to which was sometimes added an adjective, as in chorea lasciva, chorea imaginativa, malleatory chorea, chorea festinans, procursive chorea, dancing chorea, or saltatory chorea. The thesis of Manuel Leven (1831–1912) provides the phenomenological description of these various forms.[44] Charcot's Tuesday Lesson on January 17, 1888, included this caricature: *"How did Dr. de Granville call your disease? The patient: Chorea. Charcot: This word 'chorea' really seems to resolve the entire question. I ask you how the condition before you resembles chorea. To make it fit into the category of chorea, it would be necessary, alongside the already existing Sydenham's chorea and rhythmical chorea, to create a ticcing chorea."*[45] Chorea had a millennial history, which may explain the ease with which it was diagnosed. But it had not always been socially benign to exhibit abnormal movements. According to David Roth (1800–1885), Abu Al-Qasim, whose full name was Abu al-Qasim Khalaf ibn al-Abbas Al-Zahrawi, known in the West as Abulcasis, was perhaps the first to describe abnormal movements around 1100.[46] A few centuries later, in a 1566 posthumous publication of Paracelsus (1493–1541), the expression *"chorea sancti Viti ou visita"* was used to describe abnormal movements reported as contagious involuntary dances, suggesting collective hysteria or ergotism.[47] In any case, "chorea" is the Greek word for dance, and Saint Vitus is supposed to cure the sick. The persistence of the condition indicated *"the influence of an evil spirit."* Those afflicted faced the worst forms of torture until they were ready to admit *"their commerce with the devil."* The Belgian physician Jean Wier, or Johann Weyer (1515–1588), was the first to consider the victims as sick and to oppose the use of exorcism: *"He pitted the weapons of reason against the destructive prejudices of his century,"* according to Albert Regnard (1836–1903).[48] It is not surprising that the writings of Jean Wier, saved from oblivion by Alexandre Axenfeld (1825–1876), were published by Désiré-Magloire Bourneville (1840–1909) in his 1885 "Bibliothèque diabolique" collection and were considered *"the most important work of the series"* by Paul Blocq (1860–1896).[49] They denounced the harmful effects of believing in the supernatural and provided historical arguments that Bourneville, Gilles de la Tourette, and

Charcot used in their republican and anticlerical campaign at the end of the nineteenth century.[50]

Leading Up to the Seminal Description

Jumpers of Maine

In 1881, Gilles de la Tourette translated an article by the American alienist, George M. Beard (1839–1883) (Figure 9.1), "Experiments with the 'Jumpers' of Maine," which had been published in 1880 in *The Popular Science Monthly*,[51] a mainstream periodical. Beard's name remains associated with the description of neurasthenia in 1879.[52] In 1878, Beard made a brief presentation during the fourth annual meeting of the American Neurological Association; the corresponding report was twenty-five lines long in the *Journal of Nervous and Mental Disease*.[53] In his presentation, Beard described an exchange with his friend William Augustus Croffut (1835–1915). While travelling through northern

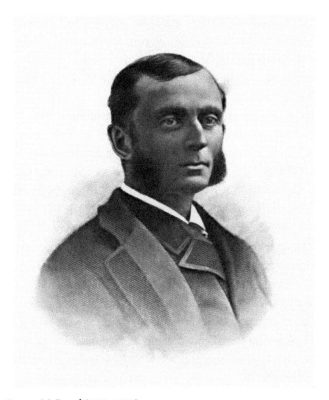

FIGURE 9.1 George M. Beard (1839–1883).
Public domain.

Maine, Croffut observed lumberjacks who, when taken by surprise, began to jump around excessively, hence the name of "Jumpers." *"It is a psychological and not a pathological state. It is not a nervous disease. It is the result of a psychical condition among a people of a low order of intellectual development."* As they jumped, they hit themselves or their entourage violently. They seemed incapable of refraining from this type of sudden, vehement reaction. Since many subjects reacted in this way in this region, Beard viewed the phenomenon as a surviving example of *"an epidemic of habits"* from the Middle Ages. Gilles de la Tourette never mentioned this 1878 presentation and its summary report, also published in London.[54]

Beard fleshed out his description, which he hoped to make scientific,[55] after going himself in June 1880 to study this population, descended from French émigrés in Québec and employed around Moosehead Lake in northern Maine. Many authors refer to an article published by Beard in *The Journal of Nervous and Mental Disease* when they cite the source used by Gilles de la Tourette. In fact, Gilles de la Tourette himself is the cause of this error. In a note in his seminal 1885 article, he wrote: *"Beard's report was published in* The Journal of Nervous and Mental Disease, *vol. VII, p. 487. We published the translation in No. 5 of vol. II, Les Archives de Neurologie, 1881, p. 146–150."* But as he had indicated in his 1881 translation, the source text appeared in *The Popular Science Monthly.* Some have contended that Gilles de la Tourette did not translate faithfully and that he considerably embellished the material. The reality is that Gilles de la Tourette did in fact translate the first-person text written by Beard in *The Popular Science Monthly,*[56] adding a French literary style, cutting out a few sentences, and omitting several proper names given by Beard. The only one that Gilles de la Tourette included is misspelled: Beard wrote Dr. Edward Steese, which Gilles de la Tourette transcribed as Dr. E. Stewe. The article published in the *Journal of Nervous and Mental Disease* is a third-person account of Beard's findings. It reads like a condensed version of the previously cited article but was published in a prestigious medical journal. Gilles de la Tourette was thus more or less faithful to the original but not to the text commonly attributed to Beard, a text that Beard probably did not write himself, even though it is the most often cited. Do authors actually read it?

Beard described young men who startled in an excessive way at the slightest stimulation but behaved normally and appropriately outside of surprising situations. They would jump and cry out at *"any sound from behind that was sharp and unexpected. . . . These phenomena suggest epilepsy, particularly in their explosive character and in the nature of the cry. The hands strike or throw with a quick, impulsive movement, which is very hard to imitate artificially. They go off like a piece of machinery; it is more like the explosion of a gun than the movement of the limbs of even an angry man; and the cry suggests that which we hear in hysteria and in epilepsy."* Aside from their violently emotional startle reflex, these men were calm and well-balanced; Beard described them as "modest, quiet, retiring." The complete description associated an exaggerated startle reflex in the Jumpers with raised arms, a piercing scream, and violent hitting, most often of themselves, with the hand directed against the head or chest. This movement was then repeated several times. This sequence occurred most often after receiving an order with sudden violence or hearing an unexpected noise. The Jumpers were lumberjacks with little education or capacity to verbalize their emotions. Beard noted similarities with hysteria: the psycho-contagious and familial aspects of the phenomenon. He also suggested a hereditary aspect. Beard did not explicitly highlight the idea of immediate and involuntary imitation, aside from the repetition of the order before its execution. It is very strange that Gilles de la Tourette did not highlight Beard's idea that the symptoms observed were probably hysterical in nature.

Latah of Malaysia

Armand de Breau de Quatrefages (1810–1892) was a physician, zoologist, and anthropologist who frequently visited Charcot at the Académie des Sciences at that time.[57] One day he said to Charcot: *"Look, I have something for you!"* Quatrefages showed Charcot an article, then gave it to Gilles de la Tourette. It was written by an English businessman and traveler, H. A. O'Brien, who described the "Latah" of Malaysia.[58] O'Brien's text was published in 1883, with additions made in 1884, in an obscure journal founded by a group of British colonial administrators.[59] Gilles de la Tourette translated this revised document. In a new article,[60] he introduced extracts from O'Brien's writings and from a very recent publication by William Hammond (1828–1900) (Figure 9.2): *"Today, we have the account of a similar state* [to the Jumpers of Maine] *which exists not in America, but in Asia, specifically Malaysia. The narrator, Mr. O'Brien, is not a physician, just someone acting on curiosity; nevertheless, he gives a good report of what he observed, abstaining from commentary. Instead of the American 'Jumping,' the term used in the Malay language is 'Latah' which may designate either the affected individual or his special state."* Gilles de la Tourette highlighted the similarities between the Jumpers of Maine and the Latah described by O'Brien: *"Persons of a peculiarly nervous organization, ranging from those who, from their mental constitution, seem absolutely subservient to another's will; down to those who appear merely of a markedly excitable temperament."* The word "Latah" can be translated by "ticklish." Upon hearing a loud or unexpected noise, a Latah will startle violently and exclaim in a manner that

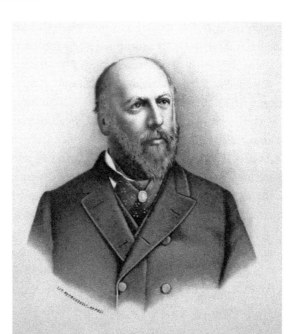

FIGURE 9.2 William Hammond (1828–1900).
Private collection of the author.

O'Brien characterized as always obscene. He or she often exteriorizes a state of panic after a sudden unforeseen stimulation. According to O'Brien, these individuals imitate the words, sounds, or movements of those around them, without being asked, all while enjoying a perfectly regular mental state in the intervals between fits. This propensity for involuntary imitation emerges as the dominant trait in O'Brien's descriptions, unlike the accounts of Beard, who never mentioned imitation. *"I have met a man several times lately who is a very strong* latah *subject. He is cook on board a local steamer, and is naturally (alas, for human nature!) the butt of all of the crew, who daily and almost hourly exercise their clumsy wit . . . at his expense. All of this skylarking, however, had a tragical ending the other day, which illustrates the point of which I am speaking. This cook was dandling his child forward one day; one of the crew came and stood before him with a billet of wood in his arms, which he began nursing in the same way as the* latah *was nursing his baby. Presently he began tossing the billet up to the awning and the cook tossed his child up also, time for time. At last, the sailor opened his hands wide apart and let the wood fall upon the deck, and the cook immediately spread out his hands away from the descending child, who never moved again after striking the boards."* Whereas the Jumping in Maine seemed only to occur in men, O'Brien told of women subjects, and most often older women who suffered from Latah. He wrote that, without any effort on his part, they *"completely abandoned themselves to* [his] *will and powers of direction."*

Miryachit in Siberia

Gilles de la Tourette copied most of the article by William Hammond, with this introduction: *"These singular facts are not limited to America or Malaysia, countries where the climate is warm; they can also be observed in Siberia, as Dr. Hammond relates with examples from the accounts of American officers."* Hammond[61] was at that time a professor of nervous and mental diseases at New York University and is still known for his seminal description of athetosis in 1871.[62] Gilles de la Tourette referred to the text published in Paris in the journal *Union Médical,*[63] entitled "Miryachit, nouvelle maladie du système nerveux." The translator is not named, but apparently translated an Italian version[64] of the original article, which was published in English in the *New York State Journal of Medicine.*[65] Whereas Hammond spelled the name of the condition *"Miryachit,"* Gilles de la Tourette wrote *"Myriachit,"* which means "to act stupidly." The description of the condition is based on an account, published in 1883,[66] of a voyage undertaken in 1882 by three American Navy officers, the lieutenant Benjamin H. Buckingham,[67] the ensign George Clayton Foulk (1856–1893),[68] and Walter McLean (1855–1930).[69] These three officers observed the unusual propensity of certain individuals in the Amur River basin in eastern Siberia to imitate the motor behavior or speech of those around them in an involuntary manner. Hammond seemed unaware that he was not the first to describe the Myriachit. It was, in fact, German physician and botanist Georg Wilhelm Steller (1709–1746),[70] who first wrote of the phenomenon, after observations during a northern expedition from 1729 to 1731. He referred to *"hysteria"* and cited the various appellations used by the peoples of the Russian Far East where these involuntary imitation behaviors were observed: *"amurakh"* (Yakuts), *"olan"* (Tougouses), *"irkunii"* (Yukaghirs/Yukagirs), *"menkeiti"* (Koryaks/Koriaks), and *"imu"* (Ainus/Aynus).[71]

Hammond drew parallels between these accounts and Beard's observations: "From this description it will at once, I think, be perceived that there are striking analogies between 'Miryachit' and this disorder of the 'Jumping-Frenchmen' of Maine. Indeed, it appears to me that if the two affections were carefully studied, it would be found that they were identical, or that, at any rate, the phenomena of the one could readily be developed into those of the other. . . . There is another analogous condition known by the Germans as Schlaftmukenheit [sic]. . . ." For this condition, Hammond gave examples of confusional states occurring when the person was purposely awakened and for which we see no link with the stress-related startle reflex and the imitation behaviors reported earlier. His descriptions suggest a sort of parasomnia categorized as "confusional arousals" of which the subject has no memory; such phenomena are frequent in children but may persist in 1–2% of adults.[72] Hammond concluded: "They all appear to be due to the fact that a motor impulse is excited by perceptions without the necessary concurrence of the volition of the individual to cause the discharge. They are, therefore, analogous to reflex actions and especially to certain epileptic paroxysms due to reflex irritations. It would seem as though the nerve-cells were very much in the condition of a package of dynamite or nitro-glycerine, in which a very slight impression is competent to effect a discharge of nerve-force. They differ, however, from the epileptic paroxysms, in the fact that the discharge is conso-nant with the perception—which is in these cases an irritation—and is hence an apparently logical act; whereas, in epilepsy, the discharge is more violent, is illogical, and does not cease with the cessation of the irritation."

In his article on the three conditions, Gilles de la Tourette continued: *"We will not attempt to interpret this bizarre state: Jumping in Maine, Latah in Malaysia, Myriachit in Siberia, and perhaps Schlaftrunkenheit in Germany. We prefer to make our own contribution to this series of related observations. In the department of our teacher, Professor Charcot, there is currently a case in many ways similar to this singular state. The subject is a 15–year-old boy, intelligent, perfectly capable of rea-soning, of sound constitution, who suffers from extreme hyperexcitability, specific tics, jolting movements of the head and trunk, after which he almost invariably and loudly pronounces the word of Cambronne [shit]. Moreover, if we speak in front of him, he faithfully echoes the last two or three words of the sentence just pronounced. This is a source of observations nearly unexplored and whose interpretation cannot be attempted until a great many facts, carefully studied, without preconceived ideas, have been collected."* Gilles de la Tourette added this note: *"Since the writing of this article, we have had the good fortune to come across another subject; the corresponding observation and three others from Mr. Charcot will be described in a forthcoming text on this matter."*[73]

Beard, O'Brien, and Hammond: Valid Introductory Material?

Gilles de la Tourette's personal behavior, as described by his contemporaries, suggests that he himself may have identified with these hyperreactive individuals who jump at the slightest stimulation. Incidentally, Gilles de la Tourette indicated that he went to London to question two famous English neurologists, Sir William Henry Broadbent (1835–1907) and John Hughlings Jackson (1835–1911), and that he met *"numerous physicians of diverse nationalities"* at the international conference of medical sciences in Copenhagen in 1884. They *"told us they had never observed similar cases, nor read descriptions of this disease."*

Turning to the articles of Beard, O'Brien, and Hammond, was Gilles de la Tourette correct in viewing them as a valid introduction to his own publication? Jumping, in the sense of startling, is a universal, stereotyped, phylogenetically old behavior that can be observed in all vertebrates. It is a reflex response to a sudden, intense, and unexpected stimulation and serves the purpose of protection or preparation for fight or flight.[74] In humans, this natural mechanism can be modified through cultural learning. Anxiety states, withdrawal from alcohol or other legal or illegal psychotropic substances, posttraumatic stress disorder, and certain affective states may increase the startle reflex, but this does not constitute a specific disease. In 1918, the Austrian pediatrician Ernst Moro (1874–1951) described a reflex present in newborns that disappears before the age of four months. Known as the *réflexe de Moro,* the clasping reflex, Moro reflex, or *Umklammerungsreflex,* it entails an extension of the four limbs, followed by their sudden flexion, after a noise, a sensation of falling, or air blown abruptly onto the face or belly.[75] In 1936, Carney Landis (1897–1962) and William Hunt (1902–1981) described the "startle response," which appears in humans as the clasping reflex disappears.[76] These reflexes, said to be archaic, are physiological reactions and resemble, in their manifestation, the response of the Jumpers in America, Asia, and Siberia.[77]

Reuben Rabinovitch (1909–1965), a neurologist in Montréal, wrote a personal and medical account of his childhood in 1965. In it, he described the arrival of lumberjacks in his childhood village in the Laurentides region north of Montréal. These men would go into the forest to cut down trees with thirty or so horses, which would sometimes kick in response to violent yelling. The lumberjacks would overcome their shock by jumping, which became a strange and comic habit. Rabinovitch agreed with physicians in the region accustomed to this behavior that it was a cultural form of hysteria.[78] In 1967, Charles Kunkle examined fifteen Jumpers entirely comparable to those described by Beard. All of them underwent a neurological examination and were found to be normal. His analysis highlighted the closed, masculine communities where they lived and their lack of education. Kunkle's diagnosis was collective neurosis.[79]

In 1986, a team of Montréal neurologists studied eight Jumpers from the Beauce region of Québec who worked in the winter as lumberjacks in the nearby forests of Maine. Although all of them described themselves as shy and ticklish, they felt quite violent by nature. In particular, they would startle when teased by others, and this reflex was always accompanied by aggressive movements directed at the tormentor. Fatigue and anxiety were found to accentuate the symptoms. They lived in groups, isolated in the forest for several months and without other social contacts, in very primitive conditions without individual beds, without changing their clothes or washing. They had little in the way of schooling. The "jumping" had started in adolescence. Several of the Jumpers had ancestors who were recognized Jumpers, but none of their own children was affected. The authors filmed the Jumpers during a "fit," and the very same behavior described by Beard can be observed. No signs of echolalia, echopraxia, or coprolalia were observed. All of them underwent a neurological examination and were found to be normal. Today, the "Jumpers of Maine" seem to have completely disappeared. This is apparently due to the fact that the poor socioeconomic conditions under which the lumberjacks once worked no longer exist. Quebecer neurologists believe that psychological and material poverty, along with a rudimentary lifestyle, explain the phenomenon of jumping and its related manifestations. They consider it a form of conversion hysteria, a form of psycho-cultural conditioning in response to stress (the hysteria of Charcot and Gilles de la Tourette!). No neurological organicity has been found.[80,81] Jumpers have been identified in different regions, in other sociocultural groups of various ethnic origins in the United States that nonetheless have similar lifestyles.[82] The phenomenon has nothing to do with motor tics; rather, it is a psychopathological condition based on cultural factors.[83] In 1980, the American Joseph Hardison recalled that in his youth, the term "goosey"[84] was applied to people who were ultra-sensitive to being tickled or teased. Hardison drew a parallel with the Jumpers of Maine.[85,86] In 1992, a review of the medical literature examined all of the psychiatric pathologies in which excessive startle reactions may occur. The list included schizophrenia, posttraumatic stress disorder, drug withdrawal, and hysteria.[87]

Holman Francis Day (1865–1935), a writer and filmmaker born in Vassalboro, Maine, penned a short story in 1902 fictionalizing the life of the jumping lumberjacks in Maine. Their miserable living conditions were made unrealistically appealing, but their behavior during jumping fits and their violent outbursts, often involving their spouses, were faithfully portrayed.[88]

Differential Diagnosis

There is a rare form of epilepsy characterized by an abnormal startle reflex. Hereditary hyperekplexia or hyperekplexia,[89] Kok disease,[90] familial startle disease, or stiff baby syndrome is characterized by "an exaggerated startle reflex." About one hundred fifty cases have been identified. Hyperekplexia is observed shortly after birth and involves a violent startle reflex in response to noises and contact, then massive and sustained hypertonia in the trunk and limbs (opisthotonos), with intense clenching of the fists followed by fits of high-frequency trembling. Newborns with this condition have an increased risk of sudden death by laryngospasm and blockpnea. The tonic fits are suggestive of convulsive fits, but the hypertonia and the startle reflex disappear during sleep and the electroencephalogram (EEG) readings remain normal. In the months following birth, hypertonia diminishes, but the startle reflex in response to the slightest stimulus persists. The acquisition of motor skills may be delayed, but intellectual development is generally normal.[91] When learning to walk, affected children toddle more markedly than healthy children. These motor difficulties increase during faster walking, in particular if acceleration is suddenly ordered by a parent, and may lead the child to fall like a log.[92] The cause of the condition may lie in an archaic center in the brainstem linked to the limbic system and may be related to impaired muscle relaxation.[93] Inheritance is autosomal dominant or recessive, and sporadic cases exist. Mutations of the gene GLRA1 (5q32) are found in certain cases but not all. This gene encodes *"the alpha1 subunit of the juvenile neuronal receptor for the inhibitory neurotransmitter, glycine. Mutations of this subunit cause a variety of dysfunctions of the neuronal chloride (Cl⁻) channel, and therefore hereditary hyperekplexia is regarded as a channelopathy."*[94,95] The mutated chlorine channel may disturb intracellular functioning of the Golgi apparatus, slowing cellular relaxation following myocyte contraction. Mutations in genes GLRB, GPHN, and SLC6A5 (4q31.3, 14q24, and 11p15.2–p15.1) have also been reported. The diagnostics are clinical, electrophysiological, and molecular.[96] The risk of developing type 1 diabetes is significantly higher in these patients.[97] It is very unlikely that the Jumpers of Maine had this complex genetic disease.

Startle epilepsy was described by Théophile Alajouanine (1890–1980) and Henri Gastaut (1915–1995) in 1955.[98] It occurs in children with brain damage in the motor cortex, most often subsequent to neonatal anoxia, and the corresponding symptomatology is stereotyped. The motor seizures with tonic features often affect only half of the body, on the side opposite the lesion. They take place immediately after the startle reflex, which is triggered by a sudden, unexpected, but slight stimulus, such as a simple touch of the skin.[99] The seizures are often pharmacoresistant and may require neurosurgical treatment.[100] This pathology certainly does not apply to the Jumpers in America, Asia, or Siberia.

Historical and Current Interpretations of Jumping, Latah, and Myriachit

The word "Latah" seems to have appeared for the first time in Malay literature in the fifteenth century, as a metaphorical form interpreted as either "love sickness" or "tickle."[101] Many cultures share the idea of a startle, and the language for it expresses the agreeable-disagreeable ambivalence of games and contact, the first steps toward the physical closeness of lovers: *Imu* in Japan, *Ikota* in Siberia, *Mali-mali* in the Philippines, *Yaun* in Vietnam, *Orgamci* or *Belenci* in Mongolia, and so forth.[102] [103] Knowledge of Latah by Europeans dates from the middle of the nineteenth century and is based on the accounts of John Turnbull Thomson (1821–1884), an English engineer involved in infrastructure projects in Malaysia,[104] and of Frederik Johannes van Leent (1829–1895), a physician and head of the Navy medical department in the Dutch East Indies, one of the first to attribute beriberi to a nutritional deficiency.[105,106] A more precise description was written in 1885 by Henry Ogg Forbes (1851–1932), a Scottish ornithologist and explorer who observed "that curious affection called by the natives 'Latah.'" His servant would jump like a jack-in-the-box upon seeing a caterpillar. Terrorized, cursing loudly, he would go into a "trance." Forbes attributed the nervousness of the inhabitants to the climate in order to explain his observations.[107] At the end of the nineteenth century, there were many medical descriptions, such as that of John Desmond Gimlette (1867–1934), who highlighted a mix of superstition and religious fervor. He saw Latah as a manifestation of hysteria expressed with local cultural acquired acceptance: *"In both cases, self-control being lost for the time being, the attention is occupied mainly by a single idea, in the 'Latah' woman by an uncontrollable desire to imitate, in which the servile portion of human nature is unconsciously displayed; in the amok man, by a reckless idea to persist in killing, in which the wild beast part of a man becomes uppermost."*[108] In the twentieth century, authors underlined colonialism's role in inciting this behavioral reaction.[109] Robert L. Winzeler, of the University of Nevada in Reno, published in 1995 a complete ethnographical and medical study on Latah, which stands as the reference work on this subject.[110]

Ardalion Ardalionowicz Tokarski (Ардалион Ардалионович Токарский, 1859–1901), after having observed numerous cases of *"meriatschenje"* in Siberia, published two observations of pathological imitation behavior in 1890.[111] In addition to his own observations, he included that of Dr. Kaschin, a Russian physician who, in 1868, around Lake Baikal, was confronted with a military corps that simultaneously repeated all of the orders received, illustrating behavioral contagion.[112] For Tokarski, Myriachit had nothing in common with the echolalia and echopraxia of what came to be known as Gilles de la Tourette syndrome. Nikolai Nikolaevich Bazhenov (often spelled Bagenoff), chief physician at the Preobrazhenskaya psychiatric hospital in Moscow, submitted a review to *Les Archives de Neurologie* in 1911 entitled *Myriatchenié et Klikouschisme,*[113] which the authors qualified as psychoneuroses the conditions described by Kaschin and Tokarski. The *"Klikouschis,"* meaning those who cry out—because they are *"possessed by the demon"* or *"have been cursed"*— exhibited attacks of *grande hystérie* (hysteria major) as described by Charcot, which Bazhenov likened to the epidemics of demonopathic *convulsionnaires,* exemplified by the Ursulines of Loudun.

Following the publication of *Jumping, Latah, Myriachit* by Gilles de la Tourette, Jose Armangué y Tuset (1849–1941), a Spanish neuropathologist, published a translated adaptation and added commentary to the effect that similar cases existed in Spain, highlighting the capacity for involuntary automatic imitation in these patients.[114]

An ethological analysis of *Jumping, Latah, Myriachit* describes these involuntary and automatic behaviors as a reaction to a visual, auditory, or tactile stimulus, which can be schematically described as "startle and imitate" with the addition, in some cases but not all, of echopraxia and echolalia. No form of tic can be likened to these startle reflexes.[115] This jumping, or, inversely, a frozen immobility, or behaviors of avoidance or aggression, are an immediate and single reaction to a stimulus, whereas tics occur without an exterior triggering factor and are, by definition, repetitive. The activity of mirror neurons, a substrate for imitating behaviors and decoding intentionality[116] that was discovered by Giacomo Rizzolatti's team at the University of Parma, explains this innate and involuntary capacity in Latahs and Myriachits to mime motor action.[117] The imitation behaviors observed in a Latah fit are accompanied by cursing directed at the tormentor. Latah seems to affect shy and introverted people whose cognitive, motor, and social development is nonetheless normal, especially middle-aged women, who reproduce the movements and gestures of their mothers.[118] Latah can thus be likened to hysteria, with specific manifestations that reflect the subjects' culture.[119] Myriachit is similar because of the behavioral imitation, but there is no cursing. It seems currently accepted to view all of these behaviors as psychiatric disturbances where the acceptance and tolerance of the social group in which they occur acts to reinforce them and favor social integration in the group. These historical documents are considered particularly valuable as anthropological studies of psychiatric conditions and of how culture influences their expression.[120,121] In 1965, Harold Stevens noted that, strangely, publications on the Jumpers disappeared after 1912. He raised the issue of translation errors in various articles that could have led Gilles de la Tourette to consider the jumping in Maine, Latah, and Myriachit as the same disease as the one he was trying to isolate, whereas Charcot drew a clear distinction.[122]

In none of the cases do these brief and isolated startle reflexes, secondary to a triggering factor outside the individual, resemble motor and phonic tics. Is the cursing the same thing as coprolalia? It is, indeed, in the medical and anthropological opinion of Ronald C. Simons,[123] whereas Robert E. Bartolomew[124] contests this view. Given the doubts expressed, it is easy to see how Gilles de la Tourette could have made a legitimate error. The imitation behaviors are harder to analyze in the accounts, but there are many situations in normal life where bodily attitudes are imitated, such as a yawn or laughter, without this necessarily constituting the echopraxia and echolalia present in Gilles de la Tourette syndrome.[125]

It is unfortunate that Gilles de la Tourette was not familiar with the remarkable thesis of the alienist Prosper Lucas (1805–1855), defended in 1833, which subtly analyzes all of the phenomena of "contagious imitation" and in which Gilles de la Tourette could have found ideas relevant to the behaviors of the Jumpers, Latahs, and Myriachits: *"Acquired similarities result from the habit of the same acts, the same feelings, the same sensations, the same ideas, in a word from one's upbringing, which over time imprints the entire organism with this character that Lavater called, in the traits and movements, the 'secondary physiognomy.' In these sympathetic propagations of nervous affection, women and those individuals they pass through like an electric shock are almost always not only controlled by the same organic conditions, but also under the yoke of the same opinions, the same superstitions, the same daily impressions, and all of the same life circumstances."*[126] A physician in Lyon, Claude Sigaud (1862–1921), in his thesis entitled *De l'échomatisme*[127] (defended in 1889 and thus subsequent to Gilles de la Tourette's seminal article) gave a psychophysiological explanation of these automatic imitation phenomena, seeing them as a cerebral automatism secondary to *"psychological poverty."*[128] He drew on the work of multiple authors, including Alfred Binet (1857–1911), Pierre Janet (1859–1947), and Théodule Ribot (1839–1916).

Introduction to the Seminal Article

As noted earlier, Gilles de la Tourette had promised at the end of his 1884 article on Jumping, Latah, and Myriachit to provide new observations in a forthcoming publication. The corresponding work was published on January 25, 1885, in the year's first issue of *Les Archives de Neurologie*, a journal founded (1880) and published by Charcot. Gilles de la Tourette had just left his position as Charcot's *interne* and was starting his last year of his *internat* with Paul Brouardel (1837–1906) at Hôpital de la Pitié in Paris. He also continued to prepare his thesis.

The new article's title referred to *"motor incoordination"*: "Étude sur une affection nerveuse caractérisée par de l'incoordination motrice, accompagnée d'écholalie et de coprolalie (Jumping, Latah, Myriachit)." He clearly wanted to highlight his affiliation with the work of Beard, O'Brien, and Hammond and did not use the word "tic."

Gilles de la Tourette's Predecessors

Gilles de la Tourette started the article by mentioning a book written by Etienne-Michel Bouteille (1732–1816) (Figure 9.3) from Manosque (Basse-Alpes region

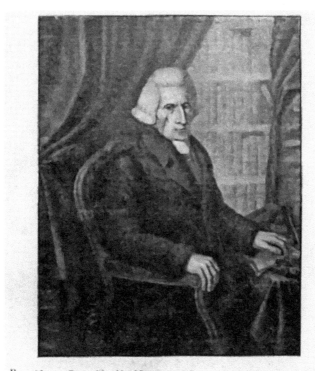

FIG. 10. — Bouteille (de Manosque). Portrait obligeamment communiqué par la famille.

FIGURE 9.3 Etienne-Michel Bouteille (1732–1816).
Private collection of the author.

of France)[129] in 1810, *Traité de la chorée ou Danse de Saint-Guy.*[130] As Gilles de la Tourette pointed out, Bouteille clearly distinguished between Sydenham's chorea and *"pseudo-choreas or false choreas,"* the latter predominated by *"involuntary movements of different body parts and grimace-inducing convulsions of the face."* Gilles de la Tourette noted that *"the disease we are going to study would have fallen into this complexus,"* which is essentially saying that the disease he was going to describe was not a chorea. He went on to indicate that the first description of involuntary movements accompanied by involuntary grunting and cursing was given by Jean-Gaspard Itard (1775–1838)[131] (Figure 9.4), in 1825.[132] Itard described various behavioral problems that today seem to lack any specific link aside from a possible psychic cause. It was his tenth case that interested Gilles de la Tourette, who presented it as the first observation of his article, highlighting it in an exaggerated fashion. Before Gilles de la Tourette, David-Didier Roth (1800–1888),[133] a Hungarian physician and disciple of Samuel-Christian Hahnemann (1755–1843), copied the observation in 1850 as part of various descriptions of abnormal movements that he called

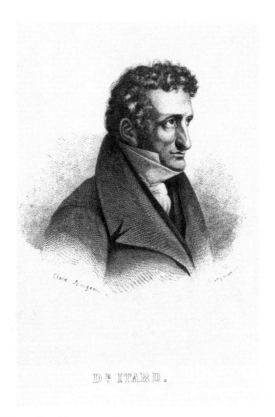

DR ITARD.

FIGURE 9.4 Jean-Gaspard Itard (1755–1838).
Private collection of the author.

"abnormal choreas," also using the word "tic" to talk about them.[134] In 1851, Stanislas Sandras (1802–1856), a physician at Hôpital Hôtel-Dieu in Paris and *agrégé* at the Faculté de Médecine, wrote a book entitled *Traité pratique des Maladies Nerveuses*, one of the first practical treatises on nervous diseases. He also copied Itard's observation, classifying it among the "partial choreas."[135] He then reported on two other clinical cases, also classified as partial chorea, even though no common points are evident. Sandras never used the word "tic," and this chapter of his book only seems relevant for having helped disseminate Itard's work, but with no new information.

Itard's patient was Mme de D (the Marquise de Dampierre, 1799–1884?), who had suffered since the age of seven from movements that *"were involuntary and convulsive, with participation of the shoulder, neck, and face muscles. The result was extraordinary contortions and grimaces. The disease had continued to progress and, the spasm affecting the organs of the voice and speech, this young person would utter bizarre cries and words devoid of meaning, but never in a state of delirium, without any disturbance of the mental faculties."* After a few years of progression, she spent nearly a year in Switzerland for treatment and returned much improved, with only the occasional tic. *"She was then married. But the marriage, rather than consolidating and completing her cure as had been hoped, caused her disease to return quite rapidly. Mme de D . . . did not have any children and was thus deprived of the favorable opportunities of the physical and moral transformation ordinarily produced by motherhood."* Itard was especially struck by the phonic tics: *"Among the continual and chaotic movements resulting from these morbid contractions, those affecting the organs of the voice and speech are the only ones worthy of our attention, as they represent an exceptional phenomenon, and constitute a most disagreeable inconvenience that deprives the patient of all of the joys of society; the disturbance they create is due to the pleasure the subject takes in social interaction. For example, in the middle of a conversation in which the subject is most interested, she suddenly, without being able to restrain herself, interrupts what she is saying or hearing with bizarre cries and words that are even more extraordinary and contrast deplorably with her intellect and her distinguished manners. These words are mostly vulgar curses, obscene epithets, and, what is no less embarrassing for her and others listening, blunt expressions of judgment or unfavorable opinions of those present in society."* Itard concluded with the idea that this pathology could be classified as a chorea: *"Between this neurosis and the one at the center of this dissertation, there is certainly no essential difference justifying a separate category amongst the numerous diseases of the brain."* The observation of the Marquise de Dampierre was reproduced in theses on chorea as the prototype of "partial choreas," for example, in the 1857 thesis of Emile Quantin.[136]

The Marquise de Dampierre: A Mystery

In the second half of the nineteenth century, attending Charcot's Lessons at Hôpital La Salpêtrière in Paris was almost compulsory for ambitious young physicians, whether from Europe or the United States. Back at home, they would translate the lessons they had heard—Charcot was more than happy to provide an introduction—in what resembled a rite of passage for those seeking fame and recognition. The example of Freud is well known. A young Italian, Giulio Melotti (1857–19?),[137] who graduated from the University of Bologna in July 1882, spent two years in Paris, from 1884 to 1886. Melotti transcribed one of Charcot's lessons on tics and on the writings of Beard, O'Brien, and Hammond[138]—*"Lezione quattordicesima"*[139]—published in Milan in 1887. There is no trace of this lesson in the complete works of Charcot, and it is likely that Melotti, rather than translating an actual lesson, combined several lessons into one, introducing information provided directly by Gilles de la Tourette, in order to give his Italian readers a detailed clinical picture of the ticcing disease.[140] Melotti also made an error that highlights the inaccuracy of his account: he wrote that Charcot said he had personally examined the Marquise de Dampierre. In fact, Charcot never treated this woman. Here is what Charcot did say, on Tuesday, December 13, 1887: *"In Parisian high society, there was a person of the most aristocratic circles who was known for uttering filthy words. I did not have the honor of knowing her; I met her one day on my way up the stairs from the Salon and I was surprised to hear her suddenly say 'shit' and 'fucking pig.'"* Gilles de la Tourette himself wrote: *"On several occasions, Professor Charcot saw this patient who, to a late age, continued to suffer from her muscular incoordination and to utter obscene words in spite of herself, even in public places, as Mr. Charcot was able to witness. The political journals announced her death, which occurred in July or August 1884, and some of them treated their readers to a list of the obscene words she used to say, in particular 'shit' and 'fucking pig.'"*

It has been impossible to safely identify who the Marquise de Dampierre really was. Since the thirteenth century, there have been many Dampierre families throughout France, but most of them "died out" in the beginning of the nineteenth century. The only Marquis de Dampierre at the time in Paris were those said to be "of Millancourt," with Elie-Louis Aymar (1787–1845), marquis, baron, Peer of France (~1827) and his wife, Marie-Charlotte d'Abadie de Saint-Germain (1789–1837). Unfortunately, neither this couple nor their close family corresponds with the patient. It is entirely possible that a girl known to be sick or disabled was purposely removed from the official genealogies. Another hypothesis is that Itard's patient was not really the Marquise de Dampierre, but another noblewoman whose name he modified so that she would not be recognized. Finally, Itard may have miscalculated her age. Since neither Charcot nor Gilles de la Tourette examined her, her name, family status, and deduced dates of birth and death may be false. Gilles de la Tourette noted that he had heard of her death without giving any precise data.

A Class of Hysteria?

In his 1859 treatise on hysteria,[141] Pierre Briquet (1796–1881), recalled the observation of a fifteen-year-old girl, which Itard had presented before the observation of the Marquise de Dampierre. Sent away to boarding school, she *"became subject to spasms that only manifested themselves when she heard the school's bell. She would slightly raise her shoulders and let out a sharp little cry. Within a few weeks, this symptom acquired such intensity that the momentary cry had degenerated into a noisy and prolonged clamor, with reverberating yells that, from afar, could have been mistaken for a dog barking. This was provoked not only by the school's bell, but also by the slightest unexpected noise and the slightest sensation of pleasure or pain, if sudden in any way. Her cries, always accompanied by a raising of the shoulders, could last for several hours without stopping, diminishing only for intervals and then bursting forth with added violence a few minutes later, finally ending with a livid tumefaction of the face, abundant transpiration, and a state of profound prostration followed by drowsiness. Irritant foot baths, mucilaginous baths, general bloodletting, application of leeches to the thighs, use of antispasmodics, insistent recommendations, and even threats to induce the patient to exercise a strong willful repression—all of these were tried without success."* Treated with no more success by Antoine Portal (1742–1842), this young patient soon had three imitators among the other boarders who reproduced her behavior and her cries in every detail. Briquet classified these cases among the hysterias with spasms of the airways, completing his demonstration with a few lines concerning the *"vulgar cursing and obscene epithets"* of the Marquise de Dampierre, based on Itard. Strangely, Gilles de la Tourette did not draw inspiration from the work of Briquet, despite the similarity of the observation of this fifteen-year-old girl who seemed to suffer from the disease he was trying to isolate.

Trousseau's Description: Twelve Years Before Gilles de la Tourette

Gilles de la Tourette mentioned very clearly that Trousseau,[142] a renowned professor (Figure 9.5), had described a clinical case while treating *"several types of choreas"* in 1862[143] and had referred specifically to tics: *"Once again, I was recently consulted by a young Englishman sent to me from Dieppe whose tic consisted in convulsive, violent movements of the head and right shoulder. . . .These tics are in*

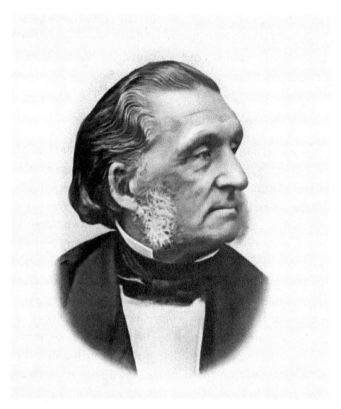

FIGURE 9.5　Armand Trousseau (1801–1867).
Private collection of the author.

some cases accompanied by a cry, the voice bursting forth more or less loudly, which is
characteristic. While on this subject, I shall mention the story that I have recounted
several times, of one of my old classmates, whom I once recognized, after twenty
years of not seeing him, while he was walking behind me, by the bark-like noise that
I had heard him make when we were students together. This cry, this yelp, this burst
of voice, a veritable laryngeal or diaphragmatic chorea, may constitute the entire
tic. In a few cases, it is not only a bursting forth of the voice, a singular cry; it is an
irresistible tendency to always repeat the same word, the same exclamation, and the
individual may even reiterate words aloud that are better to hold back. These tics are
quite often hereditary."

Trousseau precisely described a chronic disease associating multiple motor
tics and stereotyped phonic tics, given that he was able to recognize them
twenty years later. He noted their familial and hereditary character but also
that this condition did not reduce life expectancy. Gilles de la Tourette vehemently criticized the diagnosis of chorea proposed by Trousseau: *"Laryngeal*
choreas, diaphragmatic choreas—the false interpretation is too prejudicial for a

description that, as we shall see, is accurate in many details." Charles Handfield Jones (1819–1890) of Liverpool also copied Trousseau's description in 1870 without adding any new elements.[144]

Gilles de la Tourette's Observations

Among the other eight clinical cases described by Gilles de la Tourette, the second case was an observation by Pierre Marie (1853–1940), at that time *chef de clinique* (senior house officer or resident) in the La Salpêtrière department (1883–1884). The eighth case was observed by a former Charcot *interne* who became a professor in Bordeaux, Albert Pitres (1848–1928). The ninth case was recounted by Charles Féré (1852–1907), a Charcot *interne* three years before Gilles de la Tourette. In other words, Gilles de la Tourette prepared five observations himself. The article reveals a surprising fact concerning the geographical origin of the patients. Five lived in Le Havre and one in Evreux, both cities in the French region of Normandy. Gilles de la Tourette noted that the patients described in observations II and VI were treated by Dr. Gibert in Le Havre. Joseph Gibert (1829–1899) (Figure 9.6), founder of the journal *La Normandie Médicale,* would publish, between 1891 and 1893, seven articles describing attacks of hysteria using expressions such as "passionate attitudes"; he came to be known as the "Charcot of Normandy" and was in regular contact with Charcot. When Dr. Gibert's son became a student in the philosophy class of Pierre Janet (1849–1947), Janet began to spend time at Gibert's hospital where he examined Léonie Leboulanger, a "somnambulant hysteric." The study of Leboulanger was an important part of Janet's thesis, *L'automatisme psychologique, essai de psychologie expérimentale sur les formes inférieures de l'activité humaine.*[145] It was also Gibert who presented Janet to Charcot, which led to a fruitful collaboration. Rather than indicating a higher incidence of the disease in Normandy, this geographical concentration is more likely due to the fact that Gibert, a subtle and attentive clinician, played a discreet role of referring physician and sent or recommended sending these ticcers to the master at La Salpêtrière. In his lesson on January 17, 1888, Charcot noted with irony: *"I don't know why the ticcers are almost always from the seaside. We have had several from Le Havre and Rochefort."*[146] Gilles de la Tourette went to Le Havre himself, on July 15, 1884, to evaluate the progression of the disease in a young male patient examined by Pierre Marie (observation II) and released from La Salpêtrière a year prior. Three days earlier, during the same voyage, he had reexamined a boy who only had simple tics (observation V). Probably on the way home, on July 20, 1884, he saw another boy already seen by Dr. Gibert,

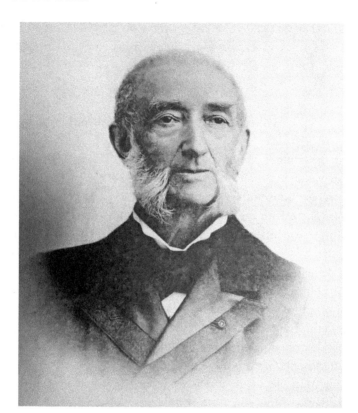

FIGURE 9.6 Joseph Gibert (1829–1899).
Private collection of K. Feltgen, with kind permission.

who had advised rest at the grand-father's home in Rouen. This boy would not see Charcot at La Salpêtrière until October 1884.

"Motor Incoordination"

Gilles de la Tourette's writings give the impression that he avoided using the word "tic," preferring the strange term of "motor incoordination": *"muscular jerks limited to muscular groups of the face and one or both upper limbs."* Was the term tic *"too trivial for this rather extravagant character"*?[147] As Georges Guinon (1859–1932) (Figure 9.7) would note: *"The involuntary movements of these patients are neither absurd nor incoordinated. On this matter, we thus cannot share the opinion of Gilles de la Tourette. What, precisely, is motor incoordination? It is still called ataxia, that is, impaired arrangement of movement. . . . Do we find anything of the sort in our patients and can the muscular jerks that we see in them be compared in any way to these highly characteristic motor problems? No, the patients are never awkward in their voluntary movements. They flex and extend their legs forcefully, hit*

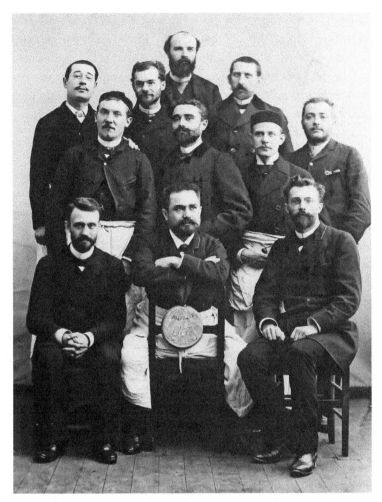

FIGURE 9.7 Seated, from left to right, Georges Guinon (1859–1932), Achille Souques (1860–1944), Emile Parmentier (1860–1940) in 1890.
Private collection of the author.

the ground squarely with their feet, are perfectly solid on their legs, and never miss a step. While it is true that they may stop walking to execute a tic, they do not throw their legs out to the sides, and they do not entangle them to the point of falling to the ground. . . . The patient's movements are not incoordinated; furthermore, they are not even illogical. Overall, and in their invariable repetition, they present a sort of arrangement that one can truly call systematic.[148] Guinon's criticisms are perfectly well founded. There can be no doubt that Gilles de la Tourette proposed this regrettable term of "motor incoordination" to bring his description closer to the cases of Jumping, Latah, and Myriachit. For example, in observation II, which included all of the clinical signs of the disease, Gilles de la Tourette used the word *"movements"* with special emphasis, never once using the word "tics" while highlighting the fact that *"all of the emotions act very keenly on* [the patient]: *he jumps when called."* In other words, he based his framework on the articles of Beard, O'Brien, and Hammond, and he wanted his descriptions to fit this framework as precisely as possible. Gilles de la Tourette employed the word "tic" only four times in his comments on the nine observations—a paradox as tics were the subject of his paper.

Evaluating the Initial Description

Do the nine observations proposed by Gilles de la Tourette describe the syndrome named for him? In fact, no. Observation IV was a description of obsessive problems (the patient, a twenty-four-year-old male, felt compelled to repeat a word or phrase when he attended a lecture and relieved this compulsion by repeating the word or words aloud when alone). The patient made a few involuntary movements (Gilles de la Tourette referred to jumping) but had no real tics nor any echolalia or coprolalia. Observation V described simple isolated tics that tended to disappear spontaneously. Observation VII told the story of a young man who had felt anxious since the traumatic events around the siege of Paris in 1871 and who exhibited a few transient tics. He would startle when surprised, similar to the Jumpers of Maine, but nothing more. As to the ninth and last observation, it involved delayed pubescence, a case of *"infantilism"* according to Gilles de la Tourette, with rhythmical movements that did not resemble tics and with no echolalia. Sometimes this male patient would utter curse words, but without real coprolalia.

The first three observations, particularly the one recounted by Itard concerning the Marquise de Dampierre, perfectly described the pathology that Gilles de la Tourette was attempting to introduce in the neurological nosology, with all clinical signs present: motor and phonic tics, associated echolalia, echokinesis, and coprolalia. The observation taken from Pitres was also entirely characteristic, but, oddly enough, Gilles de la Tourette spoke of choreoid tics and thus muddled—involuntarily—the demonstration by which he hoped to isolate "his disease" from chorea. For observation VI, Gilles de la Tourette used the word "tic" twice in his description for eye blinking. The child would say "oh, oh!" but without any other symptoms, and the progression seemed spontaneously favorable. So this case may have been nothing more than simple transient tics.

In total, four of the observations were indisputably cases of Gilles de la Tourette syndrome. In his discussion, Gilles de la Tourette perfectly described the childhood onset: between the ages of six and sixteen. He highlighted the *"utterly slow and insidious"* progression, with its periods of remission and exacerbation. He also clearly reported the capacity of patients to temporarily inhibit the exteriorization of their tics and the subsequent rebound: *"He could refrain from all his abrupt movements and stop them completely. But, immediately following this cessation, which required of him the most violent constraint of mind, the movements would return with unusual violence."* Gilles de la Tourette insisted on the echolalia: *"This is one of the most constant symptoms of their condition, and one that, in particular, most impressed the foreign authors. It is one of the first symptoms to appear after the motor incoordination, and seems to be one of the last to persist during quiescent periods. . . . This faculty of imitation, this echolalia of movements and actions is thus, in certain cases, very complete in these patients."* For the involuntary imitation of a movement, Charcot used the term *"echokinesis,"* which he coined. Pierre Marie spoke of *"echomatism."* Gilles de la Tourette insisted on the pathognomonic nature of coprolalia (his coinage) stating that *"it is never observed in other conditions. . . . Not only do patients utter obscene words; it also seems that they may exhibit a combination of echolalia, which they are often reliant on, and coprolalia.* However, *"coprolalia is not found in all subjects, in the same way that echolalia is not always present."* Finally, *"the tics are often hereditary,"* implying *"degeneration,"* which characterized the cause of neurological diseases according to the Salpêtrière School.[149] As for the prognosis, Gilles de la Tourette concluded: *"We have never seen the disease disappear completely; it may improve, but patients are not cured, and furthermore, an improvement may merely be the prelude to a new exacerbation."*

Championed by Charcot

On July 19, 1885, Paul Le Gendre gave readers of the journal *Union Médicale* a complete description of the disease, entitling his piece *"Gilles de la Tourette disease."* He began as follows: *"As the ancient proverb says, 'It is not for every man to go to Corinth'. . . and it is even less the common fate to bring a new disease to the baptismal font. While we do not know whether our colleague Gilles de la Tourette has been favored in the first case, in the second, he has most certainly deserved his good fortune, by his skillful historical evaluation and his wise clinical studies in which he pulled from the chaos of the choreas a distinct morbid entity, claiming for it a place of its own in the nosography. Mr. Charcot—and there is no better judge in such matters—declared in a clinical lesson this year that the nervous disease described by Gilles de la Tourette in* Les Archives de Neurologie *has special characteristics definite enough to legitimize the naming of this disease after our friend. It would be disrespectful on our part not to adopt the master's position, regardless of whether one is of the opinion that naming diseases for the person who first described them, or who appears to have done so, is potentially problematic, and we are among those who hold this opinion."*[150]

Georges Guinon, Forgotten Author

Georges Guinon took Gilles de la Tourette's place as Charcot's *interne* for 1885. As early as January 1886, just one year after his predecessor's seminal publication, Guinon published four new observations in *La Revue de Médecine*. Charcot's fundamental role, albeit hidden, cannot be denied; the master sought to enhance the description of this new entity and situate it precisely in the neurological nosology. Guinon described two new cases seen by Charcot in 1885 and reported by Melotti, and he wrote in his article: *"We wish to thank Mr. Charcot, who was the inspiration for this work and who helped us with his generous advice."* Who was Georges Guinon? His career was surprising. The meeting with Charcot was crucial, as it was for Gilles de la Tourette. Léon Bernard (1872–1934) wrote in his 1932 homage to Guinon: *"In all aspects of his person, his emotional as well as his intellectual being, Guinon had been absorbed by the famous personality, whose esteem he considered as the honor of his life. This memory remained alive for him, like the memory of a great love. Guinon was a simple and straightforward soul. When Charcot suddenly passed away, he faltered. Everything he had planned, all high hopes for his life came crashing down; he left the capital."*[151] The deep bereavement gave his career an unexpected and unique turn, which was unusual for a brilliant student of Charcot. Shortly after his teacher's death, he left for Normandy, where he worked as a family physician. Later, he set up his practice near the Douarnenez harbor in Brittany, where he was known as a discreet and extremely devoted physician until 1919, comforting families who lost their loved ones during World War I. In 1919, he joined Léon Bernard and the fight against tuberculosis by becoming a medical inspector for the Office Public d'Hygiène in the Seine; the new Léon-Bourgeois law had set up such offices in every French *département*. Guinon had defended his thesis on the agents that provoke hysteria[152] in 1889, with Charcot presiding over the jury. He wrote up the master's lessons from 1889 to 1893, succeeding Gilles de la Tourette as Charcot's personal secretary. In 1887, he wrote the article on convulsive tics in the monumental *Dictionnaire Encyclopédique des Sciences Médicales* of Amédée Dechambre (1812–1886).[153] In it, he noted that Gilles de la Tourette *"did in fact describe the convulsive tic disease, as we have shown in a work on this condition"*; he did not refer to motor incoordination. Guinon clearly stated: *"What is found, most often in isolation, are firstly eye blinking and then the alternating opening and closing movement of the mouth."* He then insisted on the systematic nature of involuntary movements: *"In everyone, we find a few identical tics, such as touching one's beard and spitting."*

"Idea Tics"

Acting on Charcot's wise clinical advice, Guinon added to Gilles de la Tourette's description the frequent presence of *"idées fixes,"* which Charcot called *"idea tics"*: *"Mr. Charcot called our attention to the existence in our patients of a series of psychic phenomena that we have not found noted in other, similar observations and that, if we refer to the cases we have studied, must be quite frequent in the serious forms of the tic disease. These phenomena are* idées fixes. *In absolute terms, outside the condition that interests us,* idées fixes *constitute a chapter of mental pathology, as is well known. The extent to which they can vary is common knowledge, and to cite just a few examples, we mention* la folie du pourquoi *where the patients cannot resist asking the reasons for absolutely insignificant things;* la folie du doute avec délire du toucher, *which differs slightly from simple* idées fixes *in that it leads to truly delirious ideas; arithmomania or the mania of numbers and calculations; and onomatomania, recently described by Mr. Charcot and Mr. Magnan."*[154] In 1838, Jean-Etienne Esquirol (1772–1840) had included these symptoms together with deliriums in a large group: *monomanie raisonnante* or intellectual monomania.[155] *La folie du doute* was isolated from the "monomanias" by Henri Legrand du Saulle (1830–1886) in 1875[156] and corresponds to modern-day obsessive-compulsive disorder. Guinon intuited a common pathophysiological mechanism for the disease's various symptoms: *"It is now easy to understand the link between all of these phenomena—tics, involuntary words,* idées fixes. *All three appear to be of the same family. The cause is the same; it is merely a question of degree. 1) Simple convulsive or impulsive motor representation producing facial grimaces or tics in the limbs. 2) A more complex convulsive motor representation resulting in utterance of a sound or pronunciation of a word or phrase. 3) Ordinary convulsive or impulsive ideas, either resulting in more or less complicated actions, such as counting and arranging objects on a table, or remaining limited to a conscious fact without external manifestations, such the perpetual feeling of unmotivated fear, which we have noted in one of our patients."* Through and with the help of Guinon, who added to the initial work of Gilles de la Tourette, Charcot built the complete clinical picture of the disease as we know it today. When he was finished, Guinon proposed a new term: *"convulsive tic disease, the name which, according to Professor Charcot, would be most appropriate for this condition."* This brief remark is colored by the thinly veiled spite that Guinon felt after Charcot initially named the disease for Gilles de la Tourette.

Guinon would discuss the disease again the following year, but this time formulating a personal opinion, inspired by Briquet, as a sort of challenge to Charcot. Tic disorder and hysteria could be associated and could be difficult to distinguish, given the points they had in common: *"Hysteria, among its numerous manifestations, also includes involuntary movements, in which we may include coughing, hiccupping, barking, and involuntary exclamations. These, as we have shown elsewhere, are nothing other than slightly more complex motor phenomena. . . . If we compare these phenomena to those observed in the convulsive tic disease, it is easy to see that objectively, the difference between them is far from distinct. Furthermore, as with tics, hysterical involuntary movements recur in fits. . . . It is not the movements themselves that will provide the nosological characteristic for classifying each case in the appropriate place, but rather the phenomena of all sorts that accompany them most of the time. These phenomena are all different depending on whether the subject is a hysteric or suffering from convulsive tics. Echolalia, observed in the two diseases, constitutes an exception. And in the tic disease, coprolalia is often noted, along with idées fixes, folie du doute, etc., which characterize delirium in hereditary degenerates. On the contrary, in hysteria, the well-known mental state of the patients is entirely different; most especially, neurosis will have left its mark on the patient in more or less of a lasting way. The observation of hysterical stigmata is thus of critical importance."* Guinon presented three new observations, including one given to him by Charcot. He prepared the two others during his year as an *interne* under Emile Troisier (1844–1919) at Hôpital Saint-Antoine in 1886. The first involved a hysteric girl with anarchical movements followed by prolonged lipothymias. The second and third cases were clearly convulsive ticcers in whom Guinon observed inappropriate emotional states and hemianaesthesias accompanied by a reduced visual field, which were for him indicative of hysteria. The age of onset, much earlier for tics, together with the fact that they progress over a much longer period, are arguments for differential diagnosis. *"Here we have the convulsive tic disease in hysterical subjects. And why couldn't these two neuroses be associated? Heredity, which creates in and of itself the tic disease, plays no small role in the etiology of hysteria. Moreover, don't we see similar morbid associations every day? Epilepsy often combines with hysteria to form the disease called 'hystero-epilepsy with separate crises.' Similarly, there are cases in which hysteria or the convulsive tic disease develops where the other already exists."*[157]

Maurice Lannois (1856–1942), a native of Lyon and founder of the Société française d'Oto-Rhino-Laryngologie, published his thesis on the nosography of choreas in 1886.[158] In a chapter entitled *"pseudo-choreas,"* he gave a complete, accurate clinical picture of the disease and added an observation from La Salpêtrière of a little girl whose explosive movements started at age seven: *"She is constantly crying out with a little, contained 'hum!' During fits, there is a moment where she cannot utter anything, then suddenly a barrage of words ushers forth and she has to cry out, unable to prevent herself, such that she is heard throughout the house. At this point, she sometimes cannot stop vulgar language from slipping out, the word 'shit,' for example."* Lannois wrote very clearly that it was Charcot who enriched the initial work of Gilles de la Tourette by his description of *"idea tics,"* making no mention of Guinon.

Publications Outside France

Thomas Carlton Railton in Manchester (1844–1922) published an observation in April 1886 of a man approximately forty years old with abnormal movements since the age of seven, making him an entirely typical case of the condition: *"When the lower extremity was attacked, he often kicked the toe of his boot vigorously into the ground, and usually tapped his forehead with his right hand and turned up his eyes at the same time. On other occasions he would perform the following series of movements: first, holding out his right hand, he supinated and pronated the forearm two or three times, digging his elbow into his side with each supination; then he raised his right knee and patted it several times; and lastly, he struck his nose, forehead, or the top of his head with his hand, opening his mouth and turning up his eyes, and accompanying each tap with an inarticulate cry. . . . At this period the cry was perfectly inarticulate: sometimes it was almost a squeak, sometimes like ahem, as in clearing the throat. It never occurred except at the time of one of his involuntary movements. The movements varied very much, but a particular set seemed to predominate for a certain time, to give way in turn to another series. For some time he was in the habit of making a peculiar noise with his tongue and lips, like the sound of spitting out some small thing from between the lips. Probably the disease had slowly reached this stage in the course of over twenty years, and it remained much the same for the succeeding three years of my acquaintance with him, sometimes seeming worse, the movements being larger, more perceptible, and more frequent in their occurrence; sometimes better, when they amounted only to a slight occasional jerk of the hand, or a tapping of the forehead.*

In 1882, I observed that a new phenomenon had supervened, rendering his complaint much more seriously inconvenient. Instead of the inarticulate cry, the movements were accompanied at times by a muffled sound, the purport of which could not be distinguished when it was first heard, but which became resolvable by its repetition into words never used in polite society. He would be painfully conscious of the effect upon his audience of the word or words he used, and would endeavor to turn off the obnoxious sound by continuing it either into a humming of a bar or two of music, or as a strenuous cough. . . . Such attacks formed a most painful contrast to his surroundings and to his manners, which were those of a cultivated gentleman, who, in conversation, never made use of obscene or improper language. Mr. de la Tourette, who has collected nine cases of this disease, has applied the term 'coprolalia' to this symptom, from copro = filth and lalia = to talk; and he considers that it is pathognomonic of the disease."[159]

In September 1885, Dimitri Yankowsky published a note in the journal *Vratch.*[160] Jacques Roubinovitch (1862–1950), born in Odessa and an *interne* in asylums around Paris at the time, translated the note for Gilles de la Tourette, as Jacques Catrou noted in his thesis (see later discussion). In July 1886, two American physicians, C. L. Dana and W. P. Wilkin, reported the first American case. Incidentally, they referred to another Russian publication: *"In March 1886, Dr. I. I. Pautynkhoff reported* (Russkaya Meditizina, *March 16) 'a case of imitative disease,' resembling that of Tourette's, the patient showing echolalia and echokinesis (imitation of speech and movement). Patient had defective intelligence."* They started with a discussion of echolalia and coprolalia: *"It was then noticed that when sitting quietly he would suddenly and involuntarily burst out into expressions of the most profane and obscene character; repeating them rapidly for a few movements and then stopping. A surprise or sudden noise of any kind was liable to bring on an outburst. He did not seem to understand the significance of the words used. . . . The word which he used oftenest, repeating it rapidly and automatically, was the equivalent of the French word 'merde,' which is the word quoted by Tourette as most frequently expressed by his patients. He used to be much worse mornings, and before or during his toilet would regale the house with his automatic blasphemies so loudly as to disturb the neighbors."* They continued with a description of the abnormal movements: *"When examined by us he was observed to be anemic, but fairly well grown and nourished. He has choreic movements in the face, and slight convulsive movement in legs and arms. When he is making a strong effort to repress the obnoxious words, or when he is under any restraint, the movements are more prominent. The choreic movements, as stated, affect his face and shoulders most. He had also a kind of expiratory spasm, producing a noise like a half-developed cough. If more marked, it might be put down as an illustration of laryngeal chorea."*[161] The authors then gave the complete clinical picture of the disease as Gilles de la Tourette described it in his article and repeated one of his key points: *"The coprolalia is pathognomonic of the disease, according to Tourette."* As early as 1886, Gilles de la Tourette's name was being amputated by North American authors!

Clinical Cases Presented During Charcot's Lessons

The *Leçons de Charcot*, published in 1893 and compiled by Guinon, included an "appendix" transcribing two lessons from 1886 that were omitted from the third volume of the master's works. One of them, on *"hysterical sounds,"* included a clarification on the differential diagnosis of hysteria, convulsive tic disorder, chorea, and paramyoclonus.[162] The two briefly described cases of convulsive tic disorder, already presented to students on an earlier occasion, were probably those that Melotti referred to in his article. Shortly thereafter, Charcot incorporated young patients with the disorder in his Tuesday lessons. On December 13, 1887, Charcot presented *"a young fellow aged twelve or thirteen . . . he has a tic. In front of you, he is holding back, but from time to time, he blinks, has contractions in the lower limbs which result in certain involuntary movements. Now and again he strikes the ground with his foot. If he only did that, it would be nothing serious, but sometimes he makes a sort of grunting noise: hugh! hugh! hugh! And he presents the phenomenon of coprolalia. What is coprolalia? If you are ticklish regarding the value of certain words, cover your ears. Coprolalia is the irresistible urge to pronounce the word that Victor Hugo put in the mouth of Cambronne at Waterloo and which, according to him, should take the place of the heroic phrase popularized by the legend; that is to say, the word: . . . [shit] What does this mean? you ask. Hasn't this child been raised to be polite? But of course, he has been raised as children should be. This word, he has heard it pronounced—but then, in the street one hears so many words not of one's own vocabulary! Indeed! He utters it continually, in spite of himself, by impulsion. We have often seen this condition in children. Mr. Gilles de la Tourette and Mr. Guinon have dealt with the question: this is the tic disease. When someone suffers from this disorder, he develops a series of phenomena—some of them psychic, others physical—that we have observed to combine with each other."*[163]

On January 17, 1888, Charcot examined a seventeen-year-old boy—another native of Normandy. Making the boy write and execute several movements, Charcot lectured on the differential diagnosis between "vulgar" chorea and convulsive tic disorder. His treatment consisted in hydrotherapy, *"teinture de Mars,"*[164] and *"vin de Colombo."*[165] On Tuesday, January 24, 1888, Charcot briefly presented those in attendance with two other adolescents. On February 21, 1888, Charcot began by telling a twenty-one-year-old man who suffered from tics: *"Moreover, you know that having tics in a family is not without consequences. Tics are a special mark."* What followed was a thorough interrogation on personal and family antecedents. The patient, it turned out, also had a *"folie du doute"* characterized by the fear of rabies at the sight of an animal. He had two brothers and a sister with tics: *"When there is one ticcer in a family, it is rarely an isolated case."*

In his Tuesday lesson on October 23, 1888, Charcot clearly contradicted Gilles de la Tourette: "The movements of ticcers, however complex and bizarre they may be, are not always and essentially disorganized, incoordinated, or contradictory, as is too often believed. On the contrary, they are generally systematic, to the extent that they always recur in the same way in a given subject. Moreover, very often at least, they reproduce, albeit exaggeratedly, certain automatic physiological movements that have a purpose." During this lesson, Charcot credited Gilles de la Tourette with the coinage of the word "coprolalia": "This is the remarkable phenomenon, among all of the others, that Gilles de la Tourette, in his interesting work on the tic disease, ingeniously designated using the term 'coprolalia.'" At the Tuesday lesson on June 4, 1889, Charcot refined the semiological description: "The complex tic movement is not absurd in itself. It is absurd and illogical because it is executed outside of a context, without an apparent reason. The act of scratching oneself occurs without an itch, the eyes blink in the absence of any foreign object, and so forth. In addition, tic movements are abrupt, rapid, momentary and do not have, for example, the slowness of choreic gesticulations. They are not continuous, but supervene by fits repeated at greater or lesser frequencies and lasting for greater or lesser periods, fits that patients can often, for a time, stop by an effort of will. It is also often the case that while jerking and grimacing, patients utter exclamations and entire words, quite often filthy words. You will have accumulated such specific clinical characteristics that you should be able to distinguish with certainty the tic disease from all other types of convulsive conditions."[166]

The last Tuesday lesson during which Charcot mentioned *"convulsive tic disease"* took place on June 4, 1889. He was once again teaching the difference between tics and chorea by presenting the students with a ticcer alongside a chorea patient (Huntington's chorea), both female. By way of introduction, he declared: *"You see to what extent the electric jerks of the ticcer differ profoundly from the slow and permanent gesticulations of subjects with Sydenham's chorea. Between tics and chorea, the distance is vast: do not forget this, since these conditions are sometimes wrongly given the same name, and the prognosis is quite different."* Charcot showed the opposition between the speed of the movements and highlighted the constancy of choreic writhing, whereas tics stop intermittently. The chorea patient made no sounds, whereas the ticcer *"makes from time to time expressive laryngeal noises."* The movements of the latter were chaotic and unpredictable, whereas in the former, everything was rhythmical, regular, and systematic. The ticcer started having tics at the age of twelve, whereas the other patient was *"over fifty-one"* at the time, with an age of onset at thirty-three. *"Chronic chorea is considered an incurable disease; its outcome is fatal, and the therapies are unable to stop its relentless progress, not even for a moment. This is not quite the case with the tic disease. It is also one of the most difficult conditions, to the extent that we cannot say if we ever actually cure it, but we can count on periods of cessation, often quite long, and on a certain waxing and waning, either spontaneous or brought about by appropriate therapy. Hydrotherapy, rational gymnastics, and isolation are among the approaches that may be helpful in such cases. You can now recognize the value of learning to distinguish between these two morbid states, for which the prognosis is so different."*

Breitman Introduces Degeneration Theory

On November 28, 1888, Grégoire Breitman (1859–1914),[167] a physician from the city of Ananyiv,[168] defended the first thesis on Gilles de la Tourette syndrome since the seminal article's publication, with Charcot presiding over his jury.[169] *"Alienists such as Magnan and his students Legrain and Saury see echolalia, coprolalia, and echokinesis as an episodic syndrome of* la folie des dégénérés." Paul-Maurice Legrain (1860–1939) and Honoré Saury (1854–1906),[170] disciples of Valentin Magnan (1835–1916), introduced the concept of *bouffée délirante* (brief psychotic disorder) into the psychiatric nosology. This was after both had done work on *la folie des dégénérés* (insanity in degenerates), Legrain writing his thesis[171] on the subject and Saury[172] a book. Breitman, a student alienist at the Vaucluse asylum near Paris,[173] wanted to study the heredity of involuntary imitation symptoms in order to clarify the role of "degeneration" in their genesis. This had been the accepted etiology of neuropsychiatric diseases since the work of Bénédict-Augustin Morel (1809–1873): *"As the semiology of hereditary degenerates grows more detailed, exact, and manifest, we are relegating the search for the original flaw in the various forms of alienation to a secondary position";* given that *"the aim is to find out whether, by studying the semiology of each psychic state and by grouping the signs into syndromes, we can, by deduction, demonstrate the manifestly degenerative hereditary origin."* He explained that *"under the combined influence of peripheral and central excitations, we will see degenerates, these future candidates for mental alienation, executing a series of bizarre actions, designated as 'Latah, Jumping, and Myriachit' by foreign authors."* Breitman showed, based on several observations he had collected, that echolalia, coprolalia, and echokinesis can be seen in various types of mental alienation, especially in deliriums. He invented the words *égoécholalie* and *égoéchokinésie* for when a patient would speak to himself in front of a mirror and control his movements while watching himself. For Breitman, these symptoms were related *"by the fact that they were impulses arising from an obsession."* And he categorically concluded that *"echolalia, coprolalia, and echokinesis with tics can constitute a perfectly independent morbid syndrome with a determined course, that is, tic disease or Gilles de la Tourette disease. Patients with this disease are degenerate."*

"Enhanced Habit Formation"

In 1888, Ferdinand Burot (1846–1921)[174] published his essay on the treatment of convulsive tic disorder by persuasion. He treated the young female patient studied and described by Pitres, Charcot, and Gilles de la Tourette (observation VIII).[175] This was the beginning of the psychiatrization of the disease. Burot concluded: *"The convulsive tic disease is the result of a specific cerebral excess. It is a psychic condition almost exclusively in the domain of moral treatment. This entails training the brain to operate using special instruction and brain exercises. Persuasion, which is nothing other than suggestion without sleep, is an important therapeutic agent, if methodical. It acts by increasing tenfold the will of the subject, who is then able to moderate and dominate his impulses."*[176] A few months later, Burot reported on the effect of his treatment, which he considered very successful, with the near-complete disappearance of all symptoms: *"The purpose of moral gymnastics is to destroy these vicious associations, these organized habits, to moderate the activity of the automatic sphere, and to shift the balance to benefit the psycho-intellectual sphere, which should predominate."*[177]

On November 16, 1888, in Bordeaux, Jean Urbain-Joseph Chauvreau (1863–?), a student at the Ecole de Médecine de la Marine in Rochefort, defended his thesis,[178] focused on Burot and Pitres, the latter presiding over the thesis jury. He started by describing Pitres's observation, then presented the case of a youngster he had personally observed. The child's multiple motor tics began at age three and his echolalia and coprolalia, entirely characteristic, at age five. His third observation had been presented in Toulouse, at the 1887 conference of the Association française pour l'avancement des Sciences, during the discussion following Burot's presentation on his attempts to use persuasion treatment. During this conference, Emile Duplouy (1856–1896), a Navy physician, later director of the Navy health department in Rochefort, reported on the case of a distinguished navy officer whom he had treated for four years. *"Even before entering the Ecole Navale, this officer had a convulsive tic characterized by the sudden and involuntary projection of the upper limb, with convulsions in the pharynx muscles and a guttural cry in all ways similar to a bark. These phenomena would occur when the officer approached one of his superiors, which led them to slap him frequently, at which point inappropriate words would escape the officer's lips. Hydrotherapy completely failed against this convulsive tic. The patient, always very energetic, was only able to overcome it with time. Without wishing to discourage Mr. Burot in the treatment by suggestion he is pursuing with praiseworthy perseverance that has already been rewarded by notable improvement, it is Mr. Duplouy's opinion that the aforementioned officer's cure is above all due to his advancing in age. Very pronounced in adolescence, the disease, which Mr. Duplouy readily linked to one of these most bizarre manifestations of hysteria that are sometimes observed in man, improved as the subject grew closer to the middle period of his life, and ended as soon as he had passed it."*[179] Chauvreau then included two observations provided by Gilles de la Tourette and that of Itard concerning the Marquise de Dampierre. After reviewing the clinical methods developed by Gilles de la Tourette, Guinon, and Charcot, he discussed at greater length echolalia, also observed *"during minor nervous accidents"* and in hysteria, accompanied by cries and *"barks."*

Catrou, Gilles de la Tourette's Student

On March 6, 1890, with Charcot presiding over the jury, Jacques Catrou (1865–?), a former *externe*, defended his thesis on convulsive tic disorder, in which he included Jumping, Latah, and Myriachit.[180] He started by summarizing (nearly copying) the entire beginning of the seminal article, then cited Charcot's lesson *"recorded by Mr. Melotti of Bologna"* from June 1885: *"In lesson XIV, after reviewing the history as we have already done, Mr. Charcot validated the word 'coprolalia' coined by Mr. Gilles de la Tourette and replaced the term 'motor incoordination' with 'convulsive tic.' 'There are,' he stated, 'three main elements in Gilles de la Tourette disease: the tic, echolalia, and coprolalia'. . . . Mr. Charcot also introduced in the description, a symptom of prime importance, involving the mental state of the subject. In these patients, one very often observes what he calls an 'idea tic,' such as la folie du doute, le délire du toucher, misophobia, arithmomania, and so forth."* Catrou added twenty-eight unpublished observations that Charcot and Gilles de la Tourette had sent him. He then proceeded to analyze all of the forty-five observations published to date. His first observation was taken from the letter of Yankowsky to *Vratch*. Yankowsky noted that he had worked in eastern Siberia. There he read an article on the *"Miryatschenye."* *"The word 'miryachit' or 'meryajet' means in ordinary language 'to act foolishly.' The person who acts in this manner is called 'meryascha.'"* He recounted that one evening, he examined fourteen soldiers *"in bizarre positions."* *"Some were walking, others were lying down or sitting, and all of them continued doing so, even in my presence. I asked them, 'What's wrong with you?' and all of them said in unison, 'What's wrong with you?' I asked them, 'Are you sick?' Response: 'Are you sick?' and so on. All of them answered each question together, repeating the same question. The commander of the company then arrived and noted that all of these soldiers had eaten potatoes with hempseed oil*[181] *purchased from an inhabitant of Korea. Hearing the word 'oil,' all of them began to repeat 'oil, oil, oil,' in different tones. Neither exhortations nor orders could prevent the patients from repeating the words pronounced by anyone present."* In addition to the general hilarity, Yankowsky noted either mydriasis or miosis in the patients' pupils. He began to suspect the oil, then learned that four soldiers who ate the same oil but had no symptoms did not see the oil seller, who, he was informed, was a *'meryascha.'* This explained for him the epidemic of behavioral problems, *"which proves that the 'miryachenie' is contagious."* This account confirms the hysterical nature of Myriachit (spelling used by Gilles de la Tourette). Catrou then reviewed all of the symptoms described by Gilles de la Tourette, but his thesis took a highly original turn when he argued against the theories attributing the etiology to *"degeneration"*: *"We do not subscribe in any way to the current opinion whereby all nervous pathology falls under mental degeneration aside from conditions where a physical lesion has been demonstrated."*

First German Publications

On July 27, 1889, at the Friedrich-Wilhelms-Universität in Berlin, Otto Müller (1865–?), a student of Hermann Helmotz (1821–1894) and Emil du Bois-Raymond (1818–1896) defended his thesis on tics, with as jury president Coelestin Slawyk, a pioneer in lung surgery.[182] He noted that the work of Gilles de la Tourette had generated little interest in Germany aside from a thesis defended in 1885 by Theodor von Färber, a student of Hermann Oppenheim (1857–1919).[183] Müller presented four cases of motor and phonic tics. He elaborated on Guinon's discussion of the link with hysteria and considered tics as a disease of the will for which he recommended the use of morphine and arsenic.

Heymann Hirschfeld (1860–?) described three patients with motor and phonic tics associated with echolalia and echokinesis in his thesis defended in Berlin in 1891.[184] His discussion centered on the differential diagnosis of chorea, hysteria, and paramyoclonus multiplex.[185]

In 1899, Georg Köster (1867–1932) provided two entirely characteristic observations.[186] And in the 1899 medical treatise directed by the Englishman Sir Thomas Clifford Allbutt (1836–1925, inventor of the clinical thermometer), James Samuel Risien Russell (1863–1939), born in French Guiana, paid homage to Charcot, Gilles de la Tourette, and Guinon in his chapter on tics, completely supporting their point of view.[187]

North American Contribution

The Canadian William Osler (1849–1919) gave a lesson at Johns Hopkins Hospital in Baltimore, published on December 20, 1890, during which he presented a remarkable observation of a thirteen-year-old girl with all of the symptoms described by Gilles de la Tourette, including coprolalia but not obsessional ideas. Osler nonetheless described them using a word coined by Charcot, "arithmomania," and suggested *folie du toucher*. He pointed out the difficulties of translating expressions that are apparently similar but have different meanings in French and in English: "*There is a curious disease or perhaps, more correctly, symptom group, met with chiefly in children, to which attention has been called of late by French writers, which is characterized by irregular, spasmodic movements, the utterance of involuntary explosive sounds or words, and mental defects of various sorts. It is not a very common affection in this country, and I take this opportunity to bring to your notice a case which we have been studying for the past few weeks. The cases have usually been described as chorea, or 'habit-spasm,' both of which conditions are simulated very closely by the irregular movements; certain instances also have been reported as hysteria. Unfortunately, Charcot and his pupils, Guinon and Gilles de la Tourette, have given to this ailment the name 'Maladie des tics convulsifs.' I say unfortunately, for here and in England we use the term Convulsive Tic to characterize a totally different affection, involving usually the facial muscles and of either central or peripheral origin, but not necessarily coming on in childhood and not characterized by the other features presented by the disease of which we are at present speaking; and thus it happens that if we turn to the recent editions of French books we find under 'tic convulsif' a disease very different from that described by the same name in English and American works.*"

Elsewhere in France

Dr. G. André of Toulouse noted in 1891 that "*Charcot added an important chapter to the symptomatology of convulsive tics, showing that in severe forms there were specific psychic phenomena, or idées fixes. These are what Mr. Grasset calls the 'psychic stigmata of the tic disease' or 'psychic tics.'*" André described a man of forty-five with motor tics in one arm, which he did not complain about, but he was very disturbed by his obsessional ideas, by "*searching for forgotten names*" or onomatomania[188] and by hypochondriacal ideas. The clinical picture was clearly and primarily psychiatric. While Guinon was cited, Gilles de la Tourette was not mentioned.[189]

In 1892, Raoul Brunon (1854–1929) from the city of Rouen, a friend of Charles Féré, proposed five observations of ticcers in the journal *La Normandie Médicale*. He wanted to show that many cases could be cured using a treatment that involved, every morning, "*cold lotion all over the body, then rubbing with a massage glove; pills containing belladonna extract and reduced iron (in increasing doses, up to 12 centigrams per day); a laxative every three days; physical exercise out of doors; and fewer hours of study at school."* However, his succinct descriptions leave one to suspect that none of his patients had Gilles de la Tourette syndrome.[190]

The alienist Jacques Roubinovitch (1862–1950) published an observation in 1893 of a female patient hospitalized in the department of Auguste Voisin (1829–1898) at La Salpêtrière who exhibited the complete clinical picture of Gilles de la Tourette syndrome. She had a large callus on her forehead from striking herself involuntarily. Her obsession was to break objects, driven as she was by irresistible clastic impulses, which Roubinovitch named *"krouomania."* He subscribed to Tokarski's idea whereby compulsive tic disorder and Myriachit were two distinct pathologies.[191]

Julien Noir (1866–1948) (Figure 9.8), a student of Bourneville and, like him, an editor for *Le Progrès Médical*, defended his thesis in 1893 with Victor Cornil (1837–1908) presiding over the jury. The thesis examined tics in children considered to be *"degenerates, imbeciles, and idiots"*[192] and contained numerous illustrations and photographs. Noir gave seventy-three observations

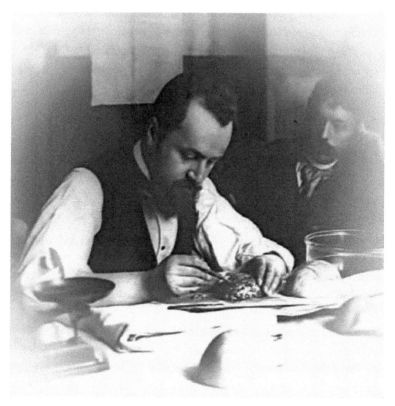

FIGURE 9.8 Julien Noir (1866–1948).
Private collection of the author.

of youngsters with mental disabilities, some of whom had tics, with echolalia, coprolalia, and echokinesis in certain cases, but these three mimetic behaviors sometimes existed without tics. Using a purely descriptive nosographical approach, he proposed four families of tics: simple motor tics; coordinated tics observed in cases of mental retardation, that is, repeated rhythmical movements (rocking, krouomania,[193] etc.); Gilles de la Tourette syndrome, Jumping, Latah, Myriachit (including echolalia, echokinesis, coprolalia); and, finally, "purely psychic tics," that is, *idées fixes*, obsessions, impulses, and so forth. None of his observations was characteristic of Gilles de la Tourette syndrome. Aside from the descriptive interest of this thesis and its underlying intellectual approach, indicative of the humanity Noir and Bourneville showed in caring for these poor patients, the work is a manifesto by colleagues of the Salpêtrière School in support of the recognition and isolation of Gilles de la Tourette syndrome, which faced opposition from detractors such as Magnan and his students André Lemoine and Nicolas Lemaire, who considered *"convulsive and psychic tics as simple stigmata of degeneration, refusing to give them their own place as a morbid entity, contrary to Gilles de la Tourette, whose ideas Catrou defended in his thesis."* Noir also presented novel ideas in the area of etiological description and research concerning repetitive and rhythmical movements having no purpose, frequently observed in people with mental disabilities. Paul Sollier (1861–1933) had initiated this study in his 1890 thesis also directed by Bourneville, with Cornil presiding over the jury.[194] The Franco-American Edouard Séguin (1812–1880),[195] a student of Itard and Esquirol (1772–1840), had not mentioned tics in his pioneering work on the treatment of "idiots." By contrast, Paul Moreau from the city of Tours (1844–1908), in one of the first pedopsychiatric treatises, entitled *La folie chez l'enfant*,[196] had described the simple and isolated tic form, citing anecdotes from Prosper Lucas and Charles Darwin (1809–1882) and agreeing with them on the role of heredity as a predisposing factor.

In 1893, Louis Chabbert (1862–1945) from Toulouse published in *Les Archives de Neurologie* four observations of patients with motor tics. The complete clinical picture of Gilles de la Tourette syndrome, with the association of phonic tics, echolalia, and coprolalia, was only present in the third observation. Chabbert observed Charcot's echokinesis but preferred the term "echocinesis." Apparently acknowledging the grounds on which Gilles de la Tourette syndrome had been isolated, he not only argued, in case after case, for the role of heredity, but also sought to highlight all possible links with hysteria.[197] His approach is reminiscent of that of Guinon.

Defended in 1894 with Jacques-Joseph Grancher (1843–1907) presiding over the jury, the thesis of Casimir Janowicz (1859–1918), born in

Kamyanets-Podilsky in what was then Poland, covered the differential diagnosis of convulsive tics, paramyoclonus multiplex, and electric chorea.[198] After describing two cases of simple transient tics, Janowicz explained the difficulties posed by the inaccurate descriptions of paramyoclonus and electric chorea—simple syndromes, still poorly defined, involving muscular spasms—whereas convulsive tic disorder had a well-established clinical picture. For Janowicz, paramyoclonus and electric chorea had a psychic origin suggesting a form of hysteria, whereas Augustin Morvan (1819–1897), in his 1890 description of fibrillary chorea ("myokimias"), explicitly described a neurological disease[199] that is now recognized as an autoimmune channelopathy known as Morvan's syndrome.

Ezio Sciamanna (1850–1905), an Italian alienist and student of Charcot and Moriz Benedikt (1835–1920), constructed a pathophysiology in 1898 around ten ticcing patients that combined tics and paranoia. Tics, for Sciamanna, were impulsive movements aimed at removing some imaginary danger. These pointless, nonadaptive actions became, by his definition, a delirium, influencing all of the individual's behaviors, preparing the way for paranoia.[200]

In 1899, Constantin Oddo (1860–1926) in Marseille set out to help practitioners differentiate tic disorder from Sydenham's chorea, but the resulting clinical picture had atrocious implications, in our view, for the patients. While chorea required a nervous heredity to develop, *"the same cannot be said for ticcers, whose hereditary past is burdened in another manner, whose flaws are more pronounced. Theirs is not only a hereditary neuropathy, but degeneration, and degeneration in its most severe form. . . . If the ticcer is not yet a degenerate, he will be, he is marked to become one. . . . Chorea patients are almost always cured; the ticcer is never cured."* The entire article follows this same vein.[201]

Gilles de la Tourette's Final Contribution

Aside from the observations he gave Catrou for his thesis, Gilles de la Tourette never published any other data on the disease named for him during Charcot's lifetime. It was not until 1899 that the transcript of one of his lessons at Hôpital Saint-Antoine was published,[202] as cited at the beginning of this chapter. A twenty-two-year-old woman came *"to ask for treatment for chorea, which seemed to explain, at least in appearance, the agitation of the muscles of her face and the left side of her body."* The abnormal movements began when she was eight years old. Periods lasting a few weeks to a few months alternated with calm periods, without *"muscular incoordination,"* but with a few residual tics in the face nonetheless. Gilles de la Tourette once again employed this awkward expression, as if not to back down and all while disowning it in the lines that followed. All of the physicians consulted had diagnosed chorea and prescribed arsenic and antipyrine. In addition to her motor tics, she had phonic tics (*hum! hum!* or *oh ah!*). *"When she grows irritated with her little boy, who is very agitated, her jerks worsen and she calls him 'pig, ass,' often including the word of Cambronne* [shit] *in her interjections. . . . I was now sure; the unanimous diagnosis of chorea should be replaced by a diagnosis of convulsive tic disease with coprolalia."* This young woman also exhibited some phobias. In his commentary, Gilles de la Tourette then recognized the contributions of Guinon and Charcot to his initial description and gave this recommendation: *"If you wish to read a good survey of the question, I urge you to consult the thesis Mr. Catrou, my student, prepared in 1890 on the convulsive tic disease, based on twenty-six unpublished observations I sent to him."* Gilles de la Tourette admitted at this point that the expression "motor incoordination" was unsuitable and acknowledged the validity of Guinon's "convulsive tics": *"jerks, or tics, to use what has become the established expression."* There followed a long section on coprolalia and echolalia, *"what can truly be deemed psychic stigmata."* While the patients could be considered to belong *"to the unbalanced group,"* Gilles de la Tourette said he *"did not care for this expression."* For him, the use of arsenic had no place in their treatment. After discussing differential diagnoses, especially regarding chorea, Gilles de la Tourette vigorously contested the view of Brissaud (see later discussion), expressed in the thesis of his student Georges Patry (1869–?)[203] and describing *"the variable chorea of degenerates"*: *"In my opinion, I shall say so immediately, this condition cannot be differentiated from the convulsive tic disease."* Fourteen years after the initial article, this clarification in 1899 presented the disease's clinical picture and course in a comprehensive fashion that remains relevant today. It was an occasion for Gilles de la Tourette to repeat the aphorism, *"once a ticcer, always a ticcer."* In 1900, when he published his last paper in *La Revue Neurologique*, he revisited the nosology of chorea in pregnant women, denying the existence of an isolated pathology; at that time, abortions were performed in such cases to save the mother and avoid the birth of a disabled child. For Gilles de la Tourette, these cases of chorea were not chorea, but either hysteria or convulsive tic disorder.[204] However, he erroneously reaffirmed once again that Sydenham's chorea did not exist after puberty and had no link with rheumatism.

The Meige and Feindel Book

In 1902, Henry Meige (1866–1940) (Figures 9.9 and 9.10) and Eugène Feindel (1862–1930) published their work on tics and their treatment.[205] In the

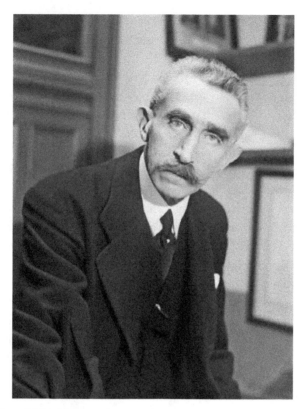

FIGURE 9.9 Henry Meige (1866–1940).
Copyright Henri Martinie / Roger-Viollet.

introduction, Brissaud was categorical: *"The authors of this book have resolutely identified the pathogenesis of tics as a mental process. The psychology of the ticcer can be easily penetrated in certain cases where the tic is equivalent to or superposed on 'other episodic stigmata of degeneration,' but the task becomes infinitely more complex when the incorrectness of psychic acts is limited to tics alone. Even under these circumstances, in examining the mental state, one always observes the insufficiency of inhibitory abilities, whose weakness allows countless unfortunate habits to form and grow entrenched over time. Such is the role of habit in the genesis of tics, revealing their similarity with all functional acts. A tic is often merely a function performed in an untimely or unsuitable manner."*

Brissaud spoke of Gilles de la Tourette syndrome as *"a lamentable neurosis"*; *"its only special feature is the somewhat systematic regularity of its progression. It is merely the superlative expression of a neuropathic and psychopathic disposition, in all ways similar to the disposition that gives rise to the most benign tics. The disease, in its initial manifestations, presents like a simple convulsive oddity that appears*

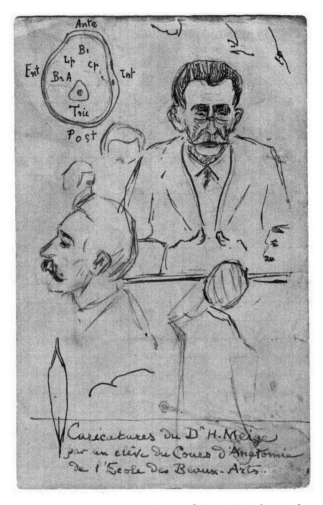

FIGURE 9.10 Henry Meige (1866–1940). A caricature of Henry Meige by a student of the School of Fine Arts, Paris, 1930.
Copyright Ecole Nationale des Beaux-arts, Paris. With kind permission.

insignificant. But when one considers that this oddity can go on indefinitely in time, spreading gradually to all limbs, accompanied by serious mental disorders that often lead to dementia, one realizes that this little symptom, this little premonitory tic at the start, always deserves to be viewed with defiance and energetically fought." This book laid the groundwork for the interference of psychoanalysis in the treatment of ticcers. The authors contested the etiopathogenic view, in all of its clairvoyance, that René Cruchet (1875–1959) (Figure 9.11) from Bordeaux proposed in 1901.

Cruchet based his reasoning on the work of Constantin von Monakow (1853–1930) and Wladimir Aleksandrowicz Muratoff, or Muratow (Владимир

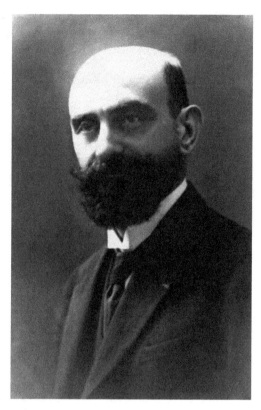

FIGURE 9.11 René Cruchet (1875–1959).
Private collection of the author.

Александрович Муратов 1865–1916) concerning athetosis and chorea. Similarly to these authors, he proposed a functional disorder *"of the cortex and basal ganglia of the brain."* [206,207] For Meige and Feindel, the tic—a coordinated movement—was evidence of a "reflex" activity of the cerebral cortex. They deduced that education (a movement oriented toward a goal) and therefore the will could overcome it. They compared the process to a baby's sucking, an innate automatism that becomes mastication, a learned automatism. They thus conceived of tics as *"the frequent repetition of a primitively voluntary movement."* In their view, the premonitory sensation associated with tics was proof that they were conscious acts, justifying their position based on Brissaud: *"The tic is a coordinated automatic act and thus of cortical origin."* They went so far as to compare tics with micturition and defecation, noting that their execution *"is preceded by a need and followed by satisfaction."* They considered the tic *"as a functional disturbance representing an act driven by an exaggerated, untimely need, followed by an excessive, inappropriate satisfaction."* Meige and Feindel used the incomplete observations reported in the seminal article of Gilles de la Tourette to posit that, alongside *"convulsive tic disease,"* there was a different clinical entity, neglected by Gilles de la Tourette but described by Brissaud: *"the variable chorea of degenerates."* This chorea *"has no uniformity in its current manifestations, or regularity in its progression, or constancy in its duration. . . . It is a neurosis that lacks symptomatic rigor as it were. . . . Do the involuntary manifestations of the syndrome warrant inclusion in the pathologies listed in the chapter on myoclonia?"*[208] It is surprising to read the following: *"Gilles de la Tourette refused to consider this condition as a chorea. For him, it is simply one of the forms of the convulsive tic disease; indeed, variable chorea does sometimes entail the utterance of explosive syllables and even coprolalia."* Brissaud seemed unaware of or unconcerned by Charcot's efforts to demonstrate the difference between chorea and tics. In any case, posterity has forgotten variable chorea and recognized Gilles de la Tourette syndrome. Meige and Feindel listed all of the medications already tried to reduce tics and stated their inefficacy, adding: *"Since ticcers have a mental state that favors all manias, one must always avoid using ether, morphine, or cocaine."* While electrotherapy and bathing in the sea were advised against, hydrotherapy was recommended, along with vigorous rubbing with a massage glove. Only *"re-education treatment"* found favor with Meige and Feindel: *"Immobilization of movements and movements of immobilization. . . . The first of these procedures consists in training the ticcer to keep the limbs and face absolutely still, photographically still, over progressively increasing time periods. . . . Parallel to imposing this discipline of immobility on patients, an effort will be made to teach them the discipline of movements. This involves making them execute slow, regular, correct movements, on command, that exercise the muscles in the region where the tic is located. . . . The adults responsible for young ticcers often lack sufficient firmness and authority to correct them, if the need arises. . . . After treatment of a tic, the task of the physician is not finished. Once the untimely movement is gone, there is still the mental state of the ticcer, which makes him easy prey for another offensive of the disease. If the mental state is sufficiently modified by re-education, then it is truly possible to hope for a definitive cure of the tic, through a firming of the will, where the congenital debility had previously allowed the tics to set in. But for some time it is wise to speak only of improvement. . . . Firmness, patience, goodness, and good sense—these are the all-powerful weapons that the physician must use to wage war on the tics. Docility, trust, and perseverance—these are the auxiliary means that the patient must provide to emerge victorious from this combat. Once this alliance is formed, the fight will begin, and will be without respite or mercy. It must be pursued unfailingly against all of the untimely habits, motor or otherwise."* After Morel, Ribot, a professor at the prestigious Collège de France and director of the influential *Revue Philosophique*, continued to develop the concept of degeneration (*"degeneration, that is, instability and psychological incoordination"*) and the associated notion of heredity, thereby providing an acceptable conceptual basis for explaining various social and asocial behaviors along with all sorts of problems, from alcoholism to depression to sterility.[209] The directive and authoritarian ideology developed by Meige and Feindel for treating tics was based on Ribot's 1883 book on diseases of the will, a best-seller in the psychological literature with its thirty-seven editions from 1883 to 1936.[210] Ribot declared: *"The voluntary faculty is closely tied to the involuntary faculty; the former rests on, and takes its force from the latter and is, by comparison, quite fragile. The education of the attention basically consists in nothing more than arousing and developing feigned perceptions and endeavoring to make them stable through repetition."* This explains why the will should make it possible to prevent outbursts of involuntary movements through sustained attention. The repetition of the adaptive movements should prevent involuntary movements because fundamentally, *"the brain is a motor organ, which is to say that many of its elements produce movement and there is not a single state of consciousness that does not contain, to some degree, motor elements."* According to Ribot, Gilles de la Tourette syndrome, like aboulia, depression, or hysteria, is *"a state of inco-ordination, lost equilibrium, anarchy, and moral ataxia that results from a constitutional impotence of the will."* It is easy to see why Meige and Feindel spoke of a fight *"without respite or mercy."* These clinical, pathogenic, and therapeutic considerations would become the accepted rule for more than half a century, making the book of Meige and Feindel, translated into English[211] and German,[212] the reference for diagnosing and treating tics. The Englishman Samuel Alexander Kinnier Wilson (1878–1937),[213] known for his description of the eponymous disease involving excess copper in the organism due to a metabolic defect,[214] adopted the theories of Meige and Feindel on tics in 1927. However, he noted the difficulty of giving a pathophysiological interpretation based on the psychopathology causing the abnormal movements, in particular tics, which were present in the sequelae of the encephalitis epidemic (Constantin von Economo, 1876–1931).[215] A recent publication casts new light on these theories based on a new physiopathological paradigm: *"Aberrant reinforcement signals to the sensorimotor striatum may be fundamental for the formation of stimulus-response associations and may contribute to the habitual behavior and tics of this syndrome."*[216]

In Medical Treatises

In the 1894 *Traité des Maladies du Système nerveux* by Joseph Grasset (1849–1918) and Georges Rauzier (1862–1920), the tic chapter used elements developed by

Letulle in the Jaccoud dictionary without presenting Gilles de la Tourette syndrome as an isolated entity.[217]

In 1902, Henri Triboulet (1864–1920) wrote the tics chapter in the *Traité de Médecine* of Brouardel and Augustin Gilbert (1858–1927). He did not distinguish transient childhood tics, leaving the reader with the impression that all ticcers have Gilles de la Tourette syndrome: *"The prognosis is always serious, due to the etiological principle: a transmittable hereditary flaw."* The discussion of differential diagnosis was more soundly structured and highlighted how to distinguish tics from chorea, hysteria, and "paramyoclonus." He recommended treating patients—as early as possible, he emphasized—with the methods of Meige and Feindel.[218]

In the so-called Charcot-Bouchard *Traité de Médecine*—actually the work of Brissaud and published in 1894—there was no chapter on tics.[219] By contrast, the *Pratique Médico-Chirurgicale* of Brissaud, Pinard, and Reclus (1909) contained a long chapter on the subject, written by Meige. The descriptions of tics were detailed, and their etiology was linked to *"neuropathic and psychopathic"* heredity. Gilles de la Tourette syndrome was reduced to banal tics associated with coprolalia, the nature of which was contested in keeping with Magnan's opinion.[220]

Psychoanalytic Inquiry

The era of psychoanalytic iatrogenesis began in 1921 with the publication of a tic theory by the Hungarian psychoanalyst Sandor Ferenczi (1873–1933) who, prior to that point, had never examined any patients,[221] basing his ideas on the account of a ticcer that formed the long first chapter of the Meige and Feindel book and was entitled *"The Confessions of a Victim to Tic."* For Ferenczi, tics were a stereotyped equivalent of onanism; ticcers were thus frustrated masturbators! Sigmund Freud (1856–1939) wrote little on tics. He was in Paris from October 1885 to February 1886, where he met Gilles de la Tourette and Guinon, and thus he must have been aware of their articles on "convulsive tics." In his study on hysteria with Josef Breuer (1842–1925), the second case was that of Frau Emmy von N.,[222] who may have been misdiagnosed by Freud and in fact suffered from Gilles de la Tourette syndrome.[223] Of course, it is not possible to establish a retrospective diagnosis with certitude. It seems probable that Freud eliminated Gilles de la Tourette syndrome as a diagnosis because his patient's tics seemed to disappear, albeit temporarily, under hypnosis, whereas "convulsive tics" were not modified. Freud was of Guinon's opinion that links existed with hysteria or that the disorder was frequently associated with convulsive tic disease.[224] After 1893, Freud never proposed any psychoanalytic explanations of the pathophysiology of tics. As for Charles-Louis Trepsat (1879–1937), in 1922, he recounted in *Le Progrès Médical* his psychoanalytic interpretation of the confession of a ticcer, a victim of onanism in childhood. Trepsat supported his case by noting that the diagnosis of tics was made by Babiński, whereas the clinical picture resembles dystonia.[225]

The Swiss psychiatrist and psychoanalyst Raymond de Saussure (1894–1971), Freud's student, stands out honorably among other psychoanalysts. He discussed the etiological role of encephalitis lethargica, described by von Economo, and presented an observation of Gilles de la Tourette syndrome in which the tics often took the form of repeated yawning: *"Despite the similarities between Gilles de la Tourette's description and Blanche's symptoms, we still hesitate to consider her yawning fits as hysterical symptoms."* For Saussure, the abnormal movements of the young patient he had treated at the Clinique de Céry (where Gilles de la Tourette died) were organic in origin, like the parkinsonian symptoms of other victims of this epidemic, and not psychological.[226]

The psychoanalyst Serge Lebovici (1915–2000) was at the other end of the spectrum and, in 1951, wrote that tics were the *"symptom signal of an obsessional psychoneurosis"*—hence the need for early treatment, which entailed *"prophylactic mental hygiene"* to avoid the development of a neurosis in adulthood.[227]

Early Modern Concepts

In 1941, André DeWulf (1903–2000) and Ludo van Bogaert (1897–1989) confirmed the validity of the conclusions of Charcot and his students, Gilles de la Tourette and Guinon, on the neurological organicity of the disease. The clinical picture for their patient was typical, with onset at age eighteen. When they began treating him at age thirty, his general condition was very impaired by advanced osseous tuberculosis. Aside from the abnormal movements, the patient had no psychiatric comorbidity. Shortly after his death following status epilepticus, they performed an autopsy: *"We undertook a detailed histological study, exploring in particular the two motor zones, the cerebellar apparatus, the red nucleus, the basal ganglia, the olivary bodies, and the anterior horns of the cervical spine. Aside from what appears to be cellular sclerosis in layers IV-V-VI in the frontal, motor, and parietal regions, we did not observe any noteworthy details. . . . What we find important in this negative examination is that it permits the conclusion that Gilles de la Tourette disease has no lesional substratum, which in turn permits us to include it among the systematized extra-pyramidal diseases."* The fact that this 1941 paper was written in Belgium under Nazi occupation and published in Switzerland may explain its lack of dissemination after the war among psychoanalysts. Nonetheless, the work gave the authors an opportunity to produce one of the first films of motor and phonic tics one month before the patient's death.[228,229] The photos of the patient that illustrated the article were reprinted in 1949 in a medical treatise published in Paris[230] (Figure 9.12).

The publications in German on this subject include the 1892 paper by Friedrich Jolly (1804–1904), a professor of psychiatry and director of the neuropsychiatric clinic at the Berlin Charité Hospital;[231] the 1896 paper by

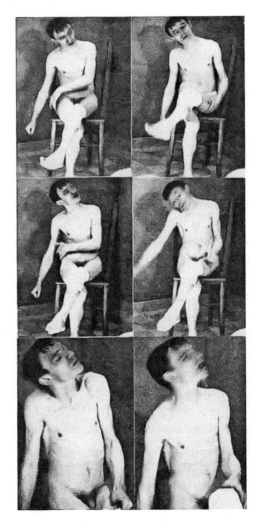

FIGURE 9.12 Patient with tic disorder, photographed by André DeWulf and Ludo van Bogaert in 1949.
Private collection of the author.

Johannes Bresler (1866–1942), who worked in an asylum in Kreuzburg (Upper Silesia), then part of Germany, currently Kluczbork (Opole Voivodeship) in Poland;[232] the 1898 paper by Hermann Wille of Münsterlingen, son of and assistant to Ludwig Wille (1834–1912), a German psychiatrist who worked in Basel, Switzerland;[233] the 1899 paper of Georg Köster (1867–1932), a professor of psychiatry and neurology in Leipzig;[234] the 1927 paper by Erwin Straus (1891–1975), a neuropsychiatrist and philosopher, assistant to Karl Bonhoeffer (1868–1948) at Berlin Charité Hospital (immigrated to Baltimore in 1938), also a critic of psychoanalysis and friend of Eugène Minkowski (1885–1972);[235] the 1927 work of Joseph Wilder (1895–1976), assistant to Otto Pötzl (1877–1962) at the university neuropsychiatric clinic of Vienna (fled to New York in 1937);[236] and the 1932 paper of Werner Runge (1882–?), a neurologist in Chemnitz.[237]

The full history of Gilles de la Tourette syndrome after World War II, especially the importance of psychoanalytic theory, particularly in the United States, is well presented in Howard Kushner's book, which stands as the reference work on this subject.[238]

Arthur and Elaine Shapiro

In a 1965 review of the literature, Diane Kelman found forty-four authentic descriptions of Gilles de la Tourette syndrome in all medical publications worldwide between 1906 and 1964. She found slightly higher incidence in males than in females, onset before age ten, and normal intelligence without any particular risk of *"degeneration"* (she used the nineteenth-century term). She confirmed the absence of any link between Jumping, Latah, Myriachit, and Gilles de la Tourette syndrome. Finally, she noted that neuroleptics seemed to reduce the symptomatology but that proper perspective was lacking to accurately assess their impact.[239] Indeed, it had only been recently, in 1961, that Jean-Noël Seignot had succeeded for the first time in effectively treating one of his patients through experimental use of haloperidol.[240] His publication did not generate immediate echoes. Then, in 1968, Arthur K. Shapiro (1923–1995) and his wife Elaine, both American psychiatrists, successfully replicated Seignot's observation. In their article, which American medical journals refused to publish, they demonstrated the efficacy of haloperidol in calming the symptomatology of Gilles de la Tourette syndrome.[241] Their work did have a large impact, first in the community of American psychiatrists and later among American neurologists. Shapiro thus became the instigator of a radical paradigm shift. This disease is organic: psychotherapy and, to an even greater degree, psychoanalysis have no role in its treatment, aside from helping patients and their families tolerate the psychoaffective repercussions of the disease. The Shapiros estimated the number of patients in the United States to be approximately 100,000 in their excellent 1978 book, which can be considered the first work since the early 1900s to comprehensively address the subject.[242] One of their colleagues, Ruth Bruun of Cornell University, described Arthur Shapiro as *"a revolutionary, willing to challenge the prevailing dogma, dynamic, charming, and relentlessly stubborn when fighting for what he thought was right and more honest than psychoanalysis then fashionable, an engaging speaker and a man of diverse interests and enthusiasms. It is extremely unusual for a couple of researchers to completely change the prevailing view of a disease, but this is exactly what they did.*[243] We salute the tenacity and perseverance of the Shapiros, who brought about a renaissance in work on Gilles de la Tourette syndrome and improved treatment for patients. Twenty years after their landmark publication, the Shapiros were able to attend a large meeting held on May 2 and 3, 1985, at Hôpital La Salpêtrière to celebrate the 100-year anniversary of the seminal article.

Gilles de la Tourette had highlighted the descriptions of some of his predecessors, notably Itard and Trousseau. However, according to Shapiro, the first description of the disease appeared in the book *Malleus Maleficarum* (often translated *Hammer of the Witches*), written by two monks, Jakob Sprenger (1436–1495) and Henricus Institoris (1430–1505), and published in 1487[244] with the approval of Pope Innocent VIII. There were several successive editions.[245] These authors described a priest with motor and phonic tics that, at the time, were considered a sign of satanic possession, to be addressed by exorcism. The 1973 American horror film *The Exorcist*, directed by William Friedkin and based on William Peter Blatty's 1971 novel of the same name, was largely inspired by the accounts in *Malleus Maleficarum*. The modern-day mother of a twelve-year-old girl with "spasms" and coprolalia, very probably a true case of Gilles de la Tourette syndrome, thinks her daughter is the victim of a possession and calls on two priests for an exorcism.

By Way of Conclusion

For Howard Kushner, the description of the disease by Gilles de la Tourette illustrates the strong role of medical fiction in the construction of a syndrome.[246] From premises that were erroneous but useful for his intellectual approach (Jumping, Latah, Myriachit) and relying on Itard's perfect, fictionalized observation of the Marquise de Dampierre, Gilles de la Tourette isolated part of the clinical symptomatology of the disease named for him. Being the fine clinician that he was, Charcot realized that the initial description was incomplete and the name given by Gilles de la Tourette (motor incoordination) inaccurate. After collecting more observations, some of which were described during the Tuesday Lessons, he tasked Guinon, Gilles de la Tourette's successor, with completing the description, especially as concerned the obsessional disturbances frequently associated with motor and phonic tics. It bears repeating that neither Gilles de la Tourette nor Charcot examined the Marquise de Dampierre, even though they made her observation emblematic of the disease they were describing.

Between 1885 and 1903, several new observations were published in France and elsewhere but, thereafter, Gilles de la Tourette syndrome, which Guinon called convulsive tic disease in refusal of the eponym, fell from prominence and seemed forgotten until the early 1960s. Apart from helping with Catrou's thesis and his own article in 1899, Gilles de la Tourette never did any further work on "his disease." Neither he nor his contemporaries seemed aware of the relevance and significance of the 1885 publication. In the 1904 biography Le Gendre wrote in memory of his friend Gilles de la Tourette, he referred to this work very briefly in a few lines and without elaboration. He did not even note that Charcot had honored Gilles de la Tourette with an eponym, whereas his other works were highlighted and presented in detail. Had Gilles de la Tourette been named Martin, or Leblanc or Guinon, would the eponym have been created? Whatever the case may be, in publishing this work as a young man, even before defending his doctoral thesis, Gilles de la Tourette is deserving of his undeniable posthumous fame.

Notes

1. Scharf JM, Miller LL, Gauvin CA, Alabiso J, Mathews CA, Ben-Shlomo Y. Population prevalence of Tourette syndrome: a systematic review and meta-analysis. *Move Dis.* 2015;30(2):221–228

2. Martino D, Madhusudan N, Zis P, Cavanna AE. An introduction to the clinical phenomenology of Tourette syndrome. In *Advances in the Neurochemistry and Neuropharmacology of Tourette Syndrome. Int Rev Neurobiol.* 2013;112:1–33.

3. Robertson MM. The Gilles de la Tourette syndrome: the current status. *Arch Dis Child Educ Pract Ed.* 2012;97(5):166–175.

4. Cath DC, Hedderly T, Ludolph AG, Stern JS, Murphy T, Hartmann A, Czernecki V, Robertson MM, Martino D, Munchau A, Rizzo R; ESSTS Guidelines Group. European clinical guidelines for Tourette syndrome and other tic disorders. Part I: assessment. *Eur Child Adolesc Psychiatry.* 2011;20(4):155–171.

5. Cavanna AE, Servo S, Monaco F, Robertson MM. The behavioral spectrum of Gilles de la Tourette syndrome. *J Neuropsychiatry Clin Neurosci.* 2009 Winter;21(1):13–23.

6. Jankovic J, Kurlan R. Tourette syndrome: evolving concepts. *Move Dis.* 2011;26(6):1149–1156.

7. Scharf JM, Yu D, Mathews CA, Neale BM, et al. Genome-wide association study of Tourette's syndrome. *Mol Psychiatry.* 2013;18(6):721–728.

8. Yu D, Mathews CA, Scharf JM, et al. Cross-disorder genome-wide analyses suggest a complex genetic relationship between Tourette's syndrome and OCD. *Am J Psychiatry.* 2015;172(1):82–93.

9. Martino D, Zis P, Buttiglione M, The role of immune mechanisms in Tourette syndrome. *Brain Res.* 2015;1617:126–143.

10. Leckman JF, Vaccarino FM. What does immunology have to do with brain development and neuropsychiatric disorders? *Brain Res.* 2015;1617:1–6.

11. Martino D, Macerollo A, Leckman JF. Neuroendocrine aspects of Tourette syndrome. *Int Rev Neurobiol.* 2013;112:239–279.

12. Kataoka Y, Kalanithi PS, Grantz H, Schwartz ML, Saper C, Leckman JF, Vaccarino FM. Decreased number of parvalbumin and cholinergic interneurons in the striatum of individuals with Tourette syndrome. *J Comp Neurol.* 2010;518(3):277–291.

13. Robertson MM, Eapen V. Tourette's: syndrome, disorder or spectrum? Classificatory challenges and an appraisal of the DSM criteria. *Asian J Psychiatry.* 2014;11:106–113.

14. Gilles de la Tourette G. La maladie des tics convulsifs. *La Semaine Médicale.* 1899;19(20):153–156.

15. DeWulf A, von Bogaert L. Etudes anatomo-cliniques des syndromes hypercinétiques complexes. Une observation anatomo-clinique de maladie des tics (Gilles de la Tourette). *Monatsschrift für Psychiatrie und Neurologie.* 1941;104(1–2):53–61.

16. JJDEM. (Jean Jourdin, docteur en médecine). *La Vraye cognoissance du cheval, ses maladies et remèdes.* Paris: Thomas de Ninville. 1647.

17. Giovanni Battista Ferraro (1528–1569). Del Tiro (1550). Reproduced in Ferraro Pirro-Antonio (ed.), *Cavallo Frenato.* Venetia: Antonio Pace. 1602.

18. Cruchet R. *Traité des torticolis spamodiques.* Paris: Masson. 1907.

19. Brissaud E. Preface. In H Meige and E Feindel (eds.), *Les tics et leur traitement.* Paris: Masson. 1902.

20. "As for the title, I formed it from two Greek words: Orthos, which means straight, free of deformity, characterized by rectitude; & Paidion, which means child."

21. Andry de Boisregard N. *L'orthopédie ou l'art de prévenir et de corriger dans les enfans, les difformités du corps. Le tout par des moyens à la portée des Peres & es Meres & des personnes qui ont des enfans à élever.* Paris: La Veuve Alix. 1741.

22. Boissier de Sauvages F. *Nosologie Méthodique dans laquelle les maladies sont rangées par classes, suivent le système de Sydenham, & l'ordre des botanistes.* Paris: Hérissant le fils. 1771.

23. Dordain G. Le concept de tic dans l'histoire des mouvements anormaux. *La Revue Neurologique.* 1986;142(11):803–807.

24. Jean-Frédéric Blumenbach (1752–1840), a professor of medicine in Göttingen, is known for his anthropological studies and also developed craniology. His physiology treatise, first published in Latin in 1787, presents a theory of multiple vital principles (fluids and solids) whose interaction is the basis for bodily activity and function.

25. Blumenbach JF. *Institutions physiologiques, traduites du Latin par JF Pugnet.* Lyon: JT. Reymann. 1797.

26. Albrecht von Haller (1708–1777), a professor of medicine in Göttingen, then in his native city of Bern; a prolific author, also a poet and naturalist, he is known for having distinguished nervous influx (sensitivity) from muscular contraction (irritability).

27. von Haller A. *Dissertation sur les parties irritables et sensibles des animaux.* Lausanne: MM. Bousquet. 1755.

28. Soulagne GA. *Essai sur le tic en général et en particulier sur le tic douloureux de la pommette.* Thèse Montpellier. G. Uzar et A. Ricard. An XII ou 1803.

29. Fothergill J. Of a painful affection of the face. *Medical Observations and Inquiries by a Society of Physicians. London.* 1773;5:129–142.

30. Pearce JM. Trigeminal neuralgia (Fothergill's disease) in the 17th and 18th centuries. *J Neurol Neurosurg Psychiatry.* 2003;74(12):1688.

31. Lewy FH The first authentic case of major trigeminal neuralgia and some comments on the history of this disease. *Ann Med Hist.* 1938;10:247–250.

32. André N. *Observations pratiques sur les maladies de l'urèthre, et sur plusieurs faits convulsifs, & la guérison de plusieurs maladies chirurgicales avec la décomposition d'un remède propre à réprimer la dissolution gangréneuse & cancéreuse, & à la réparer; avec des principes qui pourront servir à employer les différens caustique.* Paris: Delaguette, Imprimeur du Collège et de l'Acad. Roy. de chir. rue S. Jacques, à l'Olivier. 1756.

33. Sigismond Jaccoud (1830–1913).

34. Letulle M. Tics. In S Jaccoud (ed.), *Nouveau Dictionnaire de Médecine et de Chirurgie pratiques.* T35. Paris: JB. Baillière. 1883.

35. Shapiro AK, Shapiro E. Tourette syndrome: history and present status. In AJ Friedhoff and TN Chase (eds.), *Gilles de la Tourette syndrome.* Advances in Neurology, vol 35. New York: Raven Press. 1982.

36. Botrel JP. *De la chorée considérée comme une affection rhumatismale.* Thèse no. 79. Paris: Imprimerie Rignoux. 1850.

37. Sée G. De la chorée, rapports du rhumatisme et des maladies cœur avec les affections nerveuses convulsives. *Mémoires de l'Académie impériale de Médecine.* 1850;15:374–525.

38. Roger H. Recherches cliniques sur la chorée, sur le rhumatisme et sur les maladies du cœur les enfants. *Archives Générales de Médecine.* 1868;10:26–42; 148–178; 288–304; 393–421.

39. Osler W. On the general etiology and symptoms of chorea, based on the records of 410 cases at the Infirmary for Nervous Diseases. *Phila Med News.* 1887;51:437–441 / 465-470.

40. Gilles de la Tourette G, Joffroy A. Compte-Rendu de la séance de la Société de Neurologie du 7 juin 1900. *Archives de Neurologie.* 1900;10(55):65–66.

41. Huntington G. On chorea. *Med Surg Rep.* 1872;26:317–321.

42. Vassitch MV. *Etude sur les chorées des adultes.* Thèse no. 361. Paris: A. Parent. 1883.

43. Lanska DJ. The history of movement disorders. *Handb Clin Neurol.* Edinburgh, London, New York, Oxford, Philadelphia : Elsevier. 2010;95:501–546.

44. Leven M. *Pathologie générale et classification des chorées.* Paris: A. Delahaye. 1869.

45. Charcot JM. *Leçons du mardi à La Salpêtrière. Policlinique 1887–1888.* Paris: Bureaux du Progrès Médical et Delahaye & Lecrosnier. 1887–1888.

46. Roth D. *Histoire de la musculation irrésistible ou de la chorée animale.* Paris: JB. Baillière. 1850.

47. Paracelsi Th. Lib. II. *De Cavsa Et Origine Morborvm (Von vrsachen vnd herkomen der kranckheite). De Morbis Invisibilibvs (Von den vnsichtbaren kranckheiten, Jetzt newlich an tag kommen).* Gedruckt zu Cöln Durch die Erben Arnoldi Byrckmanni. 1566.

48. Regnard A. *Essais d'histoire et de critiques scientifiques à propos des conférences de la Faculté de Médecine.* Paris: Chez l'Auteur. 1865.

49. Blocq P. Sorciers et Possédés. *Gazette hebdomadaire de Médecine et de Chirurgie.* 1892;39(5):59–60.

50. Wier I. *Histoires, disputes et discours.* Paris: Bureaux du Progrès Médical. 1885.

51. Beard GM. Experiments with the "Jumpers" of Maine. *Popular Science Monthly.* 1880;18:170–178.

52. Beard GM. Neurasthenia (nerve exhaustion): with remarks on treatment. *St. Louis Med Surg J.* 1879;36:345–365.

53. Beard GM. Remarks upon "Jumpers or Jumping Frenchmen." *J Nerv Ment Dis.* 1878;5:526.

54. Anonymous. Jumping Frenchmen. *London Medical Record.* 1878;5:326.

55. Beard GM. Experiments with "Jumpers" or "Jumping Frenchmen of Maine." *J Nerv Ment Dis.* 1880;7:487–490.

56. http://en.wikisource.org/wiki/Popular_Science_Monthly/Volume_18/December_1880/Experiments_with_the_Jumpers_of_Maine

57. Melotti G. Intorno ad alcuni casi di tic convulsivo con coprolalie ed echolalia. *Riforma Medica*. Agosto 1885;1.

58. O'Brien HA. Latah. *J R Asiatic Soc (Straits Branch)*. 1883;11:143–154.

59. O'Brien HA. Latah. *J R Asiatic Soc (Straits Branch)*. 1884;12:283–284.

60. Gilles de la Tourette G. Jumping, Latah, Myriachit. *Archives de Neurologie*. 1884;8:68–74.

61. Blustein BE. *Preserve Your Love for Science: Life of William A. Hammond, American Neurologist*. Cambridge and New York: Cambridge University Press. 1991.

62. Hammond W. *A Treatrise on Diseases of the Nervous System*. New York: D. Appleton and Co. 1871.

63. Hammond W. Miryachit, nouvelle maladie du système nerveux. *L'Union Médicale*. 1884;38(59):706–708.

64. Hammond W. Miryachit, nuova malattia del sistema nervoso. *Medicina contemporanea (Napoli)*. 1884;1:126–130.

65. Hammond WA. Miryachit: a newly described disease of the nervous system and its analogues. *Br Med J*. 1884;1(1216):758–759.

66. Buckingham BH. Foulk GC, McLean W. *Observations upon the Korean Coast, Japanese-Korean ports and Siberia, made during a journey from the Asiatic Stations to the United States through Siberia and Europe, June 3 to September 8, 1882*. Information from Abroad, General Information Series Number 1. Washington DC: Office of Naval intelligence, Navy Department, Bureau of Navigation. Government Printing Office. 1883.

67. Lieutenant Benjamin H. Buckingham was part of an American military delegation that came to test the qualities of iron-nickel alloys developed by the Schneider-Creusot steel mill in 1891 and later used in American weapons due to their superiority over the alloys available up to that time. (Zapffe CA. A brief history of alloy steel. *Metal Progress*. 1948;18:459–467.)

68. George Clayton Foulk (1856–1893), a navy officer and diplomat, first served in Asia from 1877 to 1883, later represented the United States at the American legation in Korea from 1883 to 1885, and then acted as *chargé d'affaires* until 1887. After being discharged from the army, he settled in Japan where he represented American companies from 1888 to 1890. From 1890 until his death, he was a professor of mathematics at Doshisha University in Kyoto. (*The United States in Asia: A Historical Dictionary*.)

69. Walter McLean (1855–1930) would serve as the commander of the Norfolk Naval Shipyard from November 25, 1915, to February 4, 1918. He is known for having inspected several German warships and for holding them prisoner in American ports until the end of World War I (Wikipedia).

70. Nuttal M. *Encyclopedia of the Arctic*. New York: Routledge. 2004.

71. Steller GW. *Beschreibung Von Dem Lande Kamtschatka*. Frankfurt and Leipzig: JG. Flaischer. 1774.

72. Ohayon MM, Mahowald MW, Leger D. Are confusional arousals pathological? *Neurology*. 2014;83(9):834–841.

73. Gilles de la Tourette G. Étude sur une affection nerveuse caractérisée par l'incoordination motrice, accompagnée d'écholalie et de coprolalie. *Archives de neurologie*. 1885;9:19–42 / 158–200.

74. Hale ME, Long JH, McHenry MJ, Westneat MW. Evolution of behavior and neural control of the fast-start escape response. *Evolution*. 2002;56(5):993–1007.

75. Moro E. Das erste Trimenon. *Münchener medizinische Wochenschrift*. 1918;65:1147–1159; 1920;67:360.

76. Hunt WA, Landis C. Studies of the startle pattern. *J Psychol*. 1936;2(1):201–219/ 1936;2(2):339–352; 1937;4(1):199–206; 1937;3(2)339–343; 487–490.

77. Goldstein K, Landis C, Hunt WA, Clarke FM. Moro reflex and startle pattern. *Arch Neuropsychol.* 1938;40(2):322–327.

78. Rabinovitch R. An exaggerated startle reflex resembling a kicking horse. *Can Med Assoc J.* 1965;93(3):130.

79. Kunkle E. The "Jumpers" of Maine: a reappraisal. *Arch Intern Med.* 1967;119(4):355–358.

80. Saint-Hilaire MH, Saint-Hilaire JM, Granger L. Jumping Frenchmen of Maine. *Neurology.* 1986;36(9):1269–1271.

81. Saint-Hilaire MH, Saint-Hilaire JM. Jumping Frenchmen of Maine. *Move Dis.* 2001;16(3):530.

82. Kunkle EC. The "jumpers" of Maine: past history and present status. *J Maine Med Assoc.* 1965;56(9):191–193.

83. Bakker MJ, Tijssen MA. Jumping Frenchman of Maine. In K Kompoliti and L Verhagen-Metman (eds.), *The Encyclopedia of Movements Disorders.* Oxford: Academic Press. 2010.

84. "Goosey" is a familiar English word, but is not without special significance. "To goose" means to push, shake, tickle, incite, or tease. Interestingly, an equivalent exists in Hungarian: *"buta ember."*

85. Hardison JE. Are the jumping Frenchmen of Maine goosey? *JAMA.* 1980;244(1):70.

86. Massey EW. Goosey patients: relationship to jumping Frenchmen, Myriachit, Latah and tic convulsif. *N Carolina Med J.* 1984;45(9):556–558.

87. Howard R, Ford R. From the jumping Frenchmen of Maine to post-traumatic stress disorder: the startle response in neuropsychiatry. *Psychol Med.* 1992;22(3):695–707.

88. Day HF. *Pine Tree Ballads: Rhymed Stories of Unplanned Human Natur' Up in Maine.* Boston: Small, Maynard & Co. 1902.

89. Suhren O, Bruyn GW, Tuynman A. Hyperekplexia, a hereditary startle syndrome. *J Neurol Sci.* 1966;3:577–605.

90. Kok O, Bruyn G. An unidentified hereditary disease. *Lancet* 1962;279(7243):1359.

91. Koning-Tijssen MA, Brouwer OF. Hyperekplexia in the first year of life. *Move Dis.* 2000;15(6):1293–1296.

92. Thomas RH. Hyperekplexia: overexcitable and underdiagnosed. *Dev Med Child Neurol.* 2015;57(4):313

93. Dreissen YE, Bakker MJ, Koelman JH, Tijssen MA. Exaggerated startle reactions. *Clin Neurophysiol.* 2012;123(1):34–44.

94. Turecki G, Grand'Maison F, Lemieux B, Rouleau G. Hyperekplexia and the alpha1 subunit glycine receptor gene (GLRA1). *Arch Neurol.* 1996;53(9):836–837.

95. de Juan-Sanz J, Núñez E, Zafra F, Berrocal M, et al. Presynaptic control of glycine transporter 2 (GlyT2) by physical and functional association with plasma membrane Ca2+-ATPase (PMCA) and Na+-Ca2+ exchanger (NCX). *J Biol Chem.* 2014;289(49):34308–343024.

96. Bhidayasiri R, Truong DD. Startle syndromes. *Handb Clin Neurol.* Edinburgh, London, New York, Oxford, Philadelphia : Elsevier. 2011;100:421–430.

97. Fourlanos S, Neal A, So M, Evans A. Latent auto-immune diabetes in stiff-person syndrome. *Diabetes Care.* 2014;37(10):e214–e215.

98. Alajouanine T, Gastaut H. La syncinésie-sursaut et l'épilepsie-sursaut à déclenchement sensoriel ou sensitif inopiné. *Revue Neurologie (Paris).* 1955;93:29–41.

99. Alajouanine T, Gastaut H. La syncinésie-sursaut et l'épilepsie-sursaut à déclenchement sensoriel ou sensitif inopiné: considérations sur les épilepsies dites réflexes. In *Bases physiologiques et aspects cliniques de l'épilepsie.* Paris: Masson. 1958:199–231.

100. Chauvel P, Trottier S, Vignel JP et al. Somatomotor seizures of frontal lobe origin. In P Chauvel, AV Delgado-Escueta, E Halgren, and J Bancaud (eds.), *Frontal Lobe Seizures and Epilepsies. Adv Neurol.* New York: Raven press. 1992:185–232.

101. Winzeler RL. The study of Malayan Latah. *Indonesia.* 1984;37:77–104.

102. Yap PM. The Latah reaction: its pathodynamics and nosological position. *J Ment Sci.* 1952;98(413):515–564.
103. Yap P. Classification of the culture-bound reactive syndromes. *Austral NZ J Psychiatry.* 1967;1(4):172–179.
104. Thomson JT. *Some Glimpses into Life in the Far East.* London: Richardson, 1864.
105. van Leent FJ. Contributions à la géographie médicale. *Archives de Médecine Navale.* 1867;8:172–173.
106. van Leent FJ. Communication sur le béri-béri. *Congrès Périodique international des Sciences médicales.* 1880;6:170–194.
107. Forbes HO. *A Naturalist's Wanderings in Eastern Archipelago.* New York: Harper and Brothers. 1885.
108. Gimlette JD. Remarks on the etiology, symptoms and treatment of Latah, with report of two cases. *Br Med J.* 1897;2(1912):455–457.
109. Murphy HBM. *Comparative Psychiatry: The International and Intercultural Distribution of Mental Illness.* Berlin: Springer Verlag. 1982.
110. Winzeler RL. *Latah in Southeast Asia: The History and Ethnography of a Culture-Bound Syndrome.* New York: Cambridge University Press. 1995.
111. Tokarski A. Meriatschenje und maladie des tics convulsifs. *Neurologisches CentralBlatt.* 1890;9(21):662–663.
112. Tokarski A. Myriachit et maladie des tics convulsifs. *La Semaine Médicale.* 1891;11:184.
113. Bagenoff PR. Myriatchénié et Klikouchisme. *Archives de Neurologie.* 1911;2:273–274.
114. Armangué y Tuset J. *Mimicismo ó neurósis imitante ("Miryachit, Jumping, Latah").* Barcelona: Tip. de Remirez. 1884.
115. Joseph AB, Saint-Hilaire M-H. Startle syndromes. In AB Joseph and R Young (eds.), *Movement Disorders in Neurology and Neuropsychiatry,* 2nd Ed. New York: Blackwell Science; 1998:457–462.
116. Rizzolatti G, Fogassi L, Gallese V. Neurophysiological mechanisms underlying the understanding and imitation of action. *Nature Rev Neurosci.* 2001;2(9):661–670.
117. Rizzolatti G. The mirror neuron system and its function in humans. *Anat Embryol.* 2005;210(5-6):419–421.
118. Kenny MG. Latah: the logic of fear. In Wazir Jahan Karim (ed.), *Emotions of Culture: A Malay Perspective.* Singapore: Oxford University Press. 1990:123–141.
119. Aberle DF. Arctic hysteria and Latah in Mongolia. *Trans N Y Acad Sci.* 1952;14(7):291–297.
120. Simons RC. *Boo! Culture, Experience, and the Startle Reflex.* New York: Oxford University Press. 1996.
121. Simons RC. *The Culture-Bound Syndromes: Folk Illnesses of Psychiatric and Anthropological Interest.* Dordrecht, Boston, and Lancaster: D. Reidel Publishing Company. 2013.
122. Stevens H. "Jumping Frenchmen of Maine" Myriachit. *Arch Neurol.* 1965;12(3):311–314.
123. Simons RC. The interminable debate on the nature of Latah. *J Nerv Ment Dis.* 1994;182(6):339–341.
124. Bartholomew RE. Disease, disorder, or deception? Latah as habit in a Malay extended family. . *J Nerv Ment Dis.* 1994;182(6):331–8.
125. Chapel JL. Gilles de la Tourette's syndrome, Latah, Myriachit, and Jumpers revisited. *N Y State J Med.* 1970;70(17):2201–2204.
126. Lucas P. *De l'imitation contagieuse ou de la propagation sympathique des névroses et des monomanies.* Paris: Didot le Jeune. 1833.
127. *Echomatisme* was coined by Pierre Marie (1853–1940) with a meaning close to Charcot's echokinesis.
128. Sigaud Cl. *De L'échomatisme, essai de pathogénie psycho-physiologique.* Thèse Lyon, 2 décembre 1889. Lyon: Pitrat ainé. 1889.

129. Une société de Gens de Lettres. *Biographie des hommes remarquables des Basses-Alpes ou dictionnaire historique de tous les personnages de département qui se sont signalés par leur génie, leurs talents, leurs travaux, la sainteté de leur vie, leurs vertus ou leurs actes de bienfaisance, depuis les temps les plus reculés jusqu'à nos jours.* Digne: Repos Editeur-Imprimeur-Libraire. 1850.

130. Bouteille EM. *Traité de la chorée ou Danse de Saint-Guy.* Paris: Vinçard. 1810.

131. Itard was one of the first specialists on deafness in the nineteenth century and dedicated himself to the education of the deaf. This led him to handle the case of the "Wild Boy of Aveyron," who likely had autism, from 1801 to 1806.

132. Itard JG. Mémoire sur quelques fonctions involontaires des appareils de la locomotion, de la préhension et de la voix. *Archives Générales de Médecine.* 1825;3(8):385–407.

133. This Hungarian physician, widely known in Paris at the time, also distinguished himself as the "inventor of the calculator" at the French National Exposition in 1844. He had a large private art collection, and it took a week to auction it off at the Hôtel Drouot, from Friday, June 8, to Saturday June 16, 1888.

134. Roth DD. *Histoire de la musculation irrésistible ou de la chorée anormale.* Paris: JB. Baillière. 1850.

135. Sandras S. *Traité pratique des Maladies Nerveuses.* Paris: Germer Baillière. 1851.

136. Quantin E. *De la chorée.* Thèse no. 54. Paris: Imprimerie Rignoux. 4 avril 1857.

137. Giulio Melotti was born on November 18, 1857, in Bologna, son of Federico Napoleone Melotti, and he defended his thesis on July 1, 1882, in Bologna.

138. Charcot JM, Melotti G. *Nuove Lezioni sulle Malattie del sistema nervoso ed in modo particolare sull'isterismo nell'uomo.* Milano: Dottor Francesco Vallardi. 1887.

139. Charcot JM, Melotti G. *Lezione quattordicesima: Intorno ad alcuni casi di tic convulsivo con coprolalia ed ecolalia. Analogia col Jumping di Beard, il Latah della Malesia ed il Miriachit di Hammond.* Milano: Dottor Francesco Vallardi. 1887.

140. Kushner HI, Luzzatti C, Finger S. A perplexing document in the early history of Gilles de la Tourette Syndrome: Melotti's rendition of a "Lecture of Charcot" (including a complete translation from the Italian with commentary). *J Hist Neurosci.* 1999;8(1):5–20.

141. Briquet P. *Traité clinique et thérapeutique de l'hystérie.* Paris: JB. Baillière. 1859.

142. Trousseau is the first to have performed a tracheotomy in a case of asphyxiating diphtheritic croup, to associate thrombophlebitis and cancer (Trousseau sign of malignancy), and to describe contraction in the hand during hypocalcaemic tetany (Trousseau sign of latent tetany).

143. Trousseau A. *Clinique Médicale de l'Hôtel-Dieu de Paris T2.* Paris: JB. Baillière. 1862.

144. Handfield-Jones C. *Studies on Functional Nervous Disorders.* London: John Churchill and Sons. 1870.

145. In English: Psychological automatism, an experimental psychology essay on the lower forms of human activity. Pichon-Janet H. Pierre Janet, quelques notes sur sa vie. *L'Evolution psychiatrique.* 1950;15:345–355.

146. Charcot JM. *Leçons du mardi à La Salpêtrière. Policlinique 1887–1888.* Paris: Bureaux du Progrès Médical et Delahaye & Lecrosnier. 1887–1888.

147. Dugas M. La maladie des tics: d'Itard aux neuroleptiques. *Revue Neurologie (Paris).* 1986;142(11):817–823.

148. Guinon G. Sur la maladie des tics convulsifs. *Revue de Médecine.* 1886;6(1):50–80.

149. "Degeneration is the pathological state of being which, compared with that of the most immediate progenitors, is constitutionally weakened in its psychophysical resistance and only incompletely meets the biological conditions of the hereditary fight for life. This weakening corresponds to permanent stigmata which are essentially progressive, except in the case of intercurrent regeneration; when such regeneration does not occur, degeneration leads more or less rapidly to the annihilation of the species"; in Magnan V, Legrain P. *Les dégénérés.* Bibliothèque Charcot—Debove. 1895.

150. Le Gendre P. La maladie de Gilles de la Tourette. *L'Union Médicale*. 1885;40(99):109–114.

151. Bernard L. Georges Guinon. *La Presse Médicale*. 1932;39:541–542.

152. Guinon G. *Les agents provocateurs de l'hystérie*. Thèse no. 140. Paris: Bureaux du Progrès medical et A. Delahaye & Lecrosnier. 1889.

153. Guinon G. Tic convulsif. In A Dechambre (ed.), *Dictionnaire Encyclopédique des Sciences Médicales*. Paris: Masson. 1887 série 3;17:555–593.

154. Charcot JM, Magnan V. De l'onomatomanie. *Archives de Neurologie*. 1885;10(29):157–168.

155. Esquirol JE. *Des maladies mentales considérées sous les rapports médical, hygiénique et médico-légal*. Paris: JB. Baillière. 1838.

156. Legrand du Saulle H. *La folie du doute (avec délire du toucher)*. Paris: Adrien Delahaye. 1875.

157. Guninon G. Tics convulsifs et hystérie. *Revue de Médecine*. 1887;7:509–519.

158. Lannois M. *Nosographie des chorées*. Paris: JB. Baillière. 1886.

159. Railton TC. Notes of a case of involuntary muscular movements accompanied by coprolalia. *Medical Chronicle of Manchester*. April–September 1886.

160. *Vratch* ("the physician") was a medical journal published weekly in Saint-Petersburg from 1880 to 1901.

161. Dana CL, Wilkin WP. On convulsive tic with explosive disturbances of speech (so-called Gilles de la Tourette's disease). *J Nerv Ment Dis*. 1886;13(7):407–412.

162. Charcot JM. *Clinique des Maladies du Système Nerveux. Leçons du professeur, Mémoires, Notes et Observations*. Paris: Bureaux du Progrès Médical et Félix Alcan. 1893.

163. Charcot JM. *Leçons du Mardi à La Salpêtrière. Policliniques 1887–1888*. Paris: Bureaux du Progrès Médical et A. Delahaye & Emile Lecrosnier. 1887.

164. *Teinture de Mars de Zwefler* or aromatic tincture of iron acetate.

165. Colombo or Columbo, root of *Menispermum palmatum*, of the menispermaceae family, used by the Incas for digestive problems and introduced in Europe in 1771 for the treatment of diarrhea. Due to the rarity of the raw material, pharmacists often substituted gentian root, indicated "for a difficult convalescence and/or debilitated patients." *Traité de Thérapeutique et de Matière Médicale de A. Trousseau and H. Pidoux*. 1862.

166. Charcot JM. *Leçons du Mardi à La Salpêtrière. Policliniques 1888–1889*. Paris: Bureaux du Progrès Médical et E Lecrosnier & Babé. 1889.

167. Grégoire Breitman was an *externe* at the Paris Hospitals from 1885 to 1887 and went on to found a large family of French artists and politicians. http://fr.wikipedia.org/wiki/Famille_Breitman.

168. Part of Moldavia at the time, currently in the Ukraine, 160 kilometers north of Odessa.

169. Breitman G. *Contribution à l'étude de l'écholalie, de la coprolalie et de l'imitation des gestes chez les dégénérés et les aliénés*. Thèse no. 28. Paris: Ollier-Henry. 1888.

170. Howard Kushner mistakes Jules Soury (1842–1915) for Saury in his book.

171. Legrain PM. *Du délire chez les dégénérés*. Thèse no. 199. Paris: Imprimerie A. Parent. 1886.

172. Saury H. *Étude clinique sur la folie héréditaire*. Paris: A. Delahaye et E. Lecrosnier. 1886.

173. Currently the Hôpital de Santé mentale de Perray-Vaucluse, in Epinay sur Orge. http://www.perrayvaucluse.fr/etablissement/gps-perray-vaucluse-hier/de-la-gilquiniere-a-lasile-de-vaucluse-132.html

174. Navy physician, member of the Académie de Médecine, professor at the Ecole de Médecine de Rochefort.

175. Charcot was referring to the female patient in Rochefort (in Charentes).

176. Burot F. Un cas de la maladie des tics convulsifs, traité et amélioré par la persuasion. *Revue de l'Hypnotisme*. 1888;2:141–144.

177. Burot F. Sur un cas de tics convulsifs avec écholalie et coprolalie. *Revue de l'Hypnotisme*. 1888;2:330–334.

178. Chauvreau JUJ. *Les tics coordonnés avec émission brusque & involontaire de cris et de mots articulés*. Rochefort sur mer: Ch Thèze. 1888.

179. Burot F, Duplouy E. De la maladie des tics convulsifs et de son traitement par l'hypnotisme. Seizième congrès de l'Association française pour l'avancement des Sciences. *Bulletin général de Thérapeutique Médicale et Chirurgicale.* 1887;113:518–519.

180. Catrou J. *Etude sur la maladie des tics convulsifs (Jumping, Latah, Myriachit).* Thèse no. 129. Paris: Imprimerie Henri Jouve. 1890.

181. Hempseed oil is thought to contain only very small quantities of euphoria-inducing substances.

182. Müller O. *Über die als "Maladie des tics convulsifs" beschriebene Krankheit.* Berlin: von Gustav Schade. 1889.

183. Fäber Th. *Über atypische Formen und Complicationen der Chorea.* Berlin: von Gustav Schade. 1885.

184. Hirschfeld H. *Uber Maladie des Tics convulsifs.* Berlin: Buchdr. V. G. Schade. 1891.

185. Paramyoclonus multiplex is a pathology described in 1881 in Germany by Nikolaus Friedreich (1825–1882) and analysed by Pierre Marie (1853–1940) in *Le Progrès Médical* in 1886. The term has fallen out of use. At the end of the nineteenth century, several similar clinical pictures had been described in Europe and included various muscular spasms: electric chorea of Henoch-Bergeron or Dubini or Begdie; myoclonus fibrillaris of Kny; myokymia of Schultze; and familial epileptic myoclonus of Unverricht. This type of pathology is similar to Morvan's fibrillary chorea (myokimias) with, in some cases, central nervous system dysfunction, described as limbic encephalitis, whose etiopathogenesis is tied to the presence of antibodies disturbing the functioning of potassium channels (voltagegate potassium channels [VGKC] antibodies) in cases of thymoma or autoimmune pathologies such as myasthenia gravis.

186. Köster G. Ueber die Maladie des Tics impulsifs (mimische Krampfneurose). *Deutsche Zeitschrift für Nervenheilkunde.* 1899;15(3–4):147–158.

187. Risen Russel JS. The tics. In Th. Clifford Albutt (ed.), *A System of Medicine.* T7-1899. New York: Macmillan and Co. 1896–1900.

188. Obsession-impulsion involving a word or phrase invested with a beneficial or incantatory value, or considered dangerous or taboo, for oneself or a loved one; the word or words must either be pronounced or carefully avoided.

189. André G. Une observation de maladie des tics convulsifs avec onomatomanie. *Le Mercredi Médical.* 1891;2(26):325–326.

190. Brunon M. Tics et Tiqueurs. *La Normandie Médicale.* 1892;8(7):169–174.

191. Roubinovitch J. *A propos d'un cas de maladie des tics convulsifs avec mouvements par obsession.* Paris: Imprimerie Cour d'Appel. 1893.

192. Noir J. *Étude sur les tics chez les dégénérés, les imbéciles et les idiots.* Thèse no. 171. Paris: Bureaux du Progrès Médical et Félix Alcan. 1893.

193. *Krouomania* is a term coined by Roubinovitch to describe the action of hitting oneself incessantly.

194. Sollier P. *Psychologie de l'idiot et de l'imbécile: essai de psychologie morbide.* Thèse no. 66. Paris: Félix Alcan. 1890.

195. Séguin E. *Traitement moral, hygiène et éducation des idiots et autres enfants arriérés.* Paris: JB. Baillière. 1846.

196. Moreau (de Tours) P. *La folie chez les enfants.* Paris: JB. Baillière. 1888.

197. Chabbert L. De la maladie des tics (tics, chorée, hystérie: diagnostic). *Archives de Neurologie.* 1893;25(73):12–41.

198. Janowicz C. *Tic convulsif des enfants: Paramyoclonus multiplex et chorée électrique, étude critique et comparative.* Thèse no. 356. Paris: Imprimerie Henri Jouve. 1891.

199. Walusinski O, Honnorat J. Augustin Morvan (1819–1897), a little-known rural physician and neurologist. *Revue Neurologique (Paris).* 2013;169(1):2–8.

200. Sciamanna E. Sulla malattia del tic. *Rivista quindicinale di psicologia psichiatria neuropatologia.* 1898–1899:16–17.

201. Oddo C. Le diagnostic différentiel de la maladie des tics et de la chorée de Sydenham. *La Presse Médicale.* 1899;7(78):189–191.

202. Gilles de la Tourette G. La maladie des tics convulsifs. *La Semaine Médicale.* 1899;19(20):153–156.

203. Patry G. *De la chorée variable ou polymorphe.* Thèse no. 262. Paris: Imprimerie Henri Jouve. 1897.

204. Gilles de la Tourette G. Des rapports de la chorée de Sydenham avec le rhumatisme, la puberté et la chorée dite des femmes enceintes. *La Revue Neurologique.* 1900;7(12):542–547.

205. Meige H, Feindel E. *Les tics et leur traitement.* Paris: Masson. 1902. (Preceding translated passages provided by the author.)

206. Cruchet R. Le tic convulsif et ses variétés cliniques (mémoire pour la quatrième année d'internat) 1901. In R. Cruchet (ed.), *Titres et Travaux scientifiques.* Bordeaux: Gounouilhou. 1904.

207. Cruchet R. *Etude critique sur le tic convulsif et son traitement par la gymnastique.* Thèse Bordeaux. Bordeaux: Gounouilhou. 1901–1902.

208. Brissaud E. La chorée variable des dégénérés. *Revue Neurologique.* 1896;4(14):417–431.

209. Pinell P. Degeneration theory and heredity patterns between 1850 and 1900. In JP Gaudillière and I Löwy (eds.), *Heredity and Infection. The History of Disease Transmission.* London and New York: Routlegde. 2001:245–260.

210. Ribot TH. *Les maladies de la volonté.* Paris: Germer Baillière. 1883.

211. Meige H, Feindel H. *Tics and Their Treatment.* New York: William Wood and Company. 1907. (Preceding translated passages provided by the author.)

212. Meige H, Feindel H. *Der Tic, sein Wesen und seine Behandlung; nebst einer Vorrede von Professor Brissaud; Deutsche autorisierte Ausgabe von O. Giese.* Leipzig: Deuticke, 1903.

213. Broussolle E, Trocello JM, Woimant F, Lachaux A, Quinn N. Samuel Alexander Kinnier Wilson. Wilson's disease, Queen Square and neurology. *Revue Neurologique (Paris).* 2013;169(12):927–935.

214. Wilson SAK. Progressive lenticular degeneration. A familial nervous disease associated with cirrhosis of the liver. *Brain.* 1912;34:295–507.

215. Kinnier Wilson SA. The tics and allied conditions. *J Neurol Psychopathol.* 1927;8(30):93–108.

216. Delorme C, Salvador A, Valabrègue R, Roze E, Palminteri S, Vidailhet M, de Wit S, Robbins T, Hartmann A, Worbe Y. Enhanced habit formation in Gilles de la Tourette syndrome. *Brain.* 2016;139(Pt 2):605–615.

217. Grasset J, Rauzier G. *Traité Pratique des Maladies du Système Nerveux.* Montpellier: Camille Coulet and Paris: Masson. 1894.

218. Triboulet H. Tics, Maladie des tics convulsifs. In P Brouardel and A Gilbert (eds.), *Traité de Médecine et de Thérapeutique.* Tome X. Paris: JB. Baillière. 1902.

219. Charcot JM, Bouchard CJ, Brissaud E. *Traité de Médecine.* Paris: Masson. 1894.

220. Meige H. Les tics. In E. Brissaud, A. Pinard, P. Reclus. *Pratique Médico-Chiurgicale.* Paris: Masson. 1907.

221. Ferenczi S. Psycho-analytical observation on tic. *Int J Psycho-Analysis.* 1921;2:1–30.

222. Freud S. Studies in hysteria. "Frau Emmy von N." In *The Standard Edition of the Complete Psychological Works of Sigmund Freud.* London: Hogarth Press/The Institute of Psycho-Analysis. 1962.

223. Pappenheim E. Freud and Gilles de la Tourette. Diagnostic speculations on "Frau Emmy von N." *Int Rev Psycho-Analysis.* 1980;7(3):267–277. (Or, in German, *Psyche (Stuttg).* 1989;43(10):929–951.)

224. Kushner HI. Freud and the diagnosis of Gilles de la Tourette's illness. *Hist Psychiatry.* 1998;9(33):1–25.

225. Trepsat Ch. Traitement d'un tiqueur par la psychanalyse. *Le Progrès Médical.* 1922;35(16):182–184.

226. de Saussure R. Discussion sur l'étiologie d'un tic survenu quinze mois après une encéphalite léthargique atypique. *Archives suisses de Neurologie et de Psychiatrie (Schweizer Archiv für Neurologie und Psychiatrie).* 1923;12:292–317.

227. Lebovici S. *Les Tics chez l'enfant.* Paris: Presses Universitaires de France. 1951.

228. DeWulf A, von Bogaert L. Etudes anatomo-cliniques des syndromes hypercinétiques complexes. Une observation anatomo-clinique de maladie des tics (Gilles de la Tourette). *Monatsschrift für Psychiatrie und Neurologie.* 1941;104(1-2):53–61.

229. DeWulf A. *Anatomy of the Normal Human Thalamus: Topometry and Standardized Nomenclature.* Amsterdam and New York: Elsevier. 1971.

230. Lemierre A, Lenormant Ch, Pagniez Ph. *Traité de médecine. XVI, Maladies du système nerveux.* Paris: Masson. 1949.

231. Jolly F. Ueber die Sogen. Maladie des Tics convulsifs. *Charité Annalen.* 1892;17:740–753.

232. Bresler J. Beitrag zur Lehre von der Maladie des Tics convulsif (mimische Krampfneurose). *Neurologisches Centralblatt.* 1896;15:965–972.

233. Wille H. Ueber einen Fall von Maladie des Tics impulsifs. *Monatschrift für Psychiatrie und Neurologie.* 1898;4:210–226.

234. Köster G. Uber die Maladie des Tics impulsifs (mimische Krampfneurose). *Deutsche Zeitschrift für Nervenheilkunde.* 1889;15:147–158.

235. Straus E. Untersuchungen über die postchoreatischen Motilitätsstörungen, insbesondere die Beziehungen der Chorea minor zum Tic. *Monatschrift für Psychiatrie und Neurologie.* 1927;66:281–300.

236. Wilder J. Ein Fall von Maladie des Tics. In J Wilder and J Silbermann (eds.), *Beiträge zum Ticproblem.* Berlin: Karger. 1927.

237. Runge W. Beitrag zum Ticproblem. *Deutsche Zeitschrift für Nervenheilkunde* 1932;127(1-2):96–113.

238. Kushner H. *A Cursing Brain. The Histories of Tourette Syndrome.* Cambridge, MA: Harvard University Press. 1999.

239. Kelman DH. Gilles de la Tourette disease in children: a review of the literature. *J Child Psychol Psychiatry.* 1965;6:219–226.

240. Seignot JN. Un cas de maladie de Gilles de la Tourette guéri par le R1625. *Annales Médico-Psychologiques.* 1961;19:578–579.

241. Shapiro AK, Shapiro E. Treatment of Gilles de la Tourette's syndrome with haloperidol. *Br J Psychiatry.* 1968;114(508):345–350.

242. Shapiro AK, Shapiro E, Bruun RD, Sweet RD. *Gilles de la Tourette Syndrome.* New York: Raven Press. 1978.

243. Brunn RD, Bruun B. *A Mind of Its Own: Tourette's Syndrome: A Story and a Guide.* New York: Oxford University Press. 1994.

244. Institoris H, Sprenger J. *Malleus maleficarum.* Speyer: Peter Drach. 1487.

245. Sprenger J, Institoris H. *Malleus maleficarum, maleficas et earum haeresim, ut phramea potentissima conterens.* Köln: Anno XX Coloniae excudebat Joannes Gymnicus. 1520.

246. Kushner H. Medical fictions: the case of the cursing marquise and the (re)construction of Gilles de la Tourette's syndrome. *Bull Hist Med.* 1995;69(2):224–254.

10

Vibratory Medicine and Therapeutic Suspension Techniques

Pharmacopeia in general—and neurological pharmacopeia in particular—remained in its infancy until the middle of the nineteenth century. In 1838, Gaspard-Laurent Bayle (1774–1816) noted in his *Idée Générale de la thérapeutique*: *"If one considers all diseases, it is evident that, in most cases, we do not know the rational curative indication."*[1] Jean-Martin Charcot (1825–1893) was an adept of the "expectation method," as the title of his first (and unsuccessful) *agrégation* thesis in 1857 reveals.[2] This method consisted in *"observing how patients progressed, allowing nature to provide a cure, insofar as possible, with only dietary aid, and only actively intervening when symptoms indicated an opportunity for surgery or medication."*[3] By resorting to treatment only when symptoms were sufficiently explicit, Charcot revealed a skepticism influenced by the degeneration theory of Prosper Lucas (1805–1855)[4] and Bénédict-Augustin Morel (1809–1873),[5] which reinforced his fatalistic view that nervous system diseases were hereditary.[6] Charcot nonetheless had a sincere desire to relieve his patients' suffering and prescribed bromides, mercury, hyoscyamine, silver nitrate, hydrotherapy, and electrotherapy. He even created a specialized electrotherapy unit within his own department, directed by Ernest Huet (1858–1917) and Romain Vigouroux (1831–1911). Charcot is reported by Paul Berbez (1859–?) to have stated: *"You are all aware, Sirs, of how tabes neutralizes our best efforts. The apparent richness of our therapeutic arsenal masks its actual poverty. The fact that there are so many remedies for a given disease means that none of them offers all of the benefits we have every reason to demand."*[7]

Beginnings of Vibratory Medicine

In August 1892, Gilles de la Tourette published a lesson by Charcot on vibratory medicine. Charcot had examined rapid, continuous vibrations for treating specific nervous system diseases[8] and had noted: *"I have known for a long time, having been told by my patients with paralysis agitans, that travel by railway or carriage can provide great relief. Throughout the journey, the painful, tiresome sensations that nearly always accompany this disease seem to disappear almost completely. The well-being persists for a while once the journey has ended. I have often had the occasion to present these facts to students in my classes, and I have more than once voiced the hypothesis that a process reproducing all movements transmitted by a vehicle in operation would have positive effects in the treatment of Parkinson's disease."* In fact, the idea was not new. Pierre Chirac (1650–1732), a physician at Versailles during the reign of Louis XV, left a manuscript dated 1697, *Histoire des maladies de la teste*[9] (History of maladies of the head), in which he described improvement in melancholia after the patient had travelled in a mail carriage for several days. Charles-Irénée Castel, Abbot of Saint-Pierre (1658–1743) (Figure 10.1), related this anecdote in 1734 in the gazette *Le Mercure de France*: *"Skillful physicians have observed that the movement of the body in a mail carriage rolling rapidly over the cobbles for several days may be an excellent remedy for several ills attributed to melancholy, vapors, bile, and obstructions of the liver, the spleen, and other glands in the lower belly. . . . Provided that the carriage is not rolling along a bumpy road and has good suspension, the entire human body is in a condition very similar to that of an object that makes a sound when it resonates. All of the parts are slightly contracted, then extended, or friction is created at the joints, and this occurs a great number of times in a short period. If the degree of this friction does not exceed what the patient can withstand, the treatment may be useful for re-establishing harmony in the interactions between the nerves and for eliminating any aberrations."*[10] To improve upon this noisy, costly, and impractical remedy, the Abbot of Saint-Pierre proposed *"an armchair attached to a frame that produces vigorous shaking"* for home use.

With help from *"the excellent engineer-machinist Duguet,"* the Abbot of Saint-Pierre introduced the first model, known as the *"trémoussoir"* (wriggling or vibratory armchair), on December 31, 1734, and suggested that *"healthy persons could use it to replace the exercise they are unable to take, to preserve their health; others could use it to avoid bloodletting after a copious meal, as this remedy augments respiration and transpiration."* For regular physical fitness, the machine was to be used two or three days per week, for two or three hours.

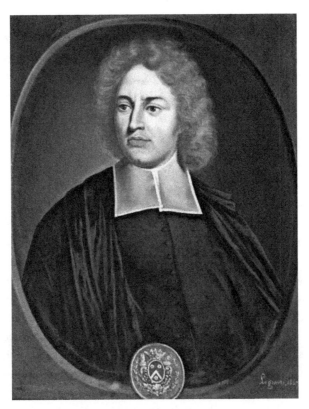

FIGURE 10.1 Charles-Irénée Castel, Abbé de Saint-Pierre (1658–1743).
Public domain.

Curative treatment, on the other hand, would involve *"rapid shaking four or five hours per day."* In 1735, Jean Astruc (1684–1766), professor at the Faculté de médecine in Montpellier, drew up an inventory of machines built since antiquity *"to shake the body, and thereby capable of replacing the exercise one gets from riding a horse or travelling in a carriage. . . . These examples and citations demonstrate the utility of a machine newly invented by an engineer, Mr. Du Guet, and baptized the 'Fauteuil de poste' (mail armchair). The objective is the same, but the use of this chair is infinitely simpler and more convenient. The user experiences the same shaking as in a mail carriage—front to back, left to right, up and down—with these different movements occurring in different ways, or several of them occurring at the same time. The user can make them as abrupt or gentle as he wishes, fast or slow, violent or weak."* [11] In 1744, Voltaire (François Marie Arouet, 1694–1778) found the treatment to his liking: *"I left for the fields, my adorable angel, rather than dining; I seated myself in the trémoussoir of the Abbot of Saint-Pierre, and now I feel a little better."*[12]

But the enthusiasm was short-lived. *"Although the Abbot tried to let the whole world know that this machine was a success and that similar models already existed in La Hague, in Germany, on the Rhine, in Berlin, Brussels, and London, the trémoussoir would be relegated for more than a century to the galleries of medical archaeology, where Mr. Charcot recently, and so fortunately, re-discovered it."* [13]

A Revival

Without citing his predecessors, Charcot thus took up an old idea: *"In 1878, in my department at La Salpêtrière, Mr. Vigouroux began testing a method I shall present to you today: the treatment of certain nervous system diseases by mechanical vibrations. Mr. Vigouroux first studied the effects of these vibrations on several hysterics. Using an enormous diapason, activated by a bow and mounted on a sounding box,* [14] *he was able to make hemi-anesthesias disappear and relax contractions almost as rapidly as with a magnet or an electrical spark. In a patient with locomotor ataxia, he calmed her painful fits by placing her legs in the sounding box."* Charcot goes on to describe the experiments of Maurice Boudet de Pâris (1849–?)[15] in which he applied a vibrating rod to the region above the orbits to relieve neuralgias or migraines, his own in particular. Charcot strongly agreed with Boudet de Pâris's hypothesis that *"the transmission of vibrations to the brain plays a role in the production of effects."* Pierre Jégu (1844–1891), a member of the audience listening to this lesson, decided to build *"an armchair with a special mechanism that transmits the rapid oscillatory movements of an anterior and lateral axis. These movements, combined and working in opposition, produce a vibration, a strong rapid shaking that resembles what one experiences in a carriage in motion, as you may judge for yourself by sitting in this armchair"* (Figure 10.2).

Jégu's sudden death interrupted his research. *"At my request, Mr. Gilles de la Tourette, my former chef de clinique, agreed to oversee and pursue the experiments."* Gilles de la Tourette recruited eight patients, who underwent *"irregular"* treatment, as Charcot was disappointed to note. *"Improvement is generally seen from the fifth or sixth shaking session, mostly for the painful phenomena that so frequently accompany Parkinson's disease. When the patient steps down from the armchair, he feels lighter, his stiffness is gone, and he can walk more easily than before. The phenomenon is nearly constant. Nights go more smoothly; a patient who used to toss and turn sleeps calmly, a source of great relief for him*[16]*. . . . We have obtained the most encouraging results, more research will be conducted, and I shall report back to you in the future with what we establish. It is already significant to be able to help those suffering from paralysis agitans, which the ordinary remedies, as you know, do little to relieve."* Charcot nonetheless acknowledged that the patients' shaking was not eliminated.

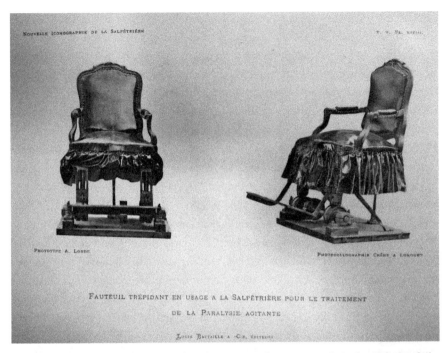

FIGURE 10.2 J-M. Charcot developed a therapeutic vibratory armchair that simulated the rhythmic shaking of a carriage.
Private collection of the author.

The Quest for a Theoretical Justification

To explain the therapeutic action of the vibrations, Vigouroux turned to physics, specifically to theories on electricity and light. *"The work of several physicists suggests that electrical action resembles the propagation of a vibratory movement; for the moment it is unimportant whether this transmission involves ether or unknown molecules. What is important is that vibration is the characteristic common to all stimulants of our nervous system. . . . What, then, is added to the understanding of a phenomenon by saying that it is vibratory in nature? One could instead ask, what isn't vibratory? Even in this vague explanatory system, a few rules ought to be observed. For example, it would be incorrect to suppose that the molecules of a body can perform outside work that is not compensated elsewhere by an equivalent loss of energy. To summarize, until now this idea of vibrations has offered us a means of comparison or schematic representation, but not an explanation. Referring to esthesiogenic elements, or the modifications they cause in the organism, it might be more appropriate to represent the various phases of oscillation, rather than chains of polarized molecules."* [17] Vigouroux used the term *"Æsthésiogène,"* coined by Paul Richer (1849–1933) in 1879 and characteristic of something that modifies sensitivity.[18]

These concepts originated in the middle of the eighteenth century. At the time, the Englishman David Hartley (1705–1757) was attempting to unite the physical and psychological realms in a neurophysiological model. The result was, of course, very speculative. His initial source of inspiration was the theory of vibrations[19] advanced by Isaac Newton (1642–1727). Hartley wanted to apply the ideas of this theory to biological life in general and human life in particular. For Hartley, the principles set forth by Newton in Latin in *Optice*[20] in 1706, and later in English in *Optiks*,[21] not only served as an interpretive framework for physical events, but also laid down the neurophysiological foundations of perception and thought: *"Is not Animal Motion perform'd by the Vibrations of this Medium, excited in the Brain by the power of the Will, and propagated from thence through the solid, pellucid and uniform Capillamenta of the Nerves into the Muscles, for contracting and dilating them? I suppose that the Capillamenta of the Nerves are each of them solid and uniform, that the vibrating Motion of the Æthereal Medium may be propagated along them from one end to the other uniformly, and without interruption: For Obstructions in the Nerves create Palsies. And that they may be sufficiently uniform, I suppose them to be pellucid when view'd singly, tho' the Reflexions in their cylindrical Surfaces may make the whole Nerve (composed of many Capillamenta) appear opake and white. For opacity arises from reflecting Surfaces, such as may disturb and interrupt the Motions of this Medium."*[21]

Hartley's theory was expressed in his book, *Observations on Man, his Frame, his Duty, and his Expectations*.[22] Published in 1749, it provided the basis for his theory of vibrations and associations and applied them to perception and thought. He proposed that sensations enter into the nervous system as vibrations (matter in motion) that give rise to localized vibrations in the brain; external objects are impressed on the sense organs, then on the nerves, and, by their intermediary, the brain, in which the infinitesimal particles are subjected to fine vibrations.[23]

Joseph Mortimer-Granville (1833–1900)

Clearly, the supposed mode of action of this "vibratory therapy" was theoretically questionable. That did not prevent Gilles de la Tourette, at Charcot's request, from building on the method and broadening its objectives. *"Mr. Gilles de la Tourette has not limited himself to monitoring how the shaking armchair works and to noting the results. He has looked for other applications of the vibratory method."* Drawing initial inspiration from the writings of Boudet de Pâris, Gilles de la Tourette perfected a technique invented in England by Joseph Mortimer-Granville (1833–1900). Mortimer-Granville used a vibrator of his own design on the skull of his patients and explained its action this way: *"The first effect of nerve-vibration, therefore, is awakening or interrupting; the second is more like tuning a violin string, or the wire of a pianoforte. Nervestretching acts in one of two ways for a time. If much force be used it disorganizes the nerve and prevents any vibration taking place in its elements, with the result, in successful cases, of giving it a new starting point when the integrity of the nerve-fibre is restored in the process of natural repair. When less force is used, the nerve is acted upon precisely as screwing and stretching act on a violin string, altering its physical capacity for vibration, and either reducing or increasing the amplitude of the waves of movement into which agitation will throw it. I doubt not that nerves of different calibres have each their proper physical capacities for vibration, and the vibrations of a nerve are, in perfect health, mathematically component and complementary parts of the vibrations of the trunk from which it springs. When a nerve becomes turgid from congestion, or is in any way swollen or attenuated, this perfect relation is disturbed, and the result is functional disorder, and probably pain. The manner in which vibration acts in the second stage or phase of its process is, I believe, explained by the law of musical concords and discords or harmonies. We interrupt by a discord, and control by substituting one set of vibrations for another. In this way, by vibrating a particular nerve daily, as nearly as possible at the same hour and for the same length of time, with a percuteur working at the same speed or number of vibrations per second, we may educate the nerve-cells or fibres, so to say, to a new rhythmical habit, and thus establish new vibratile conditions."*[24]

Helmet Designed by Georges Gaiffe (1857–1943)

In an attempt to imitate Mortimer-Granville's device, two physician friends of Gilles de la Tourette specialized in electrotherapy, Jules-Louis Larat (1857–?) and Georges-François Gautier (1857–?), began by building a vibrator consisting of an electrically activated diapason. But since this device was heavy and difficult to adjust, they turned to Georges Gaiffe (1857–1943),[25] who ran a famous medical equipment company founded by his father (Figure 10.3). Gaiffe described his contribution this way: *"The changes I made basically involve two eccentrics*[26] *turning rapidly around an axis, thereby producing vibrations. The helmet consists of a fireman's helmet in which maillechort*[27] *springs have been installed for transmitting the vibrations and fitting the helmet to any head size. A light cushion prevents the metal from injuring the patient. The vibrator is mounted on the top surface of the helmet on a little mahogany platform. It consists of a small Gramme machine*[28] *to which are attached the two eccentrics. Motor rotation at greater or lesser speeds entrains the eccentrics which, by centrifugal force, lift the helmet when they rise, whereas when lowering they apply force to the patient's head. Rapid succession of these movements produces a vibration that is transmitted to the brain and, more*

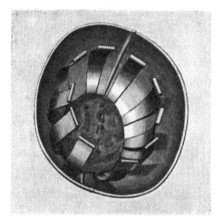
Fig. 2.–INTERIOR VIEW OF THE HELMET.

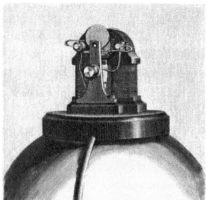
Fig. 3.–DETAILS OF THE ELECTRIC MOTOR.

FIGURE 10.3 Vibratory helmet. *Scientific American*, 1892.
Private collection of the author.

generally, to the whole person. Two bichromate elements or two accumulators are sufficient to run the device at its maximum speed. Different speeds are obtained by varying
current intensity. . . . If a more powerful motor is placed on a board, isolated from the
floor by layers of flexible rubber, and if an armchair is placed on the board, by this
simple construction we will have produced the vibratory armchair that Doctor Jégu
built, albeit not as simply, for Professor Charcot" [29] (Figure 10.4).

Use of the Helmet

Charcot gave his own description: *"It consists of a sort of helmet made of separate
strips, similar to a hat-maker's measuring device. By means of a very simple mechanism, the strips of this helmet are fitted to the subject's head during the experiment.
A small, special motor activated by a simple battery sits on a plate on top of the helmet.
On the whole, the device is easy to handle, very portable, and can run without interruption. Its construction is sturdy, making it easy to store. The little motor turns at about
6000 rotations, all very regular, producing a continuous vibration that is transmitted
all over the skull via the strips of the helmet. The entire head vibrates, as can be verified
by placing one's hands on the mastoid process. In operation, the machine makes a
continuous, soft buzzing noise, which may be of interest regarding the pathogenesis
of the results obtained. The number and amplitude of vibrations can be increased or
decreased by a simple process of adjustment. Fitted on the head of a healthy subject,
the device is perfectly tolerated and its operation causes no discomfort. After seven to
eight minutes, a feeling of numbness overcomes the entire body and almost invariably*

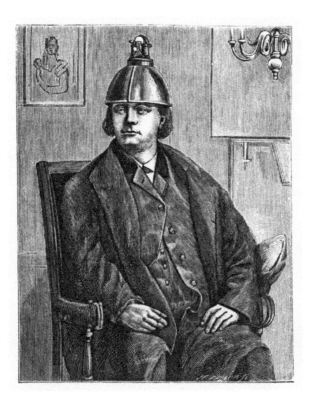

FIGURE 10.4 A vibratory helmet to shake the head and brain.
Private collection of the author.

leads to sleep. In fact, experiments have shown that a 10-minute session at around six in the evening results in calm sleep during the night that follows. Eight to ten sessions can cure insomnia when this condition is not linked to an organic affection of the brain." Charcot reported three cases of neurasthenia in which the patient was cured, as in this example: "*Vibration first eliminates cephalic symptoms, particularly vertigo and the painful vice-like sensation so specific to this affection. What indicates that the vibrations act particularly on the brain is that in this case, where spinal phenomena were predominant, pain in the lumbosacral region, weakness in the lower limbs and relative sexual impotence disappeared without the need to apply the vibrations along the spinal column. For this patient, static electricity had completely failed. In light of what I have just stated, this practice of vibration may be a powerful sedative for the nervous system.*"

Gilles de la Tourette published Charcot's lesson in *La Nouvelle Iconographie de La Salpêtrière*[30] under his name, completing it with his own findings. "*Suffice it to say that the action of the vibratory helmet has always seemed first and foremost sedative and that our best results were in cases of neurasthenic and hysterical headaches, migraine, insomnia, and in certain cases of melancholic depression. A number of experiments are still necessary to judge the method, but the results obtained so far are very encouraging, especially in light of the fact that we treated patients whose conditions had until then been resistant to the most varied medications."* Gilles de la Tourette went on to consider technical and practical aspects of the helmet, such as the average length of the sessions, individual susceptibilities, and so forth. *"Tolerance is increased with repeated sessions and with the length of the session. While the helmet seems heavy at first, once the vibrations begin, the patient has a sense of lightness and the weight of the helmet is no longer uncomfortable."*

Because of Charcot's fame, the use of vibratory therapy spread outside of France. On October 22, 1892, *Scientific American*[31] published a detailed synopsis of Charcot's lesson, referring to his *chef de clinique* as "Gillis de la Tourette." The article was illustrated with precise drawings of different configurations of the vibratory helmet. Nothing similar can be found in French publications.

Vibratory medicine has not disappeared. Only the technical aspects have been modified. Associated with acupuncture[32] or various physiotherapy methods, it no longer aims to agitate molecules but rather to stimulate proprioception to help relieve painful musculoskeletal sensations[33] or improve balance.[34] There is still no scientific proof of its efficacy.[35]

Locomotor Ataxia or Tabes

Locomotor ataxia was given its clinical description by Guillaume Duchenne de Boulogne (1806–1875) in 1858: *"Progressive abolition of movement coordination and apparent paralysis, in contrast to the integrity of muscular strength; these are the fundamental characteristics of the disease I shall describe. . . . In addition, patients were unable to remain upright without swaying or falling, nor could they walk without assistance and without throwing their lower limbs out in front of them in a more or less coordinated manner. . . . For most patients, there was abducens or oculomotor nerve palsy, or weakness or even loss of vision with pupillary inequality; these phenomena marked the beginning of movement coordination difficulties or were their precursors. These local palsies were accompanied or followed by characteristic terebrating pain that was erratic and tended to drift. Brief, lightning-like, or similar to electric shock, the pain recurred in attacks that took place throughout the body. These phenomena constituted an initial period. After a time of varying length (from several months to several years), vertigo and disturbances of balance and movement coordination appeared in a second period. At the same time, tactile or pain sensitivity (analgesia and anesthesia) was reduced or lost first in the lower limbs, or sometimes* in the upper limbs. Finally, the disease became systematic in a third period. During the course of the disease, disorders affecting the function of the rectum or bladder often occurred. . . . In all patients, intelligence remained intact; speech was not affected. . . . Usually the disease was progressive, which is to say that it ended with death." [36] As Louis Victor Marcé (1828–1864) wrote in his *agrégation* thesis: "I admit that the research of Duchenne, carried out several years after that of Landry, appears to reproduce exactly all that physiologists have written on the feeling of muscular activity. As for progressive locomotor ataxia, which the same author presented as a distinct nosographic entity, I consider this merely the morbid state following a loss of muscular feeling, a morbid state that Landry had drawn attention to in 1855." [37] Octave Landry (1826–1865) stated in 1855 that *"muscle coordination requires the sensation of muscular activity"* in his innovative dissertation, paving the way for the concepts of proprioception and stereognosis[38] and continuing research undertaken by Duchenne in 1853,[39] although Landry was unaware of this. Charles Bell (1774–1842) in 1826 in England,[40] and Friedrich-August Benjamin Puchelt (1784–1856) in 1845 in Germany,[41] had already described the difficulties with balance characteristic of ataxia but had not described the full clinical picture of the disease and its progression.

In Germany, Ernst Horn (1774–1848) provided observations to Christopher von Weidenbach[42] and Sigismund Eduard Löwenhardt (1796–1875) for their theses, defended in 1817. Von Weidenbach described the macroscopic appearance of the spinal cord using the word "tabes," which in Latin means "to disintegrate" [43] and is synonymous with "phthisis" in Greek, the term that Löwenhardt used.[44] Two years later, Gottlieb Wilhelm (Theophilus Guilelmus) Schesmer[45] described in his thesis the arthropathies occurring during tabes. Charcot published his own description in 1868.[46] In 1827, Ernst Horn had also helped his son Guillelmus Horn to write his thesis,[47] once again on the subject of tabes. While all of these theses describe gait difficulties, pain, and sexual impotence, none of them makes an explicit link between tabes and syphilis. Horn noted that the disease was more frequent in men[48] and explained this by "venereal excesses." [49] Moritz Heinrich Romberg (1795–1873), Ernst Horn's most famous student, described the complete clinical picture from 1840 to 1846 using the term *"tabes dorsalis."* [50] He added the famous eponymous sign[51] to the semiology of ataxia, seeing no other cause for it than tabes.[52] Duchenne paid him this compliment in 1872: "I am happy to acknowledge that Mr. Romberg has observed and described better than anyone most of the symptoms that occur in progressive locomotor ataxia." [53] The syphilitic etiology of progressive locomotor ataxia was proposed by Jean-Alfred Fournier (1832–1914) in 1875 but would only be accepted in the 1890s. Working with Charles Bouchard

(1837–1915), Charcot published in 1866 an anatomical-pathological description of a case whose originality, as the authors noted, lay in the fact that the disease was in a prodromal phase.[54] Charcot saw syphilis as only one possible cause among others, despite his friendship with Fournier and his admiration for the German neurologist Wilhelm Erb (1840–1921). At the 1881World Congress of Medicine in London, where Charcot was hailed, Erb declared that more than 90% of tabes patients had syphilis.[55]

A Writer's Account

Alphonse Daudet (1840–1897) left a poignant testimony, published after his death, of tabes and the suffering he endured. The first symptoms came twenty-five years after the initial contamination: *"Pain like no other: large furrows of flame cutting through and lighting up my carcass."* Daudet asked Charcot in 1884 to treat him for his "locomotor ataxia." Daudet had met Charcot, fifteen years his senior, in 1882 by the intermediary of Léon Gambetta (1838–1882) and had rapidly become a close friend, regularly invited to Charcot's Tuesday evening gatherings. He described his agony this way: *"Burning eyes. Horrible reverberating pain. And from that time onward, pins and needles in my feet, a burning sensation, high sensitivity. First a susceptibility to noise: tongs and shovel near the hearth, the sound of bells ripping through the air, the spinning of a spider's web at four o'clock in the morning."* Daudet abused morphine, acetanilide, an ancestor of paracetamol, and chloral. As with his other patients, Charcot advised Daudet to go to Lamalou in southern France for hydrotherapy, but Daudet did not derive any benefit from his time there. So Charcot recommended a new treatment.

Dr. Motchutkowsky's Suspension Technique

Charcot dedicated his January 15, 1889, lesson to the treatment of locomotor ataxia, specifically the *"suspension technique of Dr. Motchutkowsky of Odessa."*[56] Charcot's former *interne*, Fulgence Raymond (1844–1910), had made a journey to Odessa, accompanied by their student Jakow Naumowicz Onanoff (1859–1892), who had served as translator. He brought back an article that Charcot was unfamiliar with.[57] It had been published in 1883 in the Russian journal *"Vracha,"* as Charcot pronounced it (*Vratsch*, meaning "physician"), and it was later translated into English for the journal *Brain* in 1889.[58] The author, Osip Osipovich Motchutkowsky (or Motchutkovsky, 1845–1903), explained how a patient, fitted with a corset named for Lewis Sayre (1820–1900) and worn to correct scoliosis,[59] reported that the pain and motor difficulties associated with his locomotor ataxia had nearly disappeared. Berbez quoted Charcot as saying: *"The way in which the Russian physician discovered this treatment is quite extraordinary. To correct the posture of a tabes patient with scoliosis, he suspended the patient from his armpits (Serres method) and applied a plaster corset. After a few days, the patient told his physician that his searing pain was much reduced. Motchutkowsky first thought the corset was responsible for this unexpected result, but he soon realized it was in fact the suspension that had alleviated the patient's pain. He then used this treatment with a number of tabes patients and nearly all of them reported some benefit."* [60] Charcot was perfectly aware of his therapeutic impotence with regard to this disease: *"For the treatment of progressive locomotor ataxia, we are nowhere near the heights of our anatomical and clinical understanding, and it is with good reason, unfortunately, that the disease in question is generally considered incurable, at least in the vast majority of cases."* In October 1888, impressed by the article of the Odessa neurologist, Charcot decided to assign the task of testing this new therapeutic method to Gilles de la Tourette, who was then in his second year as *chef de clinique.* *"I do not think the new method will radically change the state of things, but if it proves more effective than most of the means currently at our disposal, and as innocuous in its application as the best of them, then it will no doubt be eagerly accepted."* How did suspension work? *"Naturally our confrere must have considered the theoretical question, how does suspension work? According to him, its action is based on a slight elongation of the nerve roots, and he loosely compares this to elongation of the sciatic nerve, a practice used by some surgeons a few years back. It may also act by modifications in spinal blood circulation, for which it is difficult to provide categorical explanations. Whatever the case may be, except in morbid states, suspension increases the rate of respiration while decreasing the amplitude and force of both inhalation and exhalation. Pulse rate increases and arterial pressure appears higher than normal."* Charcot went on to describe the suspension device that the drawings of Paul Richer (1849–1933) show in detail (Figure 10.5): *"In summary, Sirs, of fourteen locomotor ataxia cases treated with suspension over an average period of three months, we saw very considerable improvement in ten of those cases. And for several of the patients, there was a truly remarkable reduction in most of the spinal symptoms. In only four of the cases were the effects negligible or very slight, and in one of these cases, after a period of improvement, all symptoms worsened. No other incidents of note."* Then Charcot described improvements in gait and balance, *"bladder difficulties happily overcome,"* and the disappearance of impotence. *"If the Romberg sign disappears, it is almost always a later phenomenon. In none of the cases did we see the reappearance of the patellar reflex."* The most important result was the alleviation of pain, which frequently disappeared. *"The results obtained*

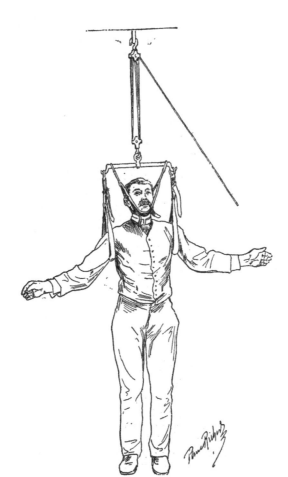

Fɪɢ. 35. — Le malade suspendu.

FIGURE 10.5 Suspension device; drawing by Paul Richer (1849–1933). Private collection of the author.

to date are, in my opinion, striking enough to be emphasized and brought to the attention of physicians interested in neuropathological studies. In my own treatment of
ataxia and with the various other therapies used, I have never observed improvement
as patent, occurring as rapidly, and in as many patients at once. But having made this
declaration, I am the first to note that we are still in the preliminary phases on several
points. Lacking sufficient experiments over a sufficiently long period, we are faced with
many questions to which we do not have the answers." Charcot then defined a key
question: "If we remain skeptical, it is not regarding the results obtained, which are
incontestable. Rather, we ask ourselves how long the improvement will last, which, of
course, the future shall reveal."

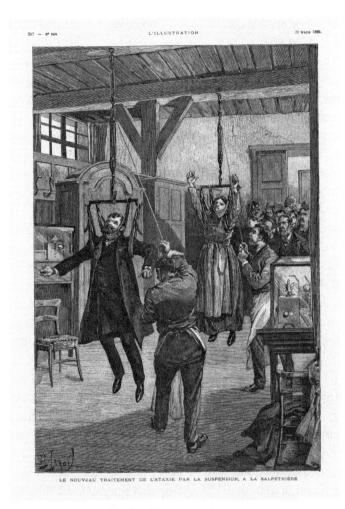

FIGURE 10.6 Locomotor ataxia treatment using suspension. *L'Illustration* (newspaper), No. 2404, March 23, 1889.
Private collection of the author.

Treatment of Locomotor Ataxia by Suspension at La Salpêtrière

The press was quick to report on this favorable opinion from the Master. For example, on March 23, 1889, *L'Illustration* devoted a full page to the Richer's drawings for the Salpêtrière lesson (Figure 10.5). On another full page, the engraver-illustrator Henri Lanos (1859–1929) captured the atmosphere of a collective suspension session with an image that is both realistic and fascinating (Figure 10.6). Within three months, 114 patients sought out suspension treatment. Charcot's approval, the publicity around the activities at La Salpêtrière, and the apparent simplicity and innocuity of the procedure led to rapid adoption of suspension therapy throughout Europe and in the United States.

In February 1889, Gilles de la Tourette noted: *"Every single day we receive requests for information on therapeutic procedure."* After overseeing more than 800 suspensions, Gilles de la Tourette decided it was *"now indispensable to examine a few technical details."* [61] He described the harness, the method for positioning it, and the precautions necessary to avoid compressing the armpits. Elevation should be slow, and the length of the session progressively increased from a few dozen seconds to a maximum of three or four minutes. He warned of the risks of daily sessions, which were not tolerated as well as sessions separated by one or two days (Figure 10.7).

Shortly thereafter, François Damaschino (1840–1889) at Hôpital Laennec, as well as Fulgence Raymond (1844–1910) and Robert-André Moutard-Martin (1850–1926) at Hôpital Saint-Antoine, began to use the method,[62] Georges-Sainfort Dujardin-Beaumetz (1833–1895) began experimenting with suspension in his department at Hôpital Cochin in 1889. He had defended his thesis on locomotor ataxia in 1862, concluding with a section on the absence of effective treatment.[63] But, very quickly, Dujardin-Beaumetz became interested in another procedure inspired by the *"gymnastic de l'opposant."*[64,65] This method, invented by Jules-Léandre Pichery (1811–?), was less brutal and had the patient participate in treatment by pulling on cables attached to counterweights and springs whose tension was adjusted by pulleys fastened to the ceiling. It was a precursor to current-day orthopedic rehabilitation techniques.[66] In 1889, Dujardin-Beaumetz helped H. Balaban (1864–?) from Odessa write his thesis, which provided translations of the observations in Motchutkowsky's seminal publication[67] and underscored the finding that the expected benefits were exhausted after around forty suspensions; symptoms could even worsen if the treatment was continued too long.

In July 1889, Gilles de la Tourette published two observations of morphine withdrawal—complete for one patient, partial for the other—after a dozen suspensions.[68] The same year, an *interne* (house officer or resident), François Aiman Raoult (1863–?), published the first literature review,[69] adding to it in 1890.[70] He listed the names of physicians who were testing this therapy, notably W. J. Morton, Charles Dana,[71] and William Hammond (1828–1900) in New York. Their results were encouraging. In Russia, B. Worotynsky, a psychiatrist in Kazan,[72] and Vladimir Bekhterev (or Bechterew, 1857–1927)[73] in Saint Petersburg also found the method beneficial to patients. Paul-Louis Ladame (1842–1919) in Geneva suspended fifteen of his patients; half of them experienced a small measure of relief, while the others abandoned the treatment or reported that their

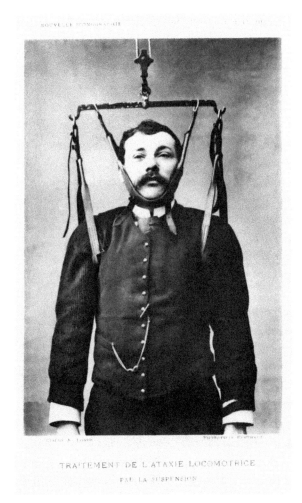

FIGURE 10.7 Locomotor ataxia treatment using suspension. *Nouvelle Iconographie de La Salpêtrière*, 1889.
Private collection of the author.

symptoms worsened.[74] A physician at West End Hospital for Nervous Diseases in London, Armand de Watteville (1846–1925),[75] translated Charcot's article after translating Motchutkowsky's article.[76] He was editor-in-chief for *Brain* starting in 1884 and one of the founders of the Neurological Society (within the Royal Society of Medicine), for which *Brain* became the official journal. Watteville added a note on his personal practice of suspensions. He improved on the equipment recommended by Charcot using a system of straps in which the tension was adjusted to the patient's weight. He believed that the physician must personally oversee all sessions.

Looking for an Explanation

Julius Althaus (1833–1900), trained in Göttingen and Berlin, heard Charcot's lessons before leaving for London, where he worked at the National Hospital for Diseases of the Nervous System including Paralysis and Epilepsy, which would later become the Maida Vale Hospital for Nervous Diseases.[77] On April 13, 1889, Althaus published an article in *The Lancet* in which he proposed a new explanation for the curative action of suspension. He wrote that the technique tore *"the meningeal adhesions that surround the posterior tracts, thus improving the conductibility of the nerve tubes, especially the most superficial tubes. This theory is apparently supported by the fact that suspension works better in recent cases than in long-standing cases and that, in the latter, it produces inflammatory phenomena. Suspension also seems to act on the sclerous, dense, and fibrous neuroglia, by loosening or breaking it, which reduces the compression on the remaining nerve tubes."*[78] Shortly thereafter, he proposed his own technical improvement aimed at more easily suspending heavy subjects by the addition of compound pulleys. After more than four hundred suspensions, he was convinced of the benefit to his patients and extended its use to Parkinson's disease, amyotrophic lateral sclerosis, and neurasthenia.[79] At the June 14, 1890, session of the Berlin psychiatric society, Léon Asher (1865–1943) reported treating twenty-three patients with suspension. Only twelve of them experienced an improvement in their mobility and sphincteric control.[80] Emanuel Mendel (1839–1907), founder of the German neurological journal *Neurologisches CentralBlatt*, treated eighty-five patients, performing more than 2,500 suspensions. He worked with his assistant Franz Rosenbaum at his Berlin-Pankow clinic and wrote: *"While it hasn't lived up to all of the promises made by French observers, suspension can be of real service to patients. After thirty to forty sessions without improvement, it is wise to stop treatment."* [81] Mendel and Albert von Eulenburg (1840–1917) tested the effects of suspension on other chronic diseases such as Parkinson's and neurasthenia.[82]

In the June 7, 1890, edition of *Le Progrès Médical*, Gilles de la Tourette reported on the treatment of five hundred patients by suspension. He was clearly committed to this therapy; no other team equaled his numbers. But Gilles de la Tourette's evaluation of the technique is not as enthusiastic as one might suppose. He noted very marked improvement in 25% of cases and incomplete improvement in 30–35%, leaving 45% of patients with few positive effects or who had abandoned the method. *"Suspension has to be tolerated. Based on our already long practice with this technique, lipothymia and syncope are the main, if not the only obstacles to this tolerance."* Gilles de la Tourette also wrote: *"The very enthusiasm the method generated turned out to be most damaging to it. Soon there was not one hydrotherapy center in France, not even one gym where this method was not applied. Most often it was left to the bath attendants, who knew nothing about medicine. Because the method has been used without discrimination for all ataxics, resulting in serious accidents and even sudden deaths, it has fallen into disrepute."* [83] For Raoult, who published the first literature review, the deaths during or just after suspension were the result of patients performing the technique at home, alone and without medical supervision.

Alphonse Daudet, In the Land of Pain

Following Charcot's advice, Daudet agreed to try suspension, hoping to alleviate his suffering. His account includes the following: *"Suspension. Sayre's device. Evening hangings of poor ataxics under Keller's supervision—sinister. The Russian hung in a seated position. Two brothers; the little dark one squirming. I remain in the air for four minutes, supported only by my jaw for two of them. Pain in my teeth. Then, coming down, when they detach me, horrible discomfort in my dorsal region and neck, as if my entire spinal cord were splitting in two. I have to squat down and straighten little by little, feeling that I must let my drawn spine reposition itself. No noticeable curative effect. Thirteen suspensions. Then I spit blood, which I attribute to congestive fatigue from the treatment."* Daudet never blamed his friend for the cruel and dangerous torture he underwent. Edmond de Goncourt (1822–1896), who had already witnessed the neurosyphilitic agony of his brother Jules (1830–1870), would later relate what his friend Daudet confided in him on January 27, 1889: *"Daudet chatted with me about his hanging before dinner. A new treatment for ataxia, imported from Russia by Charcot. For this mysterious operation, Daudet waits in the showers until everyone is gone. Then he goes secretly into a poorly lit place, pervaded by shadows. There, in the presence of Keller and another physician, the hanging takes place, lasting one minute—a long, long minute. A minute has 60 seconds, at the end of which Daudet is taken down and finds himself on the ground with intense pain in the back of the neck. 'Ah! A hanging in semi-darkness, now that's evocative!' said Daudet. 'Like a Goya!' I replied. 'Yes, a Goya! . . . And while I'm strung up in the air, if Keller happens to be alone, I recall that last year, he went mad for three months . . . what if the madness comes back and he forgets me. . . . But keep it quiet. . . . If Bloy were to find out, think of the macabre article he'd write about me in L'Evènement!'"* [84] Daudet's decline was ineluctable despite all of the suffering inflicted in the name of medicine: *"Standing before the mirror in my bathroom, what emaciation! The funny old man I've suddenly become. From forty-five to sixty-five. Twenty years I didn't live."*

Opinions Differ

As early as 1889, other authors besides Althaus contested whether the spinal cord was elongated by this technique and implicitly questioned the reported results. Paul Haushalter (1866–1925) in Nancy and his *interne* A. Adam explained their position this way: *"We view the spinal column as too solidly constructed to allow it to lengthen beyond the limits of its physiological elongation, due to the slight attraction that acts in suspension from top to bottom on the head, or to the weight of the lower segment of the body, which incidentally is supported not only by the spinal column but also by the arms and consequently by the device. As for the experiments performed on cadavers to demonstrate the extensibility of the column, we don't find them convincing. Because muscle tone no longer exists, it may be possible to see slightly more elongation than what would occur in live patients."* [85]

Gilles de la Tourette had to agree: *"Suspension does not produce significant elongation of the spinal cord. If a cadaver is suspended using a Sayre device, without auxiliary supports, it can be observed in the spinal canal previously opened along its entire length, that there is no signification modification to its content. However, since this maneuver increases the length of the spinal column by more than a centimeter, it probably has a real effect on the spinal cord and the bilateral radicular segments. But these effects are minimal, and obviously even more so when suspension is performed on a living subject, in whom the muscles around the vertebrae increase the resistance of the spinal column to the weight of the lower limbs, the only possible factor in its elongation."* [86] James Cagney, an anatomical demonstrator at the Hospital for Epilepsy and Paralysis in Regent's Park, London, arrived at clear, categorical conclusions after conducting a long series of measurements on living patients and cadavers: *"A stretching of the cord would give no rational explanation of the effects sought, but this stretching does not occur. A considerable and effective relaxation, both of the cord and its nerve-roots does occur in suspension. Relaxation is competent to account for the benefit sought. It takes place to the greatest extent in the dorsal curve, where also the tabetic lesion is always and chiefly situated, and more in the posterior than in the anterior columns of the cord. This effect is produced by the weight of the body alone, and is aided by muscular tension when the body is suspended from the axillæ. Muscular tension, like the force of gravity, acts beneficially most, if not only, in the dorsal region. Relaxation of the cord in the neck is impossible, and cervico-occipital suspension is not only dangerous and unpleasant, but unscientific and inoperative. It follows, therefore, that measures should be directed toward the dorsal region alone. For the old and infirm, the present method of suspension from the axillæ, but from the axillæ alone, will probably remain the best. No strain should ever be put upon the head."* His pathophysiological explanation cast doubt on whether inflammatory adhesions were in fact broken: *"far more efficacious must be the concomitant effect on the spinal blood-vessels and lymphatics."* [87] In Berlin, Martin Bernhardt (1844–1915) arrived a similar conclusion, writing of changes to the conditions of circulation in the cerebrospinal meninges and the spinal cord itself.[88] Contrary to Cagney, Gaétan-Hugues Dupuy-Fromy (1863–1932) recommended in his thesis that patients be suspended by their head alone, without axillary support! He thought this would facilitate *"circulation in the blood vessels to the spinal cord, by modifying the nutrition of its cells, and perhaps by making the cells that have been stretched and massaged more responsive to organic exchanges capable of renewing them."* [89] But Haushalter wrote: *"In our opinion, several of the beneficial effects obtained by suspension must be attributed, at least in large part, to a totally different cause than the dynamic, anatomical, or circulatory modifications of the rachidian nervous system that result from the effects of suspension on the spinal canal and its content."* Acknowledging improvement in only "dynamic" symptoms, the critical conclusion is unequivocal: *"Based on our observations, the improvements obtained by hanging are those that often occur spontaneously during the progression of nervous system diseases. . . . Is it not possible that the improvements result from a moral effect, produced by the suspension method, this undeniably strange treatment, a little frightening at first, very much in fashion at present, widely described and recommended? It makes a strong impression on the mind, unconsciously modifying the patient's psychic centers. By the mechanism of suggestion, it has a more or less rapid effect in the parts of the nervous system where dynamic damage has occurred."*

In contrast, David D. Stewart in Philadelphia wrote in 1891: *"After generating excessive enthusiasm in the medical profession, suspension seems to have been unfairly forgotten."* Stewart then described the disappearance of the worst symptoms in a patient.[90] Also in 1891, in *La Nouvelle Iconographie de La Salpêtrière*, Alexander Bogroff, a psychiatrist in Odessa proposed an update to the suspension technique recommended by Motchutkowsky and reviewed all articles published on this subject. He contested the position defended by Haushalter, notably the placebo effect of the technique. His own experiments on cadavers, then on living rabbits, led him to propose a vascular effect on the spinal cord, qualified as hyperemia, by creation of a negative pressure in the ependymal canal and the cerebral ventricles during suspension. To limit the dangers of the techniques initially used, Bogroff developed a pivoting traction table not requiring suspension by the neck.[91]

Endless Debate

Regardless of the criticisms, Fulgence Raymond, who had been one of the initiators for all of these experiments, stated in a lesson given a little later, in

1896, that suspension remained for him a preferred method in the systematic treatment of tabes: *"Suspension is not a curative remedy for tabes dorsalis, as some have claimed. But although it has only symptomatic value, in many cases suspension is nonetheless very salutary for some manifestations of tabes, and is a first line of treatment for searing pain, genital-urinary difficulties, and motor incoordination. Patients nearly crippled by progression of motor incoordination to the lower limbs, easily recover the use of their legs and can once again walk significant distances, without the need for support. However, and I have insisted on this point, suspension fails in many cases. There are several contraindications to its use, and it is not without danger. Finally, instrumentation is required and the technique must be learned, which means that suspension is not suitable for all physicians."* [92]

To understand the debate around attempts to explain the improvement in certain patients, it should be recalled that the absence of effective therapies against neuralgic pain, aside from morphine, led physicians to seek *"mechanical"* methods to modify nervous transmission. [93] The oldest idea consisted in *"elongating the nerves,"* as Charcot had noted. [94] The experiments conducted at the time showed that the trauma resulting from stretching the nerve inhibited its functional activity for a time. [95] In the introductory historical overview of his 1881 thesis, Edmond Wiet (1856–1921) traced these antalgic practices for treating neuralgia back to ancient times. [96] An incision was made in the skin above a nerve pathway to isolate the nerve. [97] The surgeon then manually pulled on the proximal part and, in some cases, the distal part, without causing breakage. The procedure was especially recommended for refractory cases of sciatica and trigeminal neuralgia ("tic douloureux"). The theses of Edmond Wiet (1856–1921), Florent Scheving (1855–?), [98] and Jules Chauvel (1841–1908) [99] show that physicians have never lacked for imagination in using nerve elongation (treatment of tetanus, leprosy) or paid much attention to the iatrogenic risks (treatment of athetosis, Parkinson's, transverse myelitis). Scheving concluded: *"For elongation to produce a therapeutic result, it must be performed until a persistent anesthesia is produced in the territory innervated by the elongated nerve."* In 1882, Joseph Bonnaire (1858–1918) and Henry Duret (1849–1921) founded a journal for research on nerve elongation in Europe and the United States [100]: *"This operation seems to have definitively entered our surgical habits and its results appear satisfactory in various circumstances. . . . The practical conclusion of all this experimental research appears to be that elongation causes a loss of sensitivity, if properly performed; the sensory or centrifugal current disappears. On the contrary, the motor or descending current is maintained. . . . To explain this more or less complete anesthesia, which does not affect mobility, various hypotheses have been proposed: alteration of the nerve fibers in the nerve trunks, mechanical action propagated to the nerve centers, and an effect on the peripheral endings of the nerves."*

However, certain surgeons, such as Albert Heydenreich (1849–1898) in Nancy, remained doubtful about the improvements: *"Elongation is not absolutely innocuous and success is highly variable; furthermore, when it is successful, the results are most often incomplete or temporary."*[101]

Forward Flexion of the Body

The resurgence of interest in nerve elongation in 1872 is due to the German surgeon Johann Nepomuk von Nußbaum (1829–1890),[102] a pioneer in antisepsis. Von Nußbaum sought to treat refractory cases of sciatica and neuralgia in the severed limbs of amputees who had survived the 1870–71 Franco-Prussian War.[103] In 1879, Carl Langenbuch (1846–1901)[104] had the idea to operate on an ataxic. The surgery, one of the first of its kind, was successful and the patient, initially bedridden, was able to walk again after his convalescence.[105] Amédée-René Blondeau reported on this use of the procedure in *Le Progrès Médical* in 1880: *"Nerve elongation in ataxics is a very recent operation, and it originated in Germany, where for several years various neuralgias have been treated by elongation with some degree of success. German surgeons probably came to use this procedure in ataxics because searing pain can be considered a neuralgia by organic spinal lesion. . . . In the first case, where the surgeon was Langenbuch, the two sciatic nerves were elongated, then the two femoral nerves. The results were as follows: disappearance of pain and cessation of motor incoordination. In the second case, where the surgeon was Esmach,[106] the results were even more striking: following elongation of nerves in the armpit to relieve pain in the forearm, motor incoordination disappeared completely. . . . These results inspired Dr. Debove[107] to attempt the same procedure on the patients in his department. . . . The operation was performed on November 18 by Dr. Gillette.[108] The left sciatic nerve, chosen because the pain was more violent on that side, was exposed in the posterior and middle part of the thigh. The surgeon then used his fingers to pull the nerve sharply, two times. . . . The results obtained with this patient are remarkable: the searing pain ceased completely and motor incoordination almost disappeared. However, tendon reflexes remain absent and pupil myosis has not varied. In his lectures, Charcot makes these results visible and tangible for his listeners, in keeping with an approach that has ensured his success."* [109]

Charcot examined the patient, then stated: *"What is important to note is that elongation, if the results obtained so far are confirmed, is an operation that should be of inestimable benefit to ataxics. However, we must be wary of excessive enthusiasm and not use these few successful cases as justification for elongating all ataxics; that would go beyond the goal. What is called for is prudent, scientific action, which means only operating when there are real indications.* "[110] There were also attempts to establish experimental proof in animals.[111]

As noted earlier, Gilles de la Tourette shared the pertinent viewpoint expressed by Haushalter: *"We believe that these experiments demonstrate sufficiently that the spinal canal elongation resulting from suspension, the more considerable physiological elongation caused by forward flexion of the body, and the elongation obtained by traction on the head and legs, which is used in certain treatments of vertebral deformation, are not capable of producing an elongation of the spinal cord, the nerve roots, or the pia mater and its vessels. Furthermore, we consider suspension to be ineffective at breaking the adhesions that, in tabes, can form between the pia mater and the posterior tracts. In elongation of the spinal canal, the dura mater alone undergoes an ascending movement, but the links of the pia mater and its vessels with the spinal column do not appear to us to be modified in any way. There is no basis for any comparison between the action of suspension on the spinal cord and nerves, and the immediate efficacy of surgical nerve elongation. In any case, we believe that if any modifications occur in the spinal cord, roots, and vessels during suspension due to elongation of the spinal canal, modifications that are impossible to detect in living patients or cadavers, they can just as easily be obtained by simple forward flexion of the body, as in a deep bow."*

Gilles de la Tourette paid careful attention to the counterarguments, and, in 1897, he modified his practices without abandoning them. He discouraged stretching the nerves, with which Debove had started experimenting: *"We were encouraged in this by the fact that, during the last twenty years, the treatment of this condition was dominated almost completely by this objective: to act mechanically on the diseased nervous organs. In the first period, from 1878 to 1883, many authors, both in France and abroad, tried to achieve success by nerve elongation. Currently discouraged as a general treatment method for tabes, this technique is no longer applied to the large nerve trunks, but rather to the small peripheral branches, which is the only effective therapeutic treatment for trophic accidents (ulcerated diabetic foot), as one of us recently demonstrated. . . .*[112] *Elongation of the spinal cord itself became the goal of the therapy."* Shortly thereafter, Gilles de la Tourette noted: *"It occurred to us to apply these observations to therapies used for locomotor ataxia."* [113] Next, Gilles de la Tourette traced the beginning of the use of suspension and signaled, as Raymond had, a return to these methods starting in 1895: *"We have remained constantly faithful to the principle of spinal elongation, though our ideas on the best way of achieving it have evolved, based on anatomical research that we have published. This research proves that true elongation does not require suspension, but rather bending the spinal column of our patients."* To obtain this flexion—actually, to bend his patients in half—Gilles de la Tourette had a table built on which the patient was attached by a harness at waist level. The top of the body was held by leather straps that made a figure of eight in front of and in back of the thorax. A rope attached to the shoulders and neck was slipped through pulleys and passed between the legs, which were kept straight. As the rope was progressively pulled, the trunk bent forward, the goal being to bring the shoulders in contact with the knee caps: *"The subject, forced to curve forward, feels a sensation in the lumbar region that quickly becomes painful. Tolerance generally increases during the first five or six sessions and then ceases to change. When traction is increased, the subject feels tension in the sciatic nerves on both sides. This is the best proof of an elongation of the spinal cord and the large nerve trunks that extend to the lower limbs."* Gilles de la Tourette did not even consider the elongation of the hamstrings. He performed a test on forty-seven ataxics who were neither at an initial nor an advanced stage of the disease. The patients were literally folded in half, no less than fifteen or twenty times (Figure 10.8).

They experienced an improvement after a dozen sessions, each lasting five to eight minutes. Fifty was the maximum number of sessions. For Gilles de la

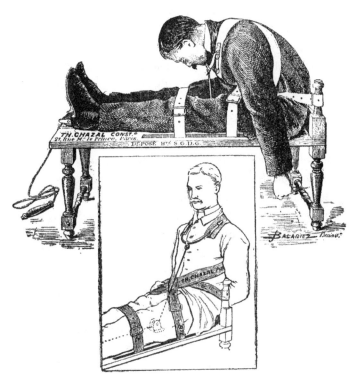

FIGURE 10.8 Gilles de la Tourette's table for elongation; patient attached by a harness at waist level.
Private collection of the author.

Tourette, this method was free of danger, unlike suspension. *"In these ataxics, flexion of the spinal column is undoubtedly the best therapeutic method, superior to all of the other mechanical methods. Our observations are the categorical demonstration."* Perhaps because of his own illness, Gilles de la Tourette had lost the prudence recommended by Charcot for interpreting results. In a brief note written in 1898 with his *chef de clinique*, Georges Gasne (1868–1910), Gilles de la Tourette reported on twenty additional patients treated on his forced flexion table, with a clear improvement for seventeen of them.[114] A translation was published in German.[115] The surgeon Antony Chipault (1833–1920) went a step further, proposing in 1900 *"a permanent elongation"* involving a plaster corset that was fitted with the patient bent at the waist.[116]

Final Analysis

In his 1898 book of therapeutic clinical lessons on nervous system diseases,[117] Gilles de la Tourette covered the diagnosis and treatment of locomotor ataxia in the tenth lesson: *"Among diseases of the spinal cord, I do not think there is any condition more frequently observed than locomotor ataxia or tabes, as it continues to be called. And there may be no condition for which the symptoms are more varied or the clinical forms more diverse, which often introduces doubt into diagnosis. For these reasons, I felt it necessary to cover this disease, while at the same time hesitating to do so. As I said at the beginning of these lessons, they always have a therapeutic conclusion. For tabes, the question remains as to whether there is such a conclusion. But as I shall show, there are few conditions for which as much ingenuity has been applied to find an effective remedy. I, myself, have endeavored to find a cure. At the very least, this has provided me with the opportunity to examine numerous ataxics."* What an admission, coming from Gilles de la Tourette himself! This lesson is in the same spirit as Charcot's lessons, which Gilles de la Tourette set out to imitate, as he stated in the book's preface. The lesson's pedagogy is excellent. Certain points, however, reveal the ambiguity of Gilles de la Tourette's opinions, especially on the syphilitic nature of tabes: *"It is certain that syphilis is very frequently, though not always, among the antecedents of tabes patients, as noted by Prof. Fournier, which has led Mr. Erb in Heidelberg to argue that tabes is always syphilitic in origin."* Heredity and above all lifestyle and exhaustion remained central to the disease's etiology: *"When syphilis exists, the ground is fertile for the development of tabes. It is very frequently the cause that provokes tabes, but is not absolutely necessary. This was the opinion of my late lamented Master, Charcot, an opinion he remained faithful to."* The contradiction becomes explicit regarding medicinal treatment: *"My opinion is that of my teacher, Prof. Fournier. I believe, as he does, that when tabes is present, especially an incipient tabes, the first treatment should be, without hesitation, mercury and iodide compounds, even if the subject is not syphilitic."*

Incidentally, in his section on semiology describing ocular disturbances, Gilles de la Tourette uses the term "Vincent's sign" for myosis and pupillary inequality. He mistakenly attributes to Napoléon-Charles Vincent (1849–1906) the description of what is generally referred to as Argyll Robertson pupils. Argyll J. Robertson (1837–1908) noted in 1869: *"I could not observe any contraction of either pupil under the influence of light, but, on accommodating the eyes for a near object, both pupils contracted."*[118] Vincent's thesis was completed later, in 1877.[119]

Gilles de la Tourette concluded his lesson this way: *"I would now be finished with my presentation of the therapies for tabes, but I have reserved a special place for a treatment method that addresses the important group of tabes phenomena, and perhaps can be said to fight the illness itself, to stop its progression by acting directly on the spinal cord, the source of the disease. I mean to speak of the treatment method by elongation of the spinal cord, which owes its invention entirely to Moczutkovski."*[120] Gilles de la Tourette goes on to describe, in detail, all of the work he personally accomplished, having been asked by the Master at La Salpêtrière in 1889 to experiment with suspension. His pride is unmistakable, even megalomaniacal. It is only in passing, and somewhat disdainfully, that he mentions the new treatment of the day, consisting of innovative rehabilitation techniques for ataxia developed by the Swiss physician Heinrich Sebastian Frenkel (1860–1931).[121] Rubens Hirschberg (1862–1920) wrote of the new treatment: *"For many years, this method has met with the most absolute indifference in the medical world. It is indeed by an ironic twist of fate that the only two methods that have yielded significant results in the treatment of tabes dorsalis—suspension and movement rehabilitation—have faced such challenges in gaining recognition. Suspension was forgotten for seven years before Professor Raymond gave it the attention it deserved. A noteworthy fact, and we also have Raymond to thank for developing the Frenkel method in France."*[122] After traveling to Heiden to learn more about this rehabilitation technique,[123] Raymond decided it was a remarkable way to help patients regain their movement capacities.[124]

This 1898 lesson was the last text Gilles de la Tourette would publish on vibratory medicine and suspension. The period during which antalgic suspension was recommended by physicians throughout the world lasted around ten years. In some cases, it brought about remission, most often brief and inevitably followed by a worsening of symptoms. And the non-negligible number of immediate deaths should not be forgotten.[125] According to Douglas Lanska, *"the disparity between early and later studies resulted from a placebo effect, from disregard of the natural history of the condition, from misdiagnosis, and from biased observation and reporting.*"[126] Russia appears to be the only country in the world where suspension is still performed today and considered an acceptable neurological therapy based on the description found by Michael Shterenshis[127] in a neurology manual for medical students.[128]

During orthopedic spinal surgery, traction is still used for realignment in cases of fractured vertebrae or in certain scolioses, but extreme caution is taken with regard to the neurological risks. Current studies on "spinal stress" during cervical fractures are slowly revealing the closely linked neuronal, synaptic, and molecular mechanisms involved in compression or traction of the spinal cord.[129] And, as always, much remains to be done.

These mechanistic treatments were not the first of their kind. Ernst Horn in Berlin,[130] building on an idea of Joseph Mason Cox (1763–1818) in Bristol,[131] England, used a bed and later a wheelchair to treat his patients, mainly suffering from mental illnesses. For Cox and Horn, disturbances in thinking arose from physical disorders that needed to be addressed by physical means; namely, centrifugal force.[132] The idea appears to have originated in 1795 with Erasmus Darwin, who regularly used centrifuges to treat delirium.[133] When subjects undergo 60 or 120 rotations per minute, they are submitted to up to 4 g of centrifugal force. The physical effects are significant and very disagreeable. These sensations were undoubtedly strange for Darwin's patients, and the resulting anxiety and discomfort must have overcome their melancholy and derangement.

Notes

1. Corvisart JN. Bayle GL. Idée Générale de la Thérapeutique. In *Encyclopédie des Sciences Médicales*. Paris: Au Bureau de l'Encyclopédie. 1838;7:604–610.
2. Charcot JM. *De l'expectation en médecine. Thèse de concours pour l'agrégation présentée et soutenue le 17 avril 1857*. Paris: Germer-Baillière. 1857.
3. Littré E. *Dictionnaire de médecine, de chirurgie, de pharmacie*. Paris: JB. Baillière. 1865.
4. Lucas P. *Traité philosophique et physiologique de l'hérédité naturelle dans les états de santé et de maladie du système nerveux: avec l'application méthodique des lois de la procréation au traitement général des affections dont elle est le principe*. Paris: JB. Baillière. 1847–1850.
5. Morel BA. *Traité des dégénérescences physiques, intellectuelles et morales de l'espèce humaine et des causes qui produisent ces variétés maladives*. Pans: JB. Baillière. 1857.
6. Pinell P. Degeneration theory and heredity patterns between 1850 and 1900. In JP Gaudillière and I Löwy (eds.), *Heredity and Infection. The History of Disease Transmission*. London and New York: Routledge. 2001:245–260.
7. Charcot JM, Berbez P. Traitement du tabes par suspension. *Gazette Hebdomadaire de Médecine et de chirurgie*. 1889;36(4):53–54.
8. Charcot JM. La médecine vibratoire. Application des vibrations rapides et continues au traitement de quelques maladies du système nerveux. Leçon recueillie par Georges Gilles de la Tourette. *Le Progrès Médical*. 1892;20(26 2è série)35:149–151.

9. Chirac P. Histoire des maladies de la teste selon le sentiment de Mr Chirac professeur de médecine et très abil praticien dans l'Université de Montpellier . . . escrites par Jacques Daveau de Saulieu en Bourgogne, achevés descrire le 8eme juillet 1697. 362 p. (BIU santé Paris, cote MS 5540).

10. Castel CI. *Fauteuil de poste. Machine pour guérir et éloigner les maladies que causent l'excès de nourriture, la vie trop sédentaire, et le défaut de transpiration suffisante.* Mercure de France dédié au Roy. Paris: Guillaume Cavelier. 1734;10(12):2879–2889.

11. Astruc J. Observation sur la Machine appelée Fauteuil de poste. *Mercure de France.* 1735;11(4):677–688.

12. Voltaire F. M. Letter, Argental, September 1744. In É Littré and LM Devic (eds.), *Dictionnaire de la langue française.* Paris: Hachette. 1883–1884.

13. Cabanes A. Un précurseur de Charcot au XVIIIᵉ, l'abbé de Saint-Pierre et son trémoussoir. *Gazette des Hôpitaux civils et militaires.* 1899;65(104):985–987.

14. This device was built for Romain Vigouroux (1831–1911) by Rudolph Koenig (1832–1901), a German-born French physicist, initially a violin maker, who, in 1855, created a workshop in Paris for making instruments to study acoustics. He conducted research into the speed of sound, vibratory movement, *diapason normal*, interference of two tones, and the characteristic notes of the different vowels. He invented several instruments, including a wave siren and the manometric flame device, which was used to visualize sound waves.

15. Boudet de Pâris M. Traitement de la douleur par les vibrations mécaniques. *Le Progrès Médical.* 1881;9(6):93–95.

16. Could Charcot be referring to the disturbances of rapid eye movement (REM) sleep in synucleinopathies?

17. Vigouroux R. Les Æsthésiogènes et la théorie des vibrations. *Le Progrès Médical.* 1880;8(36):729–731.

18. Charcot JM, Richer P. De l'influence des agents æsthésiogènes sur l'hémianesthésie et l'achromatopsie cérébrales et particulièrement du phénomène des oscillations consécutives. *Le Progrès Médical.* 1879;7(46):893–894.

19. Diffraction of light was described for the first time by a priest, Francesco Maria Grimaldi (1618–1663), in his book, *Physico-mathesis de Lumine, coloribus et iride,* published in 1665. The phenomenon of interference was first described by Newton in his *Optice* in 1706. A century would pass before the first convincing explanation, which was based on the wave theory of light of Christiaan Huygens (1629–1695).

20. Newton I. *Optice: sive de reflexionibus, refractionibus, inflexionibus & coloribus lucis libri tres.* London: Impensis Sam. Smith & Benj. Walfor. 1706.

21. Newton I. *Opticks: or a Treatrise of Reflections, Refractions, Inflections and Colours of Light* (4th edition). London: Printed for William Innys at the West-End of St. Paul's. 1730.

22. Hartley D. *Observations on Man, His Frame, His Duty, and His Expectations.* London: C. Hitch & S. Austen. 1749.

23. Glassman RB, Buckingham HW. David Hartley's neural vibrations and psychological associations. In H Whitaker, CMU Smith, and S Finger (eds.), *Brain, Mind, Medicine, Essays in Eigthteenth-Century Neuroscience.* New York: Springer. 2007:177–190.

24. Mortimer-Granville, J. *Nerve Vibration and Excitation as Agents in the Treatment of Functional Disorder and Organic Disease.* London: Churchill. 1883.

25. Georges Gaiffe (1857–1943) and his father Ladislas Adolphe Gaiffe (1832–1887) produced equipment of exceptional quality. The Maison Gaiffe was a fine example of the technical ingenuity and *savoir-faire* that still existed in France at that time. The Gaiffe name was internationally renowned, and Gaiffe was involved in manufacturing all of the most advanced, high-quality electrical and electro-medical equipment of his day.

26. In mechanical engineering, an eccentric is a mechanism that causes displacement away from or toward the axis of rotation. This enables the transformation of rotary movement into oscillatory movement.

27. Maillechort (nickel silver, German silver, Argentan, new silver, nickel brass, albata, alpaca, electrum) is an alloy of copper, nickel, and zinc that is silver in color. It was developed by two Frenchmen, Maillet and Chorier, in 1819, who gave it its name. Appreciated for its good machinability and weldability, this alloy is excellent for cold working. It is currently used to make rivets, boltwork, jewelry, and more.

28. Zénobe Gramme (1826–1901), a Belgian electrician, invented the first electric generator, known as the "Gramme dynamo," in 1868. Working with Hippolyte Fontaine (1833–1910), he demonstrated in 1873 that the dynamo was reversible, meaning that it could supply mechanical energy when connected to an electrical power source. The first electric motor was born and baptized "the Gramme machine."

29. Galante E. Casque vibratoire de MM. Les Docteurs Gilles de la Tourette, Larat et Gautier. *Revue des Instruments de Chirurgie*. 1892;2(12):1892.

30. Gilles de la Tourette G. Considérations sur la médecine vibratoire et ses applications et sa technique. *La Nouvelle Iconographie de La Salpêtrière*. 1892;5(6):265–275.

31. La Nature. Vibratory therapeutics. *Scientific American*. 1892;67(17):265.

32. Weber A, Werneck L, Paiva E, Gans P. Effects of music in combination with vibration in acupuncture points on the treatment of fibromyalgia. *J Altern Complement Med*. 2015;21(2):77–82.

33. Rodríguez Jiménez S, Benítez A, García González MA, Feliu GM, Maffiuletti NA. Effect of vibration frequency on agonist and antagonist arm muscle activity. *Eur J Appl Physiol*. 2015;115(6):1305–13012.

34. Lipsitz LA, Lough M, Niemi J, Travison T, Howlett H, Manor B. A shoe insole delivering subsensory vibratory noise improves balance and gait in healthy elderly people. *Arch Physic Med Rehabil*. 2015;96(3):432–439.

35. Orr R. The effect of whole body vibration exposure on balance and functional mobility in older adults: A systematic review and meta-analysis. *Maturitas*. 2015;80(4):342–358.

36. Duchenne (de Boulogne) G. De l'ataxie locomotrice, recherches sur une maladie caractérisée spécialement par des troubles généraux de la coordination des mouvements. *Archives Générales de Médecine*. 1858-2;Vᵉ série 12(12):641–652; 1859-1;Vᵉ série 13(1):36–62; 1859-1;Vᵉ série(2):158-181; 1859-1;V° série(4):417–451.

37. Marcé LV. *Des altérations de la sensibilité. Thèse d'agrégation*. Paris: JB. Baillière. 1860.

38. Landry O. *Mémoire sur la paralysie du sentiment d'activité musculaire*. Paris: Typographie Henri Plon. 1855.

39. Duchenne (de Boulogne) G. Recherches électro-pathologiques sur les usages de la sensibilité musculaire. *Comptes Rendus hebdomadaires des séances de l'Académie des Sciences*. 1853;37(12):950–953.

40. Bell Ch. On the nervous circle which connects the voluntary muscles with the brain. *Philo Trans R Soc*. 1826; 116:163–173.

41. Puchelt FAB. Ueber partielle Empfindungs Lähmung. *Heidelberg Medicinische Annalen*. 1844;10(4)244–265.

42. von Weidenbach C. *De Tabe Dorsuali*. Dissertatio Berolinum, typis Haynianis. 1817.

43. "Tabes, a Latin word sometimes used in French works to express any sort of consumption and weakening in the human body, whatever the organic disease from which it stems (see marasmus). Among the causes of tabes, phthisis pulmonalis and veneral excesses of all sorts are without question the most frequent. The first of these causes leads to what is known as tabes pulmonaris, the second leads to tables dorsalis." *Dictionnaire Des Sciences Médicales*. Panckoucke. 1821;54:206–207.

44. Loewenhard SE. *De myelophthisi chronica vera et notha*. Dissertatio inauguralis medica. Berlin: Typis Haynianis. 1817.
45. Schesmer TG. *Tabis Dorsualis, Adumbratio pathologica*. Dissertatio inauguralis medica. Berlin: Typis Augusti G. Schadii. 1819.
46. Charcot JM. Sur quelques arthropathies qui paraissent dépendre d'une lésion du cerveau ou de la moelle épinière. *Archives de Physiologie normale et pathologique*. 1868;1:161–178.
47. Horn G. *De tabe dorsuali Praelusio*. Berlin: Kraus. 1827.
48. Horn E. Bemerkungen über die wichtigsten Erkrankungen, Jan. *Fe*. 1813, Charité. *Neues Archiv für medizinische Erfahrung*. 1813;6:236–238.
49. Schiller F. Venery, the spinal cord, and tabes dorsalis before Romberg: the contribution of Ernst Horn. *J Nerv Ment Dis*. 1976;163(1):1–9.
50. Romberg MH. *Lehrbuch der Nervenkrankheiten des Menschen*. Berlin: Alexander Duncker. 1846; Sieveking EH (translator). A Manual of the Nervous Diseases of Man. London: Sydenham Society. 1853).
51. Pearce JMS. Romberg and his sign. *Eur Neurol*. 2005;53(4):210–123.
52. Schiller F. Staggering gait in medical history. *Ann Neurol*. 1995;37(1):127–35.
53. Duchenne (de Boulogne) G. *De l'électrisation localisée et de son application à la pathologie et à la thérapeutique par courants induits et par courants galvaniques interrompus et continus*. Paris: JB. Baillière. 1872.
54. Charcot JM, Bouchard CH. Douleurs fulgurantes de l'ataxie, sans incoordination des mouvements, sclérose commençante des cordons postérieurs de la moelle épinière. *Comptes rendus de la Société de Biologie*. 1866;3:10–19.
55. Erb W. *Ueber die etiologische Bedeutung der Syphilis für die Tabes dorsalis.Transactions of the International Medical Congress, seventh session of the International Medical Congress, London 1881*. London: JW. Kolckmann. 1881;2:32–42.
56. Charcot JM. *Du traitement de l'ataxie locomotrice par la suspension suivant la méthode du Dr Motchutkowsky. Leçons du Mardi à La Salpêtrière. Leçon du 15 janvier 1889*. Paris: Le Progrès Médical, Lecrosnier & Babé. 1889.
57. Motchutkowsky OO. Application of suspension of patients to the treatment of some disorders of the spinal cord. *Vratsch*. 1883;17–21:258–325.
58. Motchutkowsky OO. Treatment of certain diseases of the spinal cord by means suspension. *Brain*. 1889;12(3):326–345.
59. Sayre L. *Spinal Disease and Spinal Curvature, Their Treatment by Suspension and the Use of the Plaster of Paris Bandage*. London: Smith Elder & Co. 1877.
60. Charcot JM, Berbez P. Traitement du tabes par suspension. *Gazette Hebdomadaire de Médecine et de chirurgie*. 1889;36(4):53–54.
61. Charcot JM, Gilles de la Tourette G. De la technique à suivre dans le traitement par la suspension de l'ataxie locomotrice progressive et de quelques autres maladies du système nerveux. *Le Progrès Médical*. 1889;17(8):135–137.
62. Gosselin W. *De la suspension dans l'ataxie locomotrice progressive et dans deux cas de sclérose en plaques*. Thèse no. 9. Paris: Henri Jouve. 1889.
63. Dujardin-Beaumetz GS. *De l'ataxie locomotrice*. Thèse no. 32. Paris: Imprimerie Rignoux. 1862.
64. Pichery J. *Gymnastique de l'opposant*. Paris: JB. Baillière. 1880.
65. Dujardin-Beaumetz GS. De la suspension chez les tabétiques. *Bulletin général de thérapeutique médicale et chirurgicale*. 1889;117: 1–15.
66. Monet J, Quin G. De la pendaison à la rééducation motrice. *Histoire des Sciences Médicales*. 2012;46(3):235–244.
67. Balaban H. *Traitement de l'ataxie locomotrice progressive par la suspension*. Thèse no. 29. Paris: Ollier-Heny. 1889.

68. Gilles de la Tourette G. Diminution et cessation de l'usage habituel de la morphine chez deux tabétiques traités par la suspension. *Archives de Neurologie.* 1889;18(52):126–128.

69. Raoult A. Traitement de l'ataxie locomotrice et quelques autres maladies du système nerveux. *Le Progrès Médical.* 1889;17(25):469–471; *Archives de Neurologie.* 1889;18(52):129–143.

70. Raoult A. De la suspension dans le traitement des maladies du système nerveux. *Le Progrès Médical.* 1890;18(17):334–335.

71. Dana CH. The treatment of locomotor ataxia by suspension. *Boston Med Surg J.* 1889;121:429–430.

72. Worotynsky B. Ueber die Suspension als eine Behandlungsmethode bei Nervenkrankheiten. *Deutsche Zeitschrift für Nervenheilkunde.* 1895;8(1-2):75–96.

73. Bekhterev V. Ueber den Einfluss der Suspension auf die Sehstörungen bei Affectionen des Rückenmarks. *Neurologisches Centralblatt.* 1893;12(7):210–217.

74. Ladame PL. De la suspension chez les tabétiques. *Revue Médicale de la Suisse Romande.* 1889;8:347–349.

75. Obituary. Armand de Watteville. *Br Med J.* 1925;1(3350):538.

76. Motschutkovsky A. The treatment of certain diseases of the spinal cord by means of suspension (translated from the Russian by De Watteville A). *Brain.* 1889–1890;12:327–345.

77. Obituary. Julius Althaus. *Br Med J.* 1990;1:1508.

78. Althaus J. How does suspension act in locomotor ataxy? *Lancet.* 1889;133(3424):760.

79. Althaus J. Appareil modifié pour la suspension. *Le Progrès Médical.* 1889;10(1):36–37.

80. Asher L. Du traitement par la suspension. *Archives de Neurologie.* 1891;22(66):422–423.

81. Rosembaum F. Suspension dans le tabes. *Mercredi Médical.* 1890;1(18):217.

82. Eulenburg A. Mendel E. Ergebnisse der Suspensionbehandlung bei Tabes dorsalis und anderen chronischen Nervenkrankheiten. *Neurologisches Centralblatt.* 1889;8(11):313–324.

83. Gilles de la Tourette G. Modifications apportées à la technique de la suspension dans le traitement de l'ataxie locomotrice et de quelques autres maladies du système nerveux. *Le Progrès Médical.* 1890;18-1(23):457–459.

84. Goncourt (de) J, de Goncourt (de) E. *Journal, Mémoires de la vie littéraire, postface de M. Lucien Descaves. Édition définitive publiée par l'Académie Concourt.* Paris: E. Flammarion Fasquelle. 1936.

85. Haushalter P, Adam A. De la suspension dans le traitement des malades du système nerveux. *Le Progrès Médical.* 1889;17(44): 375–378 / 493–494 / 512–513.

86. Gilles de la Tourette G, Gasne G. Le traitement de l'ataxie locomotrice par l'élongation vraie de la moelle épinière. *Nouvelle Iconographie de La Salpêtrière.* 1898;11(1):18–19.

87. Cagney J. The mechanism of suspension in the treatment of locomotor ataxy. *Medical Chirurgy Transactions.* 1890;73:101–127.

88. Bernhardt M. De la suspension dans l'ataxie locomotrice. *Gazette hebdomadaire de Médecine et de Chirurgie.* 1889;36(52):846.

89. Dupuy-Fromy GHM. *De la traction cervicale graduée substituée à la suspension dans le traitement de l'ataxie locomotrice.* Thèse no. 26. Bordeaux: S.N. 1890.

90. Stewart DD. On the utility of suspension in disease of the spinal cord. *Med News.* 1891;16(974):292.

91. Bogroff A. Considérations sur le traitement des maladies du système nerveux par la méthode du docteur Motschourkovsky. *Nouvelle Iconographie de La Salpêtrière.* 1891;4:464–481 / 1892;5:18–37.

92. Raymond F. *Leçons sur les maladies du système nerveux (année 1895–1896). Leçon XXIX. Le traitement de l'incoordination motrice du tabes par la rééducation des muscles.* Paris: Octave Doin. 1897.

93. Symington J. The physics of nerve-stretching. *Br Med J.* 1882;1:770–771.

94. Keane JR. Neurectasy: the short history of therapeutic nerve stretching and suspension. *Neurology.* 1990;40:829–831.

95. Bowlby AA. Nerve-stretching: the clinical application of the operation of nerve-stretching. In *Injuries and Diseases of Nerves and Their Surgical Treatment*. London: J. & A. Churchill. 1889:332–391.

96. Wiet E. *Contribution à l'étude de l'élongation des nerfs*. Thèse no. 429. Paris: Imprimerie A. Davy. 1881.

97. Marshall J. Bradshaw Lecture on nerve-stretching for the relief or cure of pain. *Br Med J.* 1883;2:1173–1179.

98. Scheving F. *De l'élongation des nerfs*. Thèse no. 124. Paris: A. Parent. 1881.

99. Chauvel J. *De l'élongation des nerfs*. Thèse no. 943. Paris: P. Asselin. 1881.

100. Duret H, Bonnaire J. L'élongation des nerfs. *Le Progrès Médical*. 1882;10(9):163–164; (10):192–193; (12):227–228; (15):289–291; (31):603–604.

101. Heydenreich A. Résultats cliniques de l'élongation des nerfs. *La Semaine Médicale*. 1885;5:59–60.

102. von Nußbaum NJ. Blosslegung und Dehnung der Rückenmarksnerven: eine erfolgreiche Operation. *Deutsche Zeitschrift für Chirurgie*. 1872;1(5):450–465.

103. Jacquemin E. *De l'élongation nerveuse dans l'ataxie et les affections médullaires*. Thèse no. 239. Paris: A. Davy. 1883.

104. Morgenstern L. Carl Langenbuch and the first cholecystectomy. *Surg Endosc.* 1992;6(3):113–114.

105. Langenbuch C. Über Dehnung grosser Nervenstämme bei Tabes. *Berliner Klinische Wochenschrift*. 1879;16(48):709–710.

106. Freidrich von Esmarch (1823–1908) in Kiel.

107. Georges Debove (1845–1920), a former *interne* of Charcot and Paulin Eugène Gillette (1838–1886), a surgeon.

108. Paulin Eugène Gillette (1836-1886), hospital surgeon.

109. Debove G, Gillette PE. Elongation des nerfs dans l'ataxie locomotrice. *Gazette hebdomadaire de Médecine et de Chirurgie*. 1880;27(51):23.

110. Blondeau A. De l'élongation des nerfs chez les ataxiques comme traitement des douleurs fulgurantes. *Le Progrès Médical*. 1880;8(50):1015–1016.

111. Minor ML. *Contribution à l'étude expérimentale de l'élongation des nerfs*. Paris: Gauthier-Villars. 1883.

112. Chipault A. De la cure radicale du mal perforant par l'élongation des nerfs plantaires. *Gazette des Hôpitaux civils et militaires*. 1897;70:407.

113. Gilles de la Tourette G, Chipault A. Traitement de l'ataxie par l'élongation vraie de la moelle épinière. *Nouvelle Iconographie de La Salpêtrière*. 1897;10(3):144–154.

114. Gilles de la Tourette G, Gasne G. Le traitement de l'ataxie locomotrice par l'élongation vraie de la moelle épinière. *Nouvelle Iconographie de La Salpêtrière*. 1898;11(1):18–19.

115. Gilles de la Tourette G, Chipault A. Die wirkliche Dehnung des Rückenmarkes und ihre Anwendung zur Behandlung der Tabes dorsalis. *Therapeutische Wochenschrift*. 1897;4(19):459–462; 1303–1304.

116. Chipault A. De l'élongation permanente de la moelle dans l'ataxie et les myélopathies scoliogènes. *Archives de Neurologie*. 1900;10(59):421.

117. Gilles de la Tourette G. *Leçons de clinique thérapeutique sur les maladies du système nerveux*. Paris: E. Plon-Nourrit. 1898.

118. Argyll Robertson DMCL. Four cases of spinal miosis: with remarks on the action of the light on the pupil. *Edinburg Med J.* 1869;15:487–493.

119. Vincent N Ch. *Des phénomènes oculo-pupillaires dans l'ataxie locomotrice progressive et la paralysie générale des aliénés*. Thèse no. 44. Paris: Imprimerie A. Derenne. 1877.

120. Gilles de la Tourette used another spelling for "Motchutkowsky," reproducing how the name initially appeared in 1889.

121. Frenkel HS. *Ergebnisse und Grundsätze der Uebungstherapie bei der tabischen Ataxie.* Leipzig: Georg Thieme. 1896.

122. Hisrchberg R. Traitement de l'ataxie dans le tabes dorsalis par la rééducation des mouvements, méthode de Frenkel. *Archives de Neurologie.* 1896;14(9):161–185.

123. Zwecker M, Zeilig G, Ohry A. Professor Heinrich Sebastian Frenkel: a forgotten founder of rehabilitation medicine. *Spinal Cord.* 2004;42(1):55–56.

124. Raymond F. *Leçons sur les maladies du système nerveux (année 1895-1896).* Leçon XXIX. *Le traitement de l'incoordination motrice du tabes par la rééducation des muscles.* Paris: Octave Doin. 1897.

125. Weiner MF, Silver JR. Historical review: suspension therapy for the treatment of tabes dorsalis. *Eur Neurol.* 2014;72(3-4):163–172.

126. Lanska DJ, Edmonson JM. The suspension therapy for tabes dorsalis. A case history of a therapeutic fad. *Arch Neurol.* 1990;47(6):701–704.

127. Shterenshis MV. The history of modern spinal traction with particular reference to neural disorders. *Spinal Cord.* 1997;35(3):139–146.

128. Gusev YeI, Grechko VYe, Burd GS. *Nervous Diseases.* Moscow: Medicine Publishers. 1988.

129. Li K, Nicaise C, Sannie D, Hala TJ, Javed E, et al. Overexpression of the astrocyte glutamate transporter GLT1 exacerbates phrenic motor neuron degeneration, diaphragm compromise, and forelimb motor dysfunction following cervical contusion spinal cord injury. *J Neurosci.* 2014;34(22):7622–7638.

130. Horn E. *Oeffentliche Rechenschaft über mine zwoelfjaehrige Dienstfuehrung als zweiter Arzt des Koenigl. Charite Krankenhauses zu Berlin, nebst Erfahrungen über Krankenhaeuser und Irrenanstalten.* Berlin: Realschulbuchhandlung. 1818.

131. Cox JM. *Practical Observations on Insanity: In which some suggestions are offered towards an improved mode of treating diseases of the mind, and some rules proposed which it is hoped may lead to a more humane and successful method of cure; to which are subjoined remarks on medical jurisprudence as connected with diseased intellect.* London: Baldwin. 1804.

132. Harsch V. Centrifuge "therapy" for psychiatric patients in Germany in the early 1800s. *Aviation, Space, and Environmental Medicine.* 2006;77(2):157–160.

133. White JW. *A History of the Centrifuge in Aerospace Medicine.* Santa Monica: Douglas Aircraft Company, Inc. 1964.

11

Hypnotism and Analogous States

It is good to understand that there are things which cannot be understood.
—Nicolas Malebranche (1638–1715)

Written by a Doctor-in-Training

Of all the books by Gilles de la Tourette, *L'hypnotisme et les états analogues au point de vue médico-légal* was unquestionably the most successful. There were two editions, the first in 1887[1] and the second in 1889,[2] and the book was translated into German[3] and Italian.[4] The French version was prefaced by Paul Brouardel (1837–1906) and the German version by Jean-Martin Charcot (1825–1893)[5]; the Italian version included both of these prefaces, translated by Luigi Bufalini.

In November 1887, Gilles de la Tourette replaced Joseph Babiński (1857–1932) as *chef de clinique* and worked alongside Charcot. He had already published more than ten works, among them two biographies, *Théophraste Renaudot* and *Sœur Jeanne des Anges, supérieure des Ursulines à Loudun*. On August 2, 1886, he gave a speech to the Société de Médecine Légale on the subject of *"rape during hypnotism and analogous states,"* which was published in *La Semaine Médicale*[6] and simultaneously in *Le Bulletin de la Société de Médecine Légale*[7] and *Les Annales d'Hygiène Publique*.[8] Gilles de la Tourette had studied legal medicine with Brouardel and had spent part of his *internat* in Charcot's department during the period in which Charcot was focusing on hysteria. He paid tribute to his two teachers, stating: *"By inscribing the names of my two venerated masters at the beginning of this study, I fulfill a double duty of justice and acknowledgement. Mr. Charcot was the first to bring hypnotism fully into the scientific realm, and it is* to Mr. Brouardel that we owe the first complete medical-legal study of a case in this field. It is thanks to the enlightened counsel of both these men, and to the kindness of their encouragement, that I was able to successfully carry out this work." Gilles de la Tourette was uniquely prepared to introduce a scientific approach where the supernatural had reigned. To do so, he had to contend with "two different types of opinion: one denies everything and sees only phantasmagoria and charlatanism, while the other accepts everything, without sufficient control."[9]

Gilles de la Tourette's aims in writing this book were identical to those he emphasized in *Sœur Jeanne des Anges*: to fight against belief in the supernatural and to promote a secular, republican perspective. To accomplish this, he sought to unmask those who exploited the credulous. "To truly penetrate the masses, to turn them into disciples, to abuse and amaze minds, one must resort to marvels. The ordinary laws of nature must appear to have been reversed. Since these deceivers avail themselves of physiological facts to carry out their feats, it is up to physicians to explain the reality or the interpretation of these facts."[10]

Since the late seventeenth century, "magnetism" practices had spread throughout society as the universal panacea to every kind of ill. As Brouardel wrote: "Physicians no longer dared to compromise themselves by consorting with the adepts of these theories, because their theories were absolutely incomprehensible." Brouardel went on to explain the medical school's view with respect to Charcot: "Some are openly against his taking this path, which in the past has only led to disappointments or scandalous exploitation."

Background

There are four main parts to Gilles de la Tourette's book. The first part is devoted to history, the second to clinical findings, the third to therapeutic hypnotism. The fourth was of utmost importance to Gilles de la Tourette because it associated subjects on which his two masters taught: hypnotism and law. What made it innovative was threefold: it explained the delicate mission of the jurist investigating cases of rape committed while the victim was in a lethargic state, it shed light on the scandalous procedures of hypnotists at fairs, and it showed how a medical-legal expert assessment was conducted before a court of justice. Louis Beurnier (1860–1917) extolled the book in his review: "Many books have already been published on this subject, and the author admits in his preface that, during his bibliographic research, he realized that his own thoughts had already been expressed countless times. 'One cannot help but rue the fact,' he wrote, 'that the proportion of originality will be so minimal.' This is sheer modesty, and it has no place *here. Our author can rest assured; his book is original, highly and entirely original. Even if some of the facts in it have already been reported, here they are propounded from such a novel perspective, and there are so many documents, that everything seems new to the reader."*

Gilles de la Tourette introduced his book with arguments to defend it from skeptics: *"We know that the group of skeptics has not disappeared. What holds them back is moral fear, far more frequent than physical fear. They are afraid of being duped. Their intelligence, accustomed to conceiving of the unity of human understanding, struggles to accept this dislocation of nervous system characteristics and intellectual faculties. They also struggle with the reality of normal states and of trances, in which the individual differs so much from his normal self that he seems to have two separate existences. They ask themselves not why, but how these dissociations occur; finding no response, they abstain from looking further."*

To begin his history of hypnotism, Gilles de la Tourette described Franz-Anton Mesmer (1734–1815) (Figure 11.1) as more of a swindler than a therapist. The journalist Georges Montorgueil (1857–1933) reported what Gilles de la Tourette had told him: *"I know my man, for I have studied him. I have followed him step by step. I have found that this German, who claimed to be a philanthropist, was a shameless scoundrel; in six years' time, after having unsettled an entire population, he left France with six hundred thousand pounds, an enormous sum at the time. And if he was such a success, after failing so miserably in Vienna, it was because he found in Paris not only a people forever inclined to the marvelous, but also the overture to tragic circumstances. Minds were abuzz with what I shall call 'this nervous shiver, the prelude to revolution.' Neither Bailly, mayor of Paris, nor Berthollet were taken in by his deception, and Bailly in particular showed masterfully and presciently that hysterical attacks were aggravated under the influence of magnetic practices; he also noted the role of heredity."*[11] Gilles de Tourette continued to show his contempt for this "scoundrel" by publishing satirical illustrations from Mesmer's time in *La Nouvelle Iconographie de La Salpêtrière* in 1889. For the article's first illustration, "L'Apothéose de Mesmer," Gilles de la Tourette noted that *"Professor Charcot, with his natural generosity, was kind enough to send us a previously unpublished watercolor"* and then discussed the illustration's history.[12] What is curious is that it was not a watercolor but an etching. It had illustrated an anonymous book, *L'antimagnétisme ou origine, progrès, décadence, renouvellement et réfutation du magnétisme animal,* supposedly published "in London" in 1784, and which was certainly available in Parisian bookstores in the late 1800s (Figure 11.2). The illustration was a parody of Mesmer's thesis, *On the Influence of the Planets on the Human Body,* which he had defended in Vienna in 1766, as Gilles de la Tourette explained. However, he seemed unaware of the origin of this print, which had appeared on the opening page of the anonymous book, a scathing

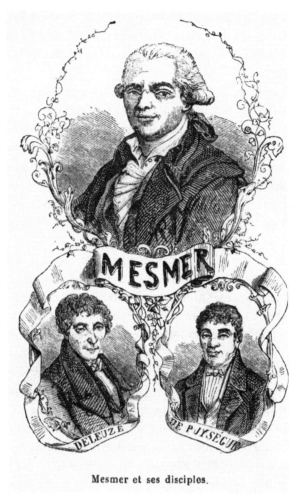

Mesmer et ses disciples.

FIGURE 11.1 Franz-Anton Mesmer (1734–1815), Joseph-Philippe-François Deleuze (1753–1835), Amand-Marc Chastenet de Puységur (1751–1825). In J. Vinchon (ed.), *Mesmer et son secret*. Paris: Amédée Legrand. 1936.
Private collection of the author.

attack whose author was in fact Jean-Jacques Paulet (1740–1826), a physician and mycologist. In it, Paulet denounced *"the magician-like imposture of magnetic healers"* and noted: *"Future generations will have difficulty believing that in the late seventeenth century, after the Lumières and their discoveries, one man, one ordinary man, was able to whip up nearly unanimous enthusiasm in Paris for several years, and almost succeeded in forming a sect."*[13]

Though Gilles de la Tourette felt nothing but hostility for Mesmer the imposter, he did acknowledge *"one thing* [that] *will argue in his favor to*

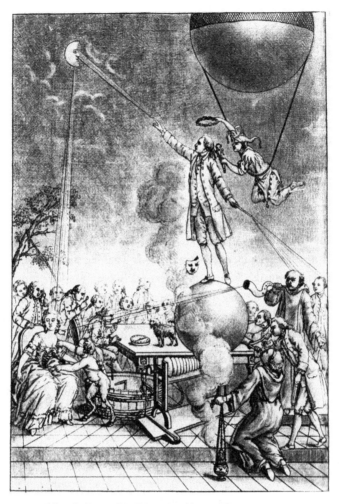

FIGURE II.2 *"L'Apothéose de Mesmer"* in *L'Antimagnétisme*, 1784.
Private collection of the author.

posterity: that he inspired, most certainly in spite of himself, the research that led Puységur to the discovery of artificial somnambulism." Gilles de la Tourette clearly esteemed Amand Marc Chastenet,[14] known by the name of Marquis de Puységur (1751–1825) (Figure 11.1),[15] for having been the first to study what would later come to be called hypnotism. *"Mesmer witnessed one of his best students making sense of the shapeless chaos that he himself had never understood. His student, whom he must have envied, isolated phenomena of the utmost importance."* Whereas Mesmer considered the convulsions he set off to be salutary, Gilles de la Tourette appreciated Puységur's prudence: *"Every time one is faced with individuals in whom magnetism produces convulsions, care must be taken not to abandon them to themselves, and moreover not to exacerbate this violent state. On the contrary, every effort must be made to calm the patient, and he must never be left alone until he has found some measure of tranquility.*" Gilles de la Tourette also held in high regard the description of catalepsy written by Jacques-Henri Petetin (1744–1808),[16] "*who had discovered, or rather, described more precisely than his predecessors, a catalepsy we could call suggestive, if we were to use a modern expression.*"[17]

Gilles de la Tourette also paid tribute to Joseph-Philippe-François Deleuze (1753–1835) (Figure 11.1) for his *Histoire critique du magnétisme animal,*[18] from which he took the description of the hypnotic state: "*The person in this state acquires a prodigious enhancement of the sensing faculty. Several of his outside organs—the organs used to see and hear—are dulled, and all of the related sensations take place internally. . . . The somnambulist has his eyes closed and does not see with his eyes. He does not hear with his ears, but he sees and hears better than a man who is awake; he sees and hears solely through those around him. He sees only what they are looking at. He looks at the objects his attention is directed towards. He is subjected to the will of his magnetizer insofar as this outside will causes him no harm and does not contradict his own ideas of justice and truth.*" This last point was important, and Gilles de la Tourette developed it further in the courtroom when faced with contradictory arguments put forth by the Nancy School of Hippolyte Bernheim (1840–1919) and by Jules Liégeois (1833–1908).[19]

José Custodio da Faria (1756–1819), better known as Abbot Faria,[20] was another precursor for Gilles de la Tourette. "*Faria was an excellent observer. A proponent of the idea that somnambulism and natural sleep were identical, he devoted himself to studying cases of prolonged sleep and was the first to have described, in no more than a few lines, the interesting condition studied by Mr. Azam, in which there exists a split personality.*"[21] Bernheim paid Faria a similar compliment: "*Faria was indisputably the first to have established the doctrine of hypnosis by suggestion and to have freed it of the useless, strange practices that had hidden the truth.*"[22] Gilles de la Tourette gave an example of Faria's practice that he himself frequently used in his "*laboratory experiments*" at La Salpêtrière: "*Faria implemented the suggestion in a 'scientific' manner (if such a word can be used) and had the patient swallow a large glass of water, transformed into an exquisite liqueur by the senses and the circumstances.*"

Gilles de la Tourette concluded by discussing his own era. He wrote of the English surgeon James Braid (1795–1860) (Figure 11.3),[23] whom he described as having inspired Charcot: "*Considering hypnotism as a series of different states arising under the influence of a single cause, he implicitly discovered the existence of the triad: lethargy, catalepsy, somnambulism. His physiological and clinical studies were to provide results of great interest to Charcot and to his school.*"

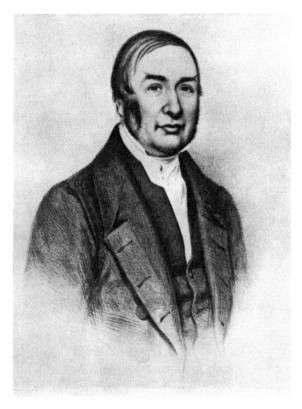

FIGURE II.3 James Braid (1795–1860).
BIU santé, Paris, Public domain.

At La Salpêtrière

After first bringing to light the work of the Bordeaux surgeon Étienne Eugène Azam (1822–1899) (Figure 11.4), who introduced the use of hypnosis in anesthesia, Gilles de la Tourette could not resist slipping in an allusion to the medical school he had attended: *"On December 19, 1859, one of our earliest and best masters, Doctor Guérineau from Poitiers, painlessly amputated a thigh at the Hôtel-Dieu in Poitiers. But hypnotism was no match against chloroform."* He referred briefly to Charles Richet (1850–1935) before referring to his master at La Salpêtrière: *"An illustrious man, one who had acquired profound knowledge of nervous system disorders over many long years, enabled hypnotism to become a veritable science, and that man is none other than Professor Charcot. It was in 1878 that his memorable lectures began at the Hospice de la Salpêtrière, lectures that were to give entirely new impetus to hypnosis studies."* The distinction relative to those who had gone before was clearly made: *"Ten years ago, Mr. Charcot began to study hypnosis once again, and to apply*

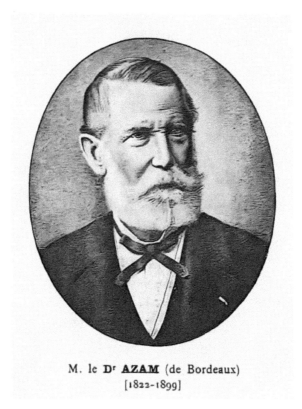

M. le Dr **AZAM** (de Bordeaux)
[1822-1899]

FIGURE II.4 Etienne-Eugène Azam (1822–1899).
Private collection of the author.

the modern method of scientific examination, using his predecessors' work but making it his own through the rigor of the critical means he brought to bear." Later in the book, Gilles de la Tourette found an opportunity to speak of himself, as he often did: *"I myself, working with P. Richer, made my own small contribution to this research during the time I was honored to be an* interne *under Professor Charcot,*[24] *and likewise, when I was an* interne *under Mr. Brouardel."*[25]

Gilles de la Tourette reviewed the many observations reported by Braid, Azam, Eugène Follin (1823–1867), Richet, and so forth, then concluded: *"It is undeniable that hysterics provide the greatest number of hypnotizable subjects."* In his view, hypnotism revealed hysteria. However, the scientific attitude that he defended required a confrontation: *"We have read the work written by the authors with opinions contrary to ours, and above all we have insisted on observing their experiments. This has only made our convictions firmer."* He pointed out that Charcot himself *"never wrote that hysterics were the only hypnotizable subjects. He simply limited himself to studying hypnotism in hysterics. . . . Let us examine the arguments put forth by the authors who today defend the opposite opinion than we do—that is, that hypnotism works perfectly in healthy subjects. . . . Among the authors who have studied hypnotism with individuals they consider healthy, let us refer to Doctor Liébault from Nancy and his pupils (we apologize for using the qualification with which they describe themselves), Mr. Bernheim and Mr. Beaunis, professors at the medical school in Nancy, and Mr. Liégeois, professor at the law school in Nancy. We shall also refer to our excellent friend, Dr. Bottey, and to Mr. Brémaud,*[26] *a first-class physician in the French Navy.*"[27] Henry-Etienne Beaunis (1830–1921) had clearly stated: "*Artificial somnambulism can be obtained with the greatest ease in a large number of subjects in whom hysteria is not present: children, the elderly, men of every constitution and every temperament.*"[28] Gilles de la Tourette distinguished Ambroise Liébault's viewpoint (1823–1904) (Figure 11.5), which he deemed acceptable and not far from his own, from that put forth by Beaunis and by Bernheim. He implicitly accused Bernheim of interpreting Liébault's results so that they would support his own theory. "*There remain the results obtained by Doctor Bottey, results that I am well placed to discuss, in that this author was an* interne *at La Salpêtrière (1884) at the same time I was, and very often we conducted experiments together.*" Fernand Bottey (1858–1900), *interne* at La Salpêtrière under Jules Luys (1828–1897) during the

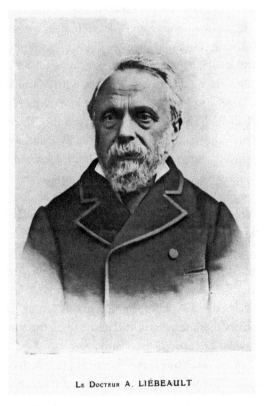

Le Docteur A. LIÉBEAULT

FIGURE 11.5 Ambroise Liébault (1823–1904).
Private collection of the author.

time Gilles de la Tourette studied under Charcot, reported a 30% rate of success in healthy subjects,[29] whereas Bernheim claimed he had hypnotized 95% of the people who had consulted him!

Unlike many of his predecessors, Gilles de la Tourette was prudent, and at no time did he attempt to provide a pathophysiological explanation of the cerebral activity in the various states he described.

Lethargy, Catalepsy, Somnambulism

Gilles de la Tourette discussed all of the hypnotization procedures: *"As for the procedures to apply, they are certainly varied; however, we shall see that their apparent variety is in fact no greater than that of the doctrines from which they arose."* For him, all of these procedures needed to be known so that they could be perfectly reproduced during medical-legal reenacts where hypnotism was involved.

Gilles de la Tourette followed this summary with a long chapter on hypnotic states, drawing heavily from the thesis and book by Paul Richer (1849–1933).[30] As he often did in his writing, he quoted several authors. In a memorandum to the Académie des Sciences on February 13, 1882, Charcot had established a classification *"of the various nervous states determined by hypnotism in hysterics,"* and Gilles de la Tourette reiterated them as follows: *"According to Charcot, there are three states in hypnotism: lethargy, catalepsy, somnambulism."*[31] To draw attention to his own research, he described his work with Marie Wittmann, better known as Blanche (1859–1913) and called the "Queen of the Hysterics." She was depicted by André Brouillet (1857–1914) in his painting, "Une leçon clinique à La Salpêtrière," which shows her being supported by Babiński. *"When Witt. . . , a hypnotizable hysteric, entered the laboratory, we directed a stream of electric light on her face. She immediately became motionless, her eyes wide open. The neuromuscular reactions that we are going to describe allowed us, by their absence, to determine that she was in a state of catalepsy. It was very easy to then bring her to a state of lethargy, then to a state of somnambulism, and to give her any relevant suggestions. . . . Unexpected and sudden closing of her eyelids, accompanied by slight pressure to the eyeballs, caused lethargy. . . . With this same patient, we obtained similar results when we concentrated directly on the sense of hearing. Unbeknownst to her, we struck a gong; the patient immediately entered a cataleptic state."* In this somewhat dull way, Gilles de la Tourette described, in detail and at length, all of the states of hypnotism per se, along with what he termed *"intermediate states."*

At times he showed a serious lack of critical perspective, citing the cases of hemi-catalepsy and hemi-lethargy described in the thesis of Edgar Bérillon (1859–1948) (Figure 11.6), a student of Victor Dumontpallier (1826–1899)

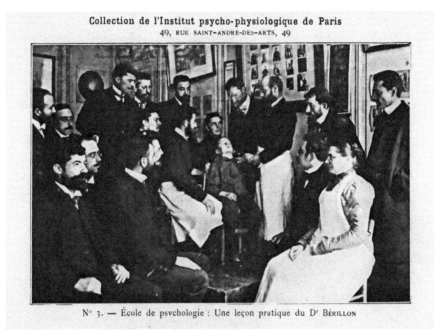

Collection de l'Institut psycho-physiologique de Paris
49, RUE SAINT-ANDRE-DES-ARTS, 49

N° 3. — École de psychologie : Une leçon pratique du D' BÉRILLON

FIGURE 11.6 A lesson by Edgar Bérillon (1859–1948).
Private collection of the author.

(Figure 11.7) at Hôpital La Pitié, entitled *De l'indépendance fonctionnelle des deux hémisphères cérébraux*,[32] and in the thesis of Gabriel Descourtis (1856–1915).[33] Gilles de la Tourette did not discuss the experiments that Bérillon always conducted with the same patients, who, whether or not Bérillon realized it, must have been entirely conditioned. Bérillon drew some striking conclusions from these experiments, whether he actually believed them or not: *"In hysterics with unilateral morbid symptoms, a single cerebral hemisphere is the primary seat of the peripheral functional disturbances"*; and, even more implausibly, *"While one experimenter speaks into the patient's left ear saying the weather is nice, the other speaks into the right ear saying the weather is rainy. The patient's face manifestly shows, on the left, a clearly characterized cheerful expression, and on the right, a most gloomy expression."* Bérillon's conclusions are peremptory: *"Since each hemisphere is complete unto itself, and since it benefits from its own specific activity, within the limits of its attributions, we can state that, from a motor, sensory, and mental standpoint, man is truly double; in other words, he possesses two organs for conceptualization, two brains."* Gilles de la Tourette only qualified the implausible conclusions reached by Bérillon as *"odd"* and even seemed to acquiesce by adding: *"Dumontpallier has shown, furthermore, that the subject could also be divided into a sub-umbilical half and a supra-umbilical half, and that there could*

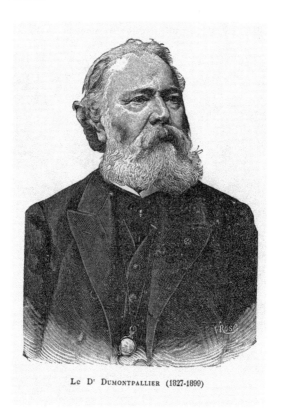

Le Dʳ Dumontpallier (1827-1899)

FIGURE 11.7 Victor Dumontpallier (1826–1899).
BIU santé, Paris with kind permission.

be alternating somnambulism, catalepsy, and lethargy." Unbelievable by today's standards!

Hypnotic Suggestion

The subject of *"hypnotic suggestion, which everyone is talking so much about these days,"* was of great interest to Gilles de la Tourette. For him, it *"formed the substratum of all medical-legal cases."* He explained: *"The experimenter can, in certain conditions, get his subject to accept ideas that can be transformed into acts—not only during sleep, but also once the subject awakens. . . . If the act suggested during sleep is performed upon waking, the subject will have absolutely no recollection of the conditions in which the suggestion was made. Nor will he be able to remember the person who made the suggestion."* This phenomenon had been noted with surprise by Puységur and Abbot Faria. Gilles de la Tourette explained how

Liébault had made it the very basis of his therapy: *"Mr. Liébault's manner of working is in some ways very naive and simple, yet one senses his deep conviction. His speech has such communicative warmth that both he and his patients are swept away by it. First, if necessary, he asks the patient what he suffers from. Then, without conducting any type of examination whatsoever, he has the patient sit, places his hand on the patient's forehead, and without even looking at him, says to the patient: 'You are going to sleep.' Immediately thereafter, he closes the patient's eyelids and assures him he is sleeping . . . and he talks. He talks unceasingly in a strong and vibrant voice, and the suggestions begin: 'You are going to get better; your digestion will be good; your sleep will be good; you will no longer cough; circulation will be free and steady; you will feel great strength in your limbs; you are going to walk with ease; and so forth.' He practically never varies this litany, which covers all illnesses. It is up to the patient to hear what applies to his case. He must make a few specific recommendations that apply to the patient's condition; however, the general recommendations take up the most time."*[34] The famous physician Emile Coué (1857–1926), one of Gilles de la Tourette's peers, based his method[35] on this approach. Gilles de la Tourette discussed all of the actions that could be achieved through suggestion and thus had to address crimes or misdemeanors that might be suggested to the patient without his knowing. He artfully contended: *"In hypnotism, one cannot be logical in every situation, and there is a significant difference between laboratory experiments, for example, and practical investigations with a specific medical-legal purpose."* There were many suggestion scenes with Blanche W. They are recounted in infinite detail and accompanied by subtle interpretations—a source of inspiration for film directors and novelists. One example is John Houston's 1962 film *Freud, the Secret Passion*, in which Sigmund Freud is in Paris and attends one of Charcot's consultations. Another example is *Augustine*, by Jacques Monod and Jean-Christophe Valat, a well-documented 2011 film that captures the atmosphere of La Salpêtrière and Charcot's lessons.

Analogous States

To avoid the risk of anachronism, recall that, in the late nineteenth century, clinical observation was the sole tool in both experimental and clinical work. For all practical purposes, there was no understanding of the physiology of sleep.[36] This helps explain what today can seem confusing. *"Pathologically, hysteria is what dominates the entire field: natural somnambulism is, by hierarchical order, a precursor of the neurosis, just as hypnotic somnambulism is a transformation of the neurosis. What this authorizes us to say is that everything is a manifestation*

of hysteria, rather than being similar to it." Today, sleepwalking[37] is considered
an occasional parasomnia event occurring in 15–30% of children before the
age of twelve. It remains a residual phenomenon in fewer than 2% of adults.
This intrinsic sleep disturbance occurs during the slow wave sleep stage and
has nothing in common with hypnotic states or hysteria. Hypnosis is an al-
tered state of consciousness with loss of both peripheral awareness and
storage of sensory information, but the subject is awake. Hypnosis continues
to be the subject of various studies. One example is the comparative study
of electroencephalograms from the waking and sleep states, potentially
useful for predicting who is hypnotizable.[38] In psychological studies, hypnosis is considered a dissociative state like that which defines schizophrenia.[39]
Most certainly inspired by Alfred Maury (1817–1892) (Figure 11.8),[40] Gilles
de la Tourette understood somnambulism to be *"a latent display of hysteria in
the child,"* in other words, an illness; whereas Joseph Frank (1771–1842) and
Friedrich A. Benjamin Puchelt (1784–1856), in their 1838 treatise, provided

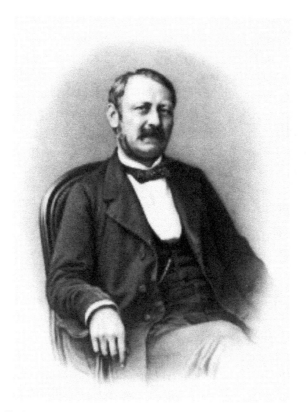

FIGURE 11.8 Alfred Maury (1817–1892).
BNF, Public domain.

a very modern definition: *"Natural somnambulism occurs when functions normally performed in the waking state are performed during otherwise normal sleep."*[41] Gilles de la Tourette did give an accurate description of natural somnambulism occurring in the first hours after the subject falls asleep, and he validated the opinion of other authors: *"Natural somnambulism is a dream in action,"* since the sleeper can be awakened using stimulation and is then amnesiac and disoriented.

Gilles de la Tourette devoted a somewhat unclear chapter to what he called "pathological somnambulism"; that is, forms with agitation and violence occurring as somnambulism set in, with aberrant eating and sexual behaviors, and also the risk of injury or death (e.g., the well-known Elpenor syndrome).[42] Gilles de la Tourette presented clinical cases based on the writings of authors such as Ernest Mesnet (1828–1898),[43] Prosper Despine (1812–1892),[44] John-Charles Bucknill (1817–1897), and Daniel Hack Tuke (1827–1895),[45] which probably discussed nocturnal epilepsy, Elpenor syndrome, and confusional arousals. Gilles de la Tourette's discussion examined medical and legal responsibility. However, none of the cases he presented had anything to do with hypnotism or hysteria.

Gilles de la Tourette borrowed widely from Azam in his discussion of *"the trance state"*—that is, *"veritable onset of prolonged somnambulism,"* the characteristics of which *"created an entirely new period of existence."* For Gilles de la Tourette: *"It is clear that individuals in a trance state have only a very relative notion of responsibility. From a legal standpoint, they are truly insane."* The observations Gilles de la Tourette addressed suggest the diagnosis of schizophrenic dissociation. The somnambulistic state he described as lasting several days, during which minor crimes could be committed, would not now be considered a sleep pathology or hysteria. However, his conclusion remains valid: *"By making this kind of knowledge more widespread, we will encourage informed examination of the facts and avoid both wrongful punishment and letting the guilty go free. Notwithstanding special circumstances, the priority is to keep these patients from harming themselves, as well as protecting society from their actions."*

Hypnosis as Medicine

Prior to discussing the dangers of non-physician use of hypnosis, Gilles de la Tourette stated a categorical opinion: *"Because hypnotism works only on neurotics, and perhaps only on hysterics, as we have demonstrated, any therapeutic action should only be used for accidents due to this pathological condition. . . . Alongside these conditions, which are only resolved by 'natura medicatrix' in addition to proper hygiene, there are others—paralyses, contractions, amauroses—whose overnight cure by hypnotization leaves no question as to their hysterical nature. As established by Briquet,*[46] *they occur as suddenly as they vanish, under the influence of a strong moral emotion, and are perfectly amenable to hypnotism, which plays the role of this emotion to the supreme degree and which cannot always be provoked anew. . . .*[47] *In these cases, hypnotism can in no way be considered as a specific; suggestion, wherever it comes from, and whether it is hypnotic or not, is responsible for the cure, as long as it is accepted."* He thus clearly agreed with the notion that the imagination could cure illnesses or their symptoms. For him, the best indication for hypnotization remained an imminent *"attack"* of hysteria. *"We have often had the opportunity to act in this way, both at La Salpêtrière and in the department headed by Professor Brouardel at Hôpital La Pitié. We know that hysterical patients most often feel their attacks coming on, and they are rarely wrong. Certain premonitory phenomena enable them to predict when an attack is going to start. . . . It is in everyone's best interest to avoid an attack; in addition to violence and nervous exhaustion, attacks may cause all sorts of hysterical complications: contractions, paralysis, and so forth."* According to Gilles de la Tourette, ideally, a state of *"lethargy"* should be reached and allowed to develop for ten to fifteen hours, with avoidance of catalepsy, the source of lasting contractions. *"Frequently hypnotized hysterical patients often experience increasingly long periods between attacks and even go several months without any hysteria."* He reported a conversation with Richer, who pointed out the following: *"For several months now I have been studying hypnotism at La Salpêtrière, and attacks of hysteria major in our patients have become much less frequent. For some patients, the times between onset are much longer. For others, their attacks have nearly, or even completely disappeared."* Could this be an inadvertent admission of a *"culture of hysteria"* at La Salpêtrière, a term coined by Bernheim of the Nancy School? For Gilles de la Tourette, hypnotic lethargy was the most effective treatment to avoid pseudo-epileptic attacks, relax contracted muscles, and circumvent paralysis. The few pages he devoted to hypnosis for anesthesia confirm his talent as a writer and a historian. He championed the work of the Scotsman James Esdaille (1808–1859),[48] founder of the Mesmeric Hospital of Calcutta in India,[49] where more than three hundred patients[50] had undergone painless operations. *"Despite the problems that hypnotism has encountered, it would have had a brilliant surgical career had chloroform not come along and forced it off the pedestal that it newly occupied. Magnetizers viewed the arrival of chloroform with regret, as it marginalized their own activity."*

Gilles de la Tourette then outlined the framework that should guide the practice of hypnosis and protect unsuspecting patients from its iatrogenic effects: *"Hypnotism must never be used other than for healing purposes. In all cases, hypnotism must be reserved solely for use with hysterics, for whom it is the only treatment likely to produce truly indisputable effects; furthermore, the actual existence of the subject's hysteria must be confirmed. Not only is hypnotism one of the most valuable therapeutic agents in the treatment of hysteria; it is also one of the best detectors of hysteria. In all cases, it would be far better to put up with temporary neuralgia than to risk convulsions and their complications, which later hypnotizations would not necessarily be able to cure."*

Dangers of Hypnotism

Gilles de la Tourette was one of the first to use the Jean-Sylvain Bailly (1736–1793) report from 1784 to provide examples of hysteria: *"These agitated persons are tormented by convulsions that are extraordinary due to their frequency, duration, and violence. . . . According to the theory of animal magnetism, it was an error to refer to this convulsive state as an 'attack,' since it was seen as a salutary event of the kind nature brings about, or that a skillful physician is able to provoke to facilitate healing."*[51] The commissioners assigned by the King to examine animal magnetism were not taken in: *"When the imagination produces convulsions, it uses violent means that are almost always destructive. Only in rare cases are such means useful at all—in desperate cases where total upheaval is required to bring about renewal. Medicine should apply these dangerous disruptions like it would a poison. Necessity is the driver and frugality the rule."* Witnessing an attack was dangerous since *"imitation, which nature appears to have made a law in us,"* induced further attacks. Gilles de la Tourette established a long list of the attacks induced by magnetizers before crowds at fairs and other gatherings and detailed the sentences handed down by the courts to punish these amateurs found guilty of inducing mental disorders. *"Great crowds heartily cheered the disastrous feats of charlatans who made their living from destroying the health of the unfortunate persons who entrusted their well-being to them."* He then recalled the words of Charcot on the subject of hypnotic suggestion: *"We must study it among ourselves, and discuss our findings with persons outside of the field of medicine only once we have been able to establish its governing laws. Until then, medicine must reign supreme in this nascent field, its absolute master and guardian, formally refusing any intrusion."*[52]

Hypnotism and the Law

Gilles de la Tourette was in his element on the subject of hypnotism and the law. *"A patient in the state of lethargy is easy prey for a lecherous magnetizer. And due to the ease with which the somnambulist accepts any kind of suggestion, he becomes, in the magnetizer's hands, an unconscious and irresponsible agent, and can even be very dangerous."* Bailly and his colleagues[53] had already noted: *"Magnetic treatment holds nothing but danger for morality. When one proposes to cure illnesses requiring long treatment, one kindles emotions that are pleasant and cherished, emotions one longs for afterwards and seeks to return to, for such feelings have natural appeal for us, and physically they contribute to our happiness. But from a moral standpoint, they are nevertheless condemnable, and made more dangerous by how easy it is to grow accustomed to them."* Gilles de la Tourette wrote at length about an expert assessment his master Brouardel had conducted following a complaint of pregnancy from a young patient in a state of lethargy after dental treatment, during which the dentist allegedly took advantage of her.[54] But Gilles de la Tourette maintained that *"one mustn't go imagining, however, that anything can be obtained from a somnambulist, even when, as we have shown, the most powerful suggestions are used. The facts we report do not allow the conclusion that these were cases of absolute automatism, contrary to the opinion of Mr. Beaunis."* His opposition to the Nancy School continued two years later, during the Eyraud-Bompard court case. Could suggestion, in and of itself, enable someone to gain ascendancy over another person? Bernheim argued that it could; Gilles de la Tourette, however, took the opposing view: *"These are all things in which hypnotism has no place."* His restriction of the scope of hypnosis was no doubt due to his determination to prove his arguments at the medical-legal level: *"Since suggestion is the scapegoat for all crimes, writers who have left us stories of misdeeds during hypnotic states should have recorded many more in the state of somnambulism, where the power of suggestion is indisputable."* He found no cases worth mentioning in the literature, which only contained "laboratory suggestion," similar to what he had experimented with. He sought to be reassuring: *"We have stirred up agitation and fears that, although fanciful, are no less dangerous, particularly in our day, neurosis having reached the most acute stage possible. Hypnotism can be enormously beneficial, and it can lead to or cause great harm, but suggestion is not the source of this harm."* Gilles de la Tourette never discussed the effects of propaganda or *"advertising"* (of which he availed himself!), although they are closely related to the effects of suggestion.

Gilles de la Tourette believed firmly in his legal principles. He hoped to demonstrate that *"regulation of hypnotism is absolutely necessary in our country"* to prevent the commercial exploitation of *"magnetism."* In order to argue his case persuasively, he revealed the following: *"For three years now, we have assiduously participated in magnetism and spiritism circles. We have consulted the most lucid somnambulists, and we have been helped in our task by devoted friends,[55] who gave unstintingly of their time and money to help us shed light on these doings that take place in the dark"* (Figure 11.9). Three hysterics he had treated at La Salpêtrière

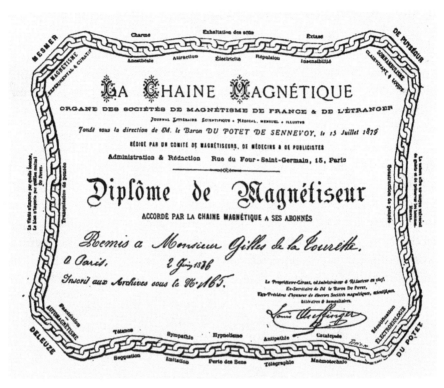

FIGURE II.9 *"Chaine magnétique"* (magnetic chain), guild card belonging to Gilles de la Tourette. Private collection of the author.

and La Charité came forward with testimony of what they had endured *"at the hands of magnetizers."* He gathered evidence—flyers, advertisements, newspaper clippings, and court rulings—and stated that: *"A person is born with somnambulism, but that person is not obligated to exploit his infirmity. On the contrary, one chooses to become a magnetizer, and does so expressly to take advantage of the gullible public by exploiting somnambulism in others."* Gilles de la Tourette drew up a long list of the guilty and castigated the *"pharmacy assistants, druggists, bone-setters, medical students in their fifteenth year—all of these second-rate characters."* He included physicians *"with degrees from foreign universities. . . . As honorability fades away, the longer the list grows."* Gilles de la Tourette wrote of sinister practices exploiting poor somnambulist women. He described a growing network of underworld figures who devised any number of ploys to lure the gullible in droves to spectacular performances and then fleece them of their belongings. Reading these descriptions at times recalls the novels of Honoré de Balzac (1799–1850). Gilles de la Tourette also criticized the creation of Societies, parodies of the established scientific societies, whose aims were *"essentially humanitarian, looking for truth and doing good."* He suggested that such vast illegal medical activity had been able to spread with the complicity of pharmacists. The numerous examples of advertising and handbills included in his book testify to the time and energy he devoted to making his case. One such example, from a *"Magnetism Clinic,"* recommended the use of somnambulism, along with magnesium, to treat refractory illnesses. Two years later, Gilles de la Tourette renewed his efforts in an article, to ensure that his message would be heard.[56]

"What are the consequences of all these practices? Accidents follow in quick succession; the resulting neurosis continues to wreak havoc." Gilles de la Tourette also discussed other European countries, describing similar practices in each. He addressed the legal and political challenges, among others, to overcome before these harmful practices could be made illegal, stating that *"love of all that is inexplicable and fear of the supernatural are innate in us."* Reading his work is of great historical interest and leads us to realize that these practices still exist, though they take different forms. Basically, nothing has really changed.

Expert Opinions Concerning Hypnotism

"How does one conduct a medical-legal investigation in a case where hypnotism appears to have been used to commit a crime or misdemeanor?" The fact that words such as "suggestion," "hypnotism," "nervous sleep," and others had become commonplace in conversation and literature was a source of concern for Gilles de la Tourette. Crimes committed in a hypnotic state were exceptional, if indeed any truly existed. Yet he asserts: *"The courts have always been busy with hysterics. . . . The true crime inherent in hypnotism and analogous states is rape."* For Gilles de la Tourette, rape was possible during hypnotic lethargy. He referred to the case that Brouardel had studied in 1878. At the end of his lengthy discussion, he recommended this approach for experts: *"After the initial physical examination of the plaintiff, which in most cases ascertains that she is hysterical, the expert should immediately seek to establish whether she is hypnotizable, and whether complete insensitivity with muscular resolution can be easily obtained—in a word, true lethargy."* It was only under these circumstances that rape could be considered. Given the risk of simulation and mythomania, great skepticism was required. As the attorney Pierre Roux-Freissineng (1863–1952) wrote in 1886: *"The man who is at the mercy of the will of others becomes the instrument or victim of all manner of fraud, of all manner of crime! Confusion and reversal of all responsibilities! Complete upheaval of civil and criminal order!"*[57] To validate

his demonstration, Gilles de la Tourette turned to observations drawn from medical journals, but he never referred to a real case in which he had been personally involved or a legal investigation for which he had given his expert opinion. This section, often quite fastidious to read, comes across more like an exercise in rhetoric than a medical text. He finished by stating: *"Theater performances and public sessions of magnetism societies must be severely prohibited, for they not only cause a host of immediate accidents; they also lead to later accidents by spreading public access to hypnotism."* At no time did Gilles de la Tourette show any remorse whatsoever for his role in dramatizing hypnotism and seeking publicity for the exhibitions at La Salpêtrière. In the early 1900s, the question of rape under hypnosis ceased to be of interest. This is undoubtedly due to the infinitesimal number of cases that the courts ever actually dealt with, in contrast to the abundant literature on the subject during a thirty-year period.[58]

Sources

Gilles de la Tourette's research and highly detailed historical fresco must have necessitated numerous documents, about which he reveals little. His scholarship did, however, draw from specific sources. He indicated several times that he had referred to Claude Burdin (1777–1858) and Frédéric Dubois (1797–1873), authors of an 1841 work, *Histoire académique du magnétisme animal,* the ideology of which undoubtedly matched his own. They had stated: *"With all of the circus acts that inevitably reappear from century to century in the history of the human mind, there is always a physician, an apostle of truth and common sense, who endeavors to lay bare the artifice and to tarnish the prestige."*[59] In our opinion, Gilles de la Tourette minimized his debt to Alexandre Bertrand (1795–1831)[60] and Alfred Maury,[61] from whose detailed works he clearly drew extensively. He did point out that Bertrand had distinguished himself at the prestigious Ecole Polytechnique, and he was likely influenced by Bertrand's book on demonic possession in Loudun, *Des possessions des religieuses de Loudun.*

Alexandre Cullerre (1849–1934) (Figure 11.10), a senior physician at La Grimaudière asylum in La Roche-sur-Yon, had published his book, *Magnétisme et hypnotisme,* just a few months before Gilles de la Tourette, whose work had an identical structure and very comparable discussions, differing only by the inclusion of a chapter on the visits he had made to observe magnetizers.[62] It seems obvious that Gilles de la Tourette drew from Cullerre's book when writing his own. He was also very familiar with the

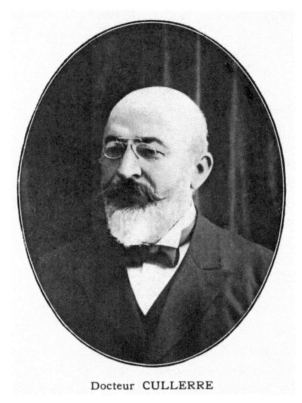

Docteur **CULLERRE**

FIGURE II.IO   Alexandre Cullere (1849–1934).
BIU santé, Paris with kind permission.

extensive *agrégation* thesis[63] written by Henri Barth (1853–1945) in 1886,[64] which included many details on the history of *"induced nervous sleep."* Barth supported the inhibition theory: *"We know through experimental evidence that exciting one point of the nervous system often has the effect of paralyzing, by means of interference, the activity of another part in relation with the first part. The mechanism of this paralysis totally escapes our understanding, but its reality cannot be doubted."* This observation laid the groundwork for the innovative concepts Paul Sollier (1861–1933) would propose in 1897.[65] Barth expressed doubt regarding the results Auguste Voisin (1829–1898) had obtained at La Salpêtrière; Voisin claimed to have calmed maniacs and patients suffering from hallucinations and delirium by inducing hypnotic sleep. To conclude, Barthes quoted Charcot: *"All of these facts need to be established. Their physiological explanation should be made known to the general public in order to convince the world that the supernatural plays absolutely no part. There is only a series of nervous phenomena that physicians, and only physicians, must study. If this were respected, magnetizers would no longer have a clientele."*

Following Publication

Paul Magnin (1854–1913), another of Dumontpallier's students, spoke very highly of Gilles de la Tourette's book in the new *Revue de l'Hypnotisme*, while also drawing attention to his own work.[66] Magnin's friend, Louis Beurnier (1860–1917), writing in *Les Archives de Médecine*, gave well-deserved praise for the chapter recounting Gilles de la Tourette's visits to observe magnetizers.[67] Albert Charrin (1856–1907) also praised the book in *Les Annales d'hygiène publique et de médecine légale*: *"It is important, from the social standpoint, to come to the aid of justice, to keep it from going off course, from lending an ear to erroneous fables, from confusing scientific doctrine worthy of the name with the chicanery and sleight-of-hand performed by exploiters of public credulity. This is just what Mr. Gilles de la Tourette has sought to do. A former interne of Professors Charcot and Brouardel, he could not have been better prepared for the task he undertook; it is only fair to acknowledge how successfully he has completed it."*[68] Writing in the *Bulletin général de thérapeutique médicale et chirurgicale*, Albert Deschamps (1859–?) went into detail on the book's various chapters and emphasized that lawmakers should read it. He also praised Gilles de la Tourette, the writer: *"The author has taken us on an excursion through the cesspools of charlatanism. The result is what a modern-day novelist would term a human document, but at least this document is supported by acute observation."*[69] Edouard Brissaud (1852–1909) wrote a long, detailed, and laudatory report in *La Gazette Hebdomadaire de Médecine et de Chirurgie*, concluding with the humor he was known for:[70] *"Gilles de la Tourette has shown that criminal suggestion is no source of security for the author of such suggestion. His arguments are well chosen and finely presented; the reader can do nothing better than adopt his conclusions and be guaranteed a good night's sleep."*[71] Bottey, the research associate of Gilles de la Tourette, wrote an incisive review in *Le Progrès Médical* in which he emphasized the conceptual antagonism that separated Gilles de la Tourette and the Nancy School: *"Monsieur Liégeois had tried to turn suggestion into a sword of Damocles hanging over society. Gilles de la Tourette put suggestion back in its proper place, showing through reasoning and facts that it offers no special security to the person using it. . . . The book, based on a wide array of facts and documents, filled with observations, should be read from cover to cover. There are practical lessons to be learned on every page."* Le Gendre couldn't help but applaud his friend's work, especially the chapter describing his direct observations of magnetizers: *"The so-called offices of somnambulists and the inner workings of societies for magnetism and spiritism hold no further secrets for Mr. Gilles de la Tourette, who tells us all about his excursions into their strange world. We agree wholeheartedly with him that laws must be passed to closely monitor all the ways in which magnetism can be exploited. . . . Themis, do not let your sword rust in its scabbard! And you my esteemed colleague, continue to provide us with useful, well-written books like the ones you have penned up till now. For though they may not be easy to criticize, they are a sheer pleasure to read."*[72]

Six years later, in December 1893, when an attempt was made on Gilles de la Tourette's life, journalists did not fail to look back on his categorical positions on hypnotism with some degree of irony. For example, in *L'Est Républicain* of December 9, 1893, one journalist wrote: *"The papers have been focusing on a crime with unusual circumstances, even more interesting in light of the recent controversy over hypnotism. Is this a crime of hypnosis? It would be strange indeed if Doctor Gilles de la Tourette, one of Charcot's disciples and thus opposed to the possibility of criminal suggestion, were himself the victim of criminal suggestion. A few days ago, we published a conversation between one of our journalists and Dr. Liébault, along with a few considerations on Dr. Mesnet's book, allowing readers to judge for themselves. Kamper's revolver almost changed things dramatically. We are told that suggestion wasn't involved and that Kamper simply suffers from hallucinations. That way, Doctor Gilles de la Tourette, once recovered, will not have to admit the failure of his doctrine, but his positions may well be compromised."*[73] The debate, which set proponents of *"free will"* against those who believed in *"innate determinism,"* filled the papers and literature of the time. This conflict was a by-product of the general acceptance, by the Salpêtrière School among others, of the concept of degeneration developed by Bénédict-Augustin Morel (1809–1873).[74]

In 1889, Richer and Gilles de la Tourette were assigned with writing the *"Hypnotism"* entry in the *Dictionnaire des Sciences Médicale.*[75] They began by expressing their dissatisfaction with an 1873 article entitled *Mesmérisme* by the *"lamented"* Amédée Dechambre (1812–1886), who had questioned the reality of hypnotism. They then condensed the bulk of Gilles de la Tourette's 1887 book into sixty-three pages. Certain paragraphs were copied verbatim from the book.

In his 1893 biography of Charcot, Paul Peugniez (1859–1943) wrote that the master, wary following the Eyraud-Bompard case, had advised Gilles de la Tourette against publishing a third edition of his treatise. Quoting Gilles de la Tourette, Peugniez wrote: *"When I told him I intended to prepare the third edition of my* Traité de l'hypnotisme, *he said with some sadness: 'Wait. The time has not yet come for those truly interested in science to speak of this issue once again.' "*[76]

Additional Information

Presented here is a translation of the preface by Jean-Martin Charcot to the German version of Gilles de la Tourette's book

My dear Sirs,

In introducing the book written by my student Doctor Gilles de la Tourette, a work you would be well advised to present to the specialists in your country, I shall briefly discuss the reasons that explain, in my opinion, the success with which this book has met. This translation into German bears further witness to its achievement.

Several years after the first experiments conducted on hypnotism at Hôpital La Salpêtrière, some decided to step off the beaten path in order to widen the field of their research. Consequently, a host of different states were attributed to hypnotism, and many of these states did not, in truth, present all of the somatic phenomena that, in my opinion, are essential to the genuinely scientific description of this nervous state in which affected patients find themselves.

For some, of course, the individual is "sleeping," but they cannot prove this assertion in a way that excludes all possible simulation. For example, they are not capable of proving the absence of trickery or anything else unrelated to hypnotism. However, a small number of symptoms have been noted that seem to justify assuming that the individual has truly fallen asleep, despite the fact that we cannot say, in every case, which stage of hypnotic sleep is involved. And from a strictly medical standpoint, this is indispensable. Unlike the authors I refer to above, Dr. Gilles de la Tourette has based his work on proven data.

Without underestimating the psychic phenomena, he has justifiably used all of the somatic stigmata as his guideline. From this perspective, he has clearly shown that a medical-legal expert opinion must be based on reliable symptoms that legitimize the final decision.

The medical examiner must be a keen and prudent observer, more perceptive than even the jurist. Insofar as possible, his diagnosis must be irrefutable, a perfect reflection of the relevant laws. His opinion must take into account the entire set of positive phenomena whereby any simulation is excluded, for expert opinions weigh heavily in the court's ruling. The greatest homage I can pay the book translated herein is that every single page reflects the serious work undertaken to provide experts with the resources they need to avoid errors, which in many cases could be fatal.

Paris, June 27, 1888

Jean Martin Charcot, member of the Académie des Sciences

Notes

1. Gilles de la Tourette G. *L'hypnotisme et les états analogues au point de vue médico-légal, les états hypnotiques et les états analogues, les suggestions criminelles, cabinets de somnambules et sociétés de magnétisme et de spiritisme, l'hypnotisme devant la loi* (préface de M. le Dr P. Brouardel). Paris: E. Plon-Nourrit. 1887.

2. Gilles de la Tourette G. *L'Hypnotisme et les états analogues au point de vue médico-légal* (préface de M. le Dr P. Brouardel). 2nd édition. Paris: Plon-Nourrit. 1889.

3. Gilles de la Tourette G. *Der Hypnotismus und die verwandten Zustände vom Standpunkte der gerichtlichen Medicin. (Préface de JM. Charcot.)* Hamburg: Richter. 1889.

4. Gilles de la Tourette G. *L'ipnotismo e gli stati analoghi sotto l'aspetto medico-legale. Con prefazioni dei Professori Brouardel e Charcot; Versione italiana del Dott. Luigi Bufalini.* Milano: L. Vallardi. 1888.

5. Translated at the end of this chapter.

6. Gilles de la Tourette G. Le viol dans l'hypnotisme et les états analogues. *La Semaine Médicale.* 1886;6(31):310.

7. Gilles de la Tourette G. Le viol dans l'hypnotisme et les états analogues. *Bulletin Société de Médecine Légale.* 1887;9:380–399.

8. Gilles de la Tourette G. Le viol dans l'hypnotisme et les états analogues. *Annales d'hygiène publique et de médecine légale.* 1886;16(3ᵉ série):445–464.

9. Beurnier L. Bibliographie l'hypnotisme et les états analogues. *Archives Générales de Médecine.* 1888; 65-série7(23):120–124.

10. Burdin CL, Dubois F. *Histoire académique du magnétisme animal.* Paris: JB Baillière. 1841.

11. Montorgueil G. La mort du Docteur Gilles de la Tourette. *L'Éclair.* 24 mai 1904.

12. Gilles de la Tourette G. Documents satiriques sur Mesmer. *Nouvelle Iconographie de La Salpêtrière.* 1889;2(1):59–65; 1889;2(2):103–106.

13. Anonyme (Paulet JJ). *L'antimagnétisme ou origine, progrès, décadence du magnétisme animal.* A Londres. 1784.

14. His first name is indeed Amand and not Armand, as is too often written.

15. Chastenet AM, dit Marquis de Puységur. *Mémoires pour servir à l'histoire et à l'établissement du magnétisme animal.* A Londres, 1784.

16. Petetin JH. *Electricité animale, prouvée par la découverte des phénomènes physiques et moraux de la catalepsie hystérique, et de ses variétés, et par les bons effets de l'Electricité artificielle dans le traitement de ces maladies.* Paris: Chez Brunot-Labbe et Gautier-Bretin / Lyon: Chez Reymann et Cie. 1808.

17. Petetin JH. *Mémoire sur la découverte des phénomènes que présentent la catalepsie et le noctambulisme: Symptômes de l'affection hystérique essentielle, avec des recherches sur la cause physique de ces phénomènes.* Première partie. Lyon. 1787; and Petetin JH. *Mémoire sur la découverte des phénomènes de l'affection hystérique essentielle et sur la méthode curative de cette maladie.* Seconde partie. Lyon. 1787.

18. Deleuze JPF. *Histoire critique du magnétisme animal.* Paris: Mame. 1813.

19. Gilles de la Tourette G. L'épilogue d'un procès célèbre. *Le Progrès Médical.* 1891;19-1(5): 89–96.

20. Faria JC. *De la Cause du sommeil lucide, ou Étude de la nature de l'homme. Bramine, Docteur en théologie et en philosophie. Membre de la Société Médicale de Marseille.* Paris: 1819.

21. Étienne Eugène Azam (1822–1899), a surgeon from Bordeaux, was interested in psychology and thus took as a patient a woman referred to as "Félida," whom he treated over a long period. In eight years' time, he published three books on this patient, who presented "alternating personalities," a condition similar to what was later called multiple personality disorder or dissociative identity disorder, the reality of which is now highly disputed.

22. Bernheim H. *De la suggestion dans l'état hypnotique et dans l'état de veille.* Paris: Octave Doin. 1884.

23. Braid J. *Neurypnology; or, The Rationale of Nervous Sleep: Considered in Relation with Animal Magnetism. Illustrated by numerous cases of its successful application in the relief and cure of disease.* London: Churchill. 1843.

24. Gilles de la Tourette G, Richer P. Sur les caractères cliniques des paralysies psychiques expérimentales. *Comptes Rendus hebdomadaires des Séances et Mémoires de la Société de Biologie.* 1884;36:198–200.

25. Gilles de la Tourette G. Le viol dans l'hypnotisme et les états analogues. *Bulletin Société de Médecine Légale.* 1886;9:380–399.

26. Paul Brémaud (1846–1905), chief Navy physician in Brest.

27. Brémaud P. *Des Différentes Phases de l'hypnotisme et en particulier de la fascination.* Paris: Cerf. 1884.

28. Beaunis HE. *Le noctambulisme provoqué; études physiologiques et psychologiques.* Paris: Baillière. 1886.

29. Bottey F. *Le magnétisme animal, étude clinique et expérimentale sur l'hypnotisme ou sommeil nerveux provoqué chez les sujets sains.* Paris: Plon-Nourrit. 1884.

30. Richer P. *Etude descriptive de la grande attaque hystérique ou attaque hystéro-épileptique et des principales variétés.* Thèse no. 179. Paris: Adrien Delahaye. 1879.

31. Charcot JM. Physiologie pathologique. Sur les divers états nerveux déterminés par l'hypnotisation chez les hystériques. *Comptes rendus de l'Académie des sciences.* 1882;94:403–405.

32. Bérillon E. *De l'indépendance fonctionnelle des deux hémisphères cérébraux.* Thèse no. 360. Paris: A. Davy. 1884.

33. Descourtis G. *De fractionnement des opérations cérébrales et en particulier de leur dédoublement dans les psychopathies.* Thèse no. 190. Paris: A. Davy. 1882.

34. Delboeuf J. Le magnétisme animal: à propos d'une visite à l'Ecole de Nancy. *Revue de Belgique.* 1888;60:241–260; 386–408.

35. Guillemain H. *La méthode Coué, histoire d'une pratique de guérison au XXᵉ siècle.* Paris: L'univers historique. Le Seuil. 2010.

36. Langlet JB. *Etude critique sur quelques points de la physiologie du sommeil.* Paris: Louis Leclerc. 1872.

37. A somnambulist is someone who walks in their sleep.

38. Madeo D, Castellani E, Santarcangelo EL, Mocenni C. Hypnotic assessment based on the recurrence quantification analysis of EEG recorded in the ordinary state of consciousness. *Brain Cogn.* 2013;83(2):227–233.

39. Cleveland JM, Korman BM, Gold SN. Are hypnosis and dissociation related? New evidence for a connection. *Int J Clin Exp Hypnotism.* 2015;63(2):198–214.

40. Maury A. *Le sommeil et les rêves, études psychologiques sur ces phénomènes et les divers états qui s'y rattachent.* Paris: Didier et Cie. 1862.

41. Frank J, Puchelt FAB. *Traité de pathologie médicale.* Paris: Chez M. Gautret, P. Mellier. 1838–1845.

42. In Greek mythology, Elpenor, one of Ulysses's companions, fell asleep near a temple dedicated to Circe. When it was time to leave, he was not yet fully awake and fell from the terrace to his death.

43. Mesnet E. Etudes sur le noctambulisme envisagé au point de vue pathologique. *Archives Générales de Médecine.* 1860;37(2):147–173.

44. Despine P. *Étude scientifique sur le noctambulisme, sur les phénomènes qu'il présente et sur son action thérapeutique dans certaines maladies nerveuses, du rôle important qu'il joue dans l'épilepsie, dans l'hystérie et dans les névroses dites extraordinaires.* Paris: F. Savy. 1880.

45. Bucknill JC, Tuke DH. *A Manual of Psychological Medicine Containing the Lunacy Laws, the Nosology, Etiology, Statistics, Description, Diagnosis, Pathology and Treatment of Insanity: With an Appendix of Cases.* London: J. and A. Churchill. 1879.

46. Pierre Briquet (1796–1891).

47. Here, Gilles de la Tourette described catharsis, a concept used by Sigmund Freud to refer to consciously recalling a repressed idea.

48. Waltraud E. Esdaile, James (1808–1859). In *Oxford Dictionary of National Biography*. New York: Oxford University Press. 2004.

49. Esdaille J. *Mesmerism in India, and Its Practical Application in Surgery and Medicine*. London: Longman, Brown, Green, and Longmans. 1846.

50. Pulos L. Mesmerism revisited: the effectiveness of Esdaile's techniques in the production of deep hypnosis and total body hypnoanesthesia. *Am J Clin Hypnosis*. 1980; 22(4):206–211.

51. Bailly JS, Lavoisier A, Bory de Saint Vincent JB, Franklin B, Le Roy JB *Rapport des commissaires chargés par le Roi de l'examen du magnétisme animal*. Paris: Imprimerie Royale 1784.

52. Peugniez P. *J-M Charcot (1825–1893)*. Amiens: Imprimerie Picarde. 1893.

53. Antoine Lavoisier (1743–1794), Jean-Baptiste Bory de Saint-Vincent (1778–1846), Benjamin Franklin (1706–1790), Jean-Baptiste Le Roy (1719–1800), Michel Joseph Majault (1714–1790).

54. Brouardel P. Accusations de viol accompli pendant le sommeil hypnotique. Relation médico-légale de l'affaire Lévy, dentiste à Rouen. *Annales d'hygiène et de médecine légale* 1879;50(1):39–67.

55. Gabriel Legué and Th. Belin. See Chapter 14 on *Sœur Jeanne des Anges, supérieure des Ursulines de Loudun*.

56. Gilles de la Tourette G. Dangers de l'hypnotisme et interdiction des représentations théâtrales. *Bulletin Société de Médecine Légale*. 1889;10:252–255.

57. Roux-Freissineng P. *L'hypnotisme dans ses rapports avec le droit*. La Conférence des Avocats de Marseille. Marseille: Imprimerie de Barlatier-Feisat. 1886.

58. Letrou-Bertaut ML. *Femmes violées et hypnotisme: un problème de la psychiatrie médico-légale à la fin du XIXᵉ siècle*. Thèse Caen. 1994.

59. Burdin Cl, Dubois F. *Histoire académique du magnétisme animal*. Paris: JB. Baillière. 1841.

60. Bertrand A. *Du magnétisme animal en France et des jugements qu'en ont portés les Sociétés savantes*. Paris: JB. Baillière. 1826.

61. Maury A. *Le sommeil et les rêves, études psychologiques sur ces phénomènes et les divers états qui s'y rattachent*. Paris: Didier et Cie. 1862.

62. Cullerre A. *Magnétisme et hypnotisme, exposé des phénomènes observés pendant le sommeil nerveux provoqué*. Paris: JB. Baillière. 1886.

63. 1886 *agrégation*: Brissaud (toxic paralyses), Lannois (nosography of choreas), Ballet (interior language and various forms of aphasia), Grenier (localizations in nervous diseases without appreciable lesions), and more.

64. Barth H. *Du sommeil non naturel, ses diverse formes*. Thèse présentée au concours d'agrégation. Paris: Asselin et Houzeau.1886.

65. Sollier P. *Genèse et nature de l'hystérie. Recherches cliniques et expérimentales de psycho-physiologie*. Paris: F. Alcan. 1897.

66. Magnin P. Revue Critique: L'hypnotisme et les états analogues au point de vue médico-légal par M. le Dr. Gilles de la Tourette. *Revue de l'hypnotisme*. 1887;1(5):176–179.

67. Beurnier L. Bibliographie: L'hypnotisme et les états analogues au point de vue médico-légal. *Archives Générales de Médecine*. 1888;65:120–124.

68. Charrin A. Bibliographie: L'hypnotisme et les états analogues. *Annales d'hygiène publique et de médecine légale*. 1887;58:555–558.

69. Deschamps A. Bibliographie: L'hypnotisme et les états analogues. *Bulletin général de thérapeutique médicale et chirurgicale*. 1887;113:40–41.

70. Poirier J. *Le docteur Édouard Brissaud (1852–1909): un neurologue d'exception dans une famille d'artistes*. Paris: Hermann. 2010.

71. Brissaud E. Neurologie Médico-légale. L'hypnotisme et les états analogues au point de vue médico-légal. *Gazette Hebdomadaire de Médecine et de Chururgie*. 1886; 33(53):859–862.

72. Le Gendre P. Bibliothèque: L'hypnotisme et les états analogues au point de vue médico-légal. *L'Union Médicale*. 1887; 40(16): 188–190.

73. Goulette L. Encore l'hypnotisme. *L'Est Républicain,* 9 décembre 1893;10(1944):1.

74. Plas R. Hysteria, hypnosis, and moral sense in French 19th-century forensic psychiatry: the Eyraud-Bompard Case. *Int J Law Psychiatry.* 1998;21(4):397–407.

75. Richer P, Gilles de la Tourette G, Hypnotisme. In A Dechambre (ed.), *Dictionnaire encyclopédique des sciences médicales*. 1889; série 4 tome 15 (HYL—INH):67–132.

76. Peugniez P. *J-M Charcot (1825–1893)*. Amiens: Imprimerie Picarde. 1893.

$$\mathcal{L} \; 12 \; \mathcal{L}$$

Clinical and Therapeutic Treatise on Hysteria

Hystérie Normale

Hysteria, what crimes are committed in your name!

—Georges Gilles de la Tourette

ONTRARY TO WHAT is commonly believed, hysteria still exists today, in the twenty-first century. The international classification of "mental illnesses"[1] has tended to discourage medical use of the word "hysteria" since 1980,[2] replacing it with other terms such as "dissociative syndrome"[3] or "conversion syndrome,"[4] which underscore the persistence of a dualistic concept of body and mind.[5] Progress in investigative neurological techniques[6] has revealed that the condition is as frequent, if not more frequent, than previously estimated.[7] [8] For more than a century, Freudianism perpetuated the secular approach to femininity through hysteria. By contrast, Jean-Martin Charcot (1825–1893) and his School focused on this pathology as an essential means of furthering neurological understanding. The best example is the most famous and widely used of the clinical signs for neurological examinations, the Babiński sign,[9] described by Joseph Babiński (1857–1932), who considered it the best way to distinguish between an organic condition and a psychogenic one. For a number of phenomena—including epilepsy, abnormal movements, consciousness, memory, and pain—hysteria served as a mirror, gradually making it possible to define a detailed clinical picture of organic conditions and to propose a pathophysiology of the diseases it simulated.[10]

The concepts underlying the theory of evolution of Charles Darwin (1809–1882) provide one of the best ways to understand the reasons behind hysteria and its eternal renewal. In 1907, Edouard Claparède (1873–1940) took an ethologist's approach to summarize the phylogenetic parallel between hysteria and the protective behavioral inhibition in response to a predator: *"Hysterical reactions are defense reactions or phenomena symbolizing a defense. But for the most part, these reactions are used in the normal individual only in the rudimentary state; some of them may only be the reviviscence of ancestral reactions whose biological utility is only evident in animals that manifest them."*[11]

According to Paul Le Gendre (1854–1936) (Figure 12.1), Gilles de la Tourette was able to complete his three-volume hysteria treatise in less than three years (1890–1893) because it allowed him to overcome personal difficulties: *"To numb himself, Gilles de la Tourette found nothing better than to work even more relentlessly, never passing up an opportunity to take on additional projects. This perhaps explains the ambition for which he was so criticized. He undertook more and more studies, most of which were aimed at a complete treatise on hysteria."*[12] There

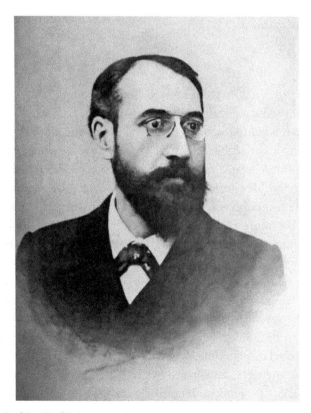

FIGURE 12.1 Paul Le Gendre (1854–1936).
Private collection of the author.

can be no doubt that, for Gilles de la Tourette, this publication was the most important of all. In his later writings, he always advised his readers to refer to it. Charcot, in his 1891 preface, presented it as follows: *"In a way, this treatise was completed under my immediate direction. It reproduces, as faithfully as possible, my teachings and the work subsequently undertaken by my students. I would go even further: while reading the work of Gilles de la Tourette before it was printed, I was surprised on several occasions to find ideas of mine I considered absolutely personal, that I thought I never talked about, which, in any case, had never been published. Mr. Gilles de la Tourette, who was my interne and my chef de clinique at La Salpêtrière and has been affiliated with the department for nearly eight years, carefully noted day after day what I thought or said about hysteria, based on clinical observations. He worked tirelessly to compile a work which, I believe, fills a gap in today's scientific knowledge."* A German translation of the first 1891 volume was published in 1894 in Leipzig and Vienna.[13]

Normal or Interparoxysmic Hysteria

The first volume was published on November 5, 1891,[14] with the curious title of *Hystérie normale ou inter-paroxystique* (Normal or interparoxysmic hysteria). Gilles de la Tourette wrote that, since Charcot had taken an interest in the disease, *"it became possible to attribute laws of evolution to hysteria, a particular determinism that was bound to affirm itself sooner or later, and make of what had been an 'elusive proteus,' a real disease, stable in its very incoherence, an incoherence that is more apparent than real and which, in every case, ignorance has especially exaggerated."* Gilles de la Tourette was thus following in Charcot's footsteps. He distinguished the permanent stigmata, the subject of the first volume, from what they gave rise to, the paroxysms and attacks that were the subject of the following two volumes, entitled *Hystérie pathologique ou paroxystique* (Pathological or paroxysmic hysteria), published in January 1895.[15] Charcot paid him this fine tribute in the preface: *"In the study of hysteria, Gilles de la Tourette has introduced an element of precision, something palpable that will singularly illuminate the diagnosis of difficult cases; at the same time, he has established the reality of clinical phenomena."*

For the initial historical part, Gilles de la Tourette expressed his thanks for the guidance of Alexandre Laboulbène (1825–1898), who had held the Chair of the Medical History since 1879. He also thanked the surgeons Aristide Verneuil (1823–1895) and Jean-François Le Dentu (1841–1926), with whom he was an *externe*, for the use of their laboratories to study *"related cutaneous or surgical questions."* He acknowledged Alfred Fournier (1832–1914), despite

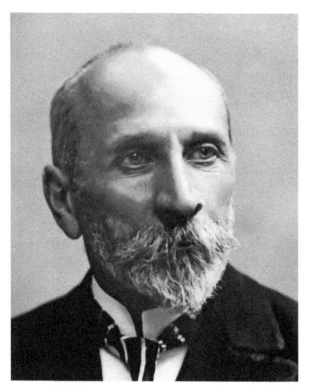

FIGURE 12.2 Paul Richer (1849–1933).
Private collection of the author.

his disagreement with Fournier's view that tabes and general paralysis were syphilitic in origin. His treatise included several drawings from the thesis[16] and the book[17] of Paul Richer (1849–1933) (Figure 12.2), important sources of inspiration: *"He simply added a new expression of his friendship to the many he had already bestowed upon us."* He omitted (voluntarily?) to cite his many borrowings, some almost plagiaristic, from *Traité des Névroses* by Alexandre Axenfeld (1825–1876), in its posthumous second edition (1883), which was completed by Axenfeld's student, Henri Huchard (1844–1910).[18]

Historical Considerations

Gilles de la Tourette's initial chapter on the history of hysteria does not go into much depth. In it, he wrote: *"The extremely precious knowledge that we possess on hysteria at this time in history we owe to our eminent Master, Professor Charcot, and to our friend, Mr. Paul Richer, whose names appear on every page of this work."* He had in fact chosen to incorporate within each chapter his very numerous historical references, specifically selected according to the relevant subject. Gilles de la Tourette began his general history with a summary of the 1887 book by Charcot and Richer, *Les démoniaques dans l'art*, from which he borrowed some of the illustrations.[19] As he stated himself, he wished to move swiftly to the early nineteenth-century authors. He used citations from Etienne Georget (1795–1828) and subscribed to his judgments. *"The empty dissertations of Louyer-Villermay were soon to be correctly evaluated by Georget."*[20] He expressed admiration for Jean-Louis Brachet (1789–1858)[21] and especially for Pierre Briquet (1796–1881),[22] considering them worthy predecessors for Charcot.

He devoted a long section to clarifying the term *"hystero-epilespy,"* concluding with a citation from Charcot's lesson on March 19, 1889: *"In the past, my respect for tradition led me to keep the term 'hystero-epilepsy,' but I admit that it is bothersome, because it is absurd. Here is a patient suffering from two very different conditions brought together in one name. There is not the slightest similarity between epilepsy and hystero-epilepsy, even when the latter involves mixed attacks."*[23] Gilles de la Tourette naturally supported this view: *"This is why we shall never use the term 'hystero-epilepsy,' but rather 'hysteria,' the only term that is truly rational."*

Etiology and Triggering Agents

"Heredity is the primordial agent of hysteria." Fatalistically, the daughter of a hysterical mother would be hysterical herself; the fact that an ascendant suffered from a "nervous condition" explained the case under study. A person so marked by heredity would be victim to a "triggering agent" that would set off hysteria. Gilles de la Tourette referred to the book of Charles Féré (1852–1907), *La famille névropathique.*[24] *"The continuity of the germinative plasma"* explained the inexorable transmission of defects and disorders whose ultimate result could be none other than *"degeneration,"*[25] as it was defined by Prosper Lucas (1805–1855)[26] and Bénédict-Augustin Morel (1809–1873).[27] These ideas generated much interest at the end of the nineteenth century.

To list the triggering agents of hysteria, Gilles de la Tourette used elements from the thesis of Georges Guinon (1859–1932),[28] his successor as Charcot's secretary. First among these agents was *"violent moral emotions,"* whose role in the development of hysteria *"had always been acknowledged, and their importance became even greater when the mental state of hysterics, characterized by suggestibility, was recognized."* Gilles de la Tourette went on to list the following influences, with relevant observations and discussion: trauma; acute and chronic infectious diseases (tuberculosis); diseases of the genitalia; lead poisoning or addiction to alcohol, tobacco, or morphine; and all nervous diseases (tabes, epilepsy, tic disorder, myopathy).

Permanent Hysterical Stigmata

For Charcot, certain somatic and psychic symptoms found outside of an attack were indicative of hysteria. Foremost among them were disturbances of sensibility, especially partial or total anesthesia; Charcot considered these to be constant markers of hysteria. Gilles de la Tourette thus immersed his readers in *"diabolical possessions"* in order to show that, in previous centuries, insensitivity to pain was considered the sign of a pact with the devil. As an example, he enumerated the torments endured by Urbain Grandier in Loudun.

Charcot had stated: *"Hemianesthesia is a clinical symptom of hysteria that is all the more important by virtue of its being more or less permanent."* At this point, Gilles de la Tourette entered into a seemingly endless discussion, given all of the various details he wove in, taken from several doctoral theses defended before Charcot in Paris, Albert Pitres (1848–1928) in Bordeaux, or Joseph Grasset (1849–1918) in Montpellier. He seemed to have set himself the task of citing all of the works on hysteria since Charcot had taken an interest in the matter. Or perhaps there was a hidden challenge. As early as 1864, Charles Lasègue (1816–1883) noted: *"This cutaneous anesthesia, so clearly observed in hysterics, has particular aspects that we have perhaps not sufficiently examined. First of all, it is admittedly strange that this sort of phenomenon went unnoticed for so long, given that it must have caused great inconvenience. . . . However, experience shows that hysterics not yet informed by the investigations of a physician make no mention of anesthesia."*[29] The suggestion was that anesthesia was not as pathognomonic as the Salpêtrière School claimed. *"The patient maintains her sense of touch even though a pinprick is not felt,"* which Lasègue explained this way: *"It is likely that hysterics, whose normal state has so many other peculiarities, acquire through their disease a sort of dullness that makes them less receptive via certain sensory modalities."*

Gilles de la Tourette then expanded on the experiments conducted by Victor Burq (1823–1884) on *"metallotherapy and metalloscopy."* He highlighted the role played by Charcot, Jules Luys (1828–1897), and Victor Dumontpallier (1826–1899) as members of the expert committee named by the Société de Biologie, which at the time was headed by Claude Bernard (1813–1878). The committee validated the observed action of metals in the recovery of sensitivity in anesthetized areas or in the inversion of the half of the body anesthetized, referred to as the "transfer phenomenon." In transcribing a lesson given by Charcot in 1879, Richer coined the term "aesthésiogène" (esthesiogenic) to qualify these metallic agents and their surprising powers: *"Although the mechanism governing these successive displacements of sensitivity is obscure, their study itself is not without interesting implications. And it is rational to ask if the consecutive oscillations are not the pathological paratygm [sic] of some physiological law that is still unknown."*[30] This physiological law is probably what underlies the placebo effect, already masterfully described in 1800 by the English physician John Haygarth (1740–1827) (Figure 12.3).[31] As *chef de clinique* under Charcot, Babiński continued work on esthesiogenic materials, studying how magnets could be used to transfer one patient's hysterical manifestation to another patient.[32] *"Following the work of the Société de Biologie committee, which validated Burq's discovery, numerous observers shared their findings and a great number of esthesiogenic agents came to light, including static electricity, hot or cold water, vesicants and mustard plasters, certain ores or mineral salts (such as iron sulfide, calcium fluoride, sulfate, and iron carbonate), wood (Hoggard), jaborandi*

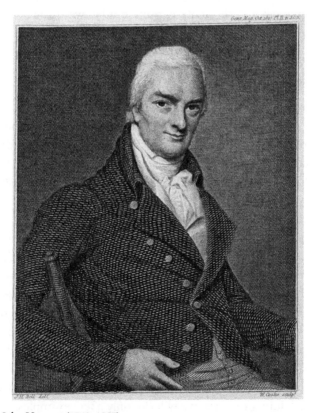

FIGURE 12.3 John Haygart (1740–1827).
The National Library of Medicine (the public domain).

as sub-cutaneous injections, amyl nitrite as inhalations, and so forth." Gilles de la Tourette was referring to Haygarth, which he misspelled[33] and whose work he clearly did not read. Otherwise, he would have understood that the use of wood in Haygarth's experiments was to establish the effects of the imagination and nothing more. Further on, Gilles de la Tourette noted: "*It was then that Hughes Bennet[34] and Hack Tuke[35]abandoned physical theories, considering that the imagination was the sole cause of the esthesiogenic action. However, this psychic theory does not account for the positive results perfectly obtained*" (by Charcot). For three pages, Gilles de la Tourette defended the existence of an organic mechanism not yet understood and refuted a psychic cause, which for Haygarth was the imagination.

Hysterical Hyperesthesias and Hysterogenic Zones

Physiological knowledge of sensitivity was still tenuous when Gilles de la Tourette wrote this chapter. The first studies exploring the physiology of sensitivity and the tests of its various modes were the work of Ernst Heinrich Weber (1795–1878) in Leipzig,[36] Albrecht von Haller (1708–1777) in Bern,[37] Johannes Müller (1808–1858) in Koblenz,[38] and Octave Landry (1826–1865) in Paris.[39] In 1835, Filippo Pacini (1812–1883) described the corpuscles that would be named for him; Georg Meissner (1829–1905) described his in 1852, and Wilhelm Krause (1833–1910) described his in 1859. In 1875, Friedrich Sigmund Merkel (1845–1919) described the skin cells that would be named for him. Decisive progress was made by Gilles de la Tourette's contemporaries Hermann von Helmholtz (1821–1894), Alfred Goldscheider (1858–1935), Henry Donaldson (1857–1938), Magnus Blix (1849–1904), Max von Frey (1852–1932), Henry Head (1861–1940), and Louis Ranvier (1835–1922). Gilles de la Tourette had not yet assimilated their findings.[40] He distinguished between anesthesia and hyperesthesia, but dysesthesias, hyperpathia, and allodynia were not differentiated. For Gilles de la Tourette, all of these disturbances of sensitivity were signs of hysteria, the prime etiology. He noted that "*disturbances in sensitivity most often involve psychic territories rather than what can strictly be referred to as nervous territories.*" Charles Sherrington (1857–1952) did not begin to develop the notion of the dermatome until 1890, which he would not precisely establish before 1898.[41]

Gilles de la Tourette included a vast catalogue of the disturbances in sensitivity observed during hysteria; we will cite only a few examples.

Past and Present

The hysterical arthralgia par excellence was pseudocoxalgia, although gonalgia was the most frequent for Charcot. The causes were *"almost always psychic in origin."* The distinguishing clinical criterion was pain that the patient described as highly acute, with variable positioning and deformation that simulated shortening of the limb and total ankylosis. *"There is something excessive, exaggerated."* In *"tuberculosis of the hip,"* functional impotence occurs progressively, whereas it is immediately complete in hysteria. Finally, certain disturbances currently considered functional are very similar to Gilles de la Tourette's descriptions, aside from the localization now in the lumbar or cervical spine rather than the hip. Parallels can be drawn between these cases and those described by Gustave Eugène Joseph Buet (1854–?) in his thesis on hysterogenic zones, defended on February 21, 1881, before Charcot. Buet described *"myosalgias,"* pain resulting from pressure applied to the spinous processes, and *"grooves,"* involving *"muscular hyperexcitability: by pressing a muscle through the skin, a contraction is provoked."*[42] Buet's thesis is in some ways similar to current-day attempts to depict a "new pain entity," such as fibromyalgia.

Ovary Compressor

"We owe the discovery of hysterogenic zones to Professor Charcot. In 1873, in his Lessons on Nervous System Diseases, the eminent professor of La Salpêtrière described the ovarian hyperesthesia of hysterics. He showed that in many cases, the hysterical attack is preceded by an aura that starts in the ovarian region, and that pressure applied in this region may, in certain patients, cause a convulsive attack; moreover, very frequently, hysterical convulsions can be instantly stopped by sudden pressure in the hyperesthesized ovarian region." This is what brought the infamous *"ovary compressor"* into use (Figure 12.4). The ambivalence of the underlying reasoning is clear; any link between hysteria and the uterus was denied, but brutal compression techniques were used on young female patients. In reality, Charcot was following in the footsteps of Thomas Willis (1621–1675), who wrote in 1668: *"It is certain that the convulsive spasm that comes from the belly is stopped, and that its rise to the neck and head is prevented, by compression of the abdomen, using the arms to enlace the body, or tightly wrapped sheets."*[43]

It should be noted that ovulation in mammals was brought to light by Karl Ernst von Baer (1792–1876) in 1827.[44] Charles Négrier (1792–1862) described the ovulatory cycle in women in 1840[45] and posited that the cyclical variations in the emotional and affective state of many women were a consequence

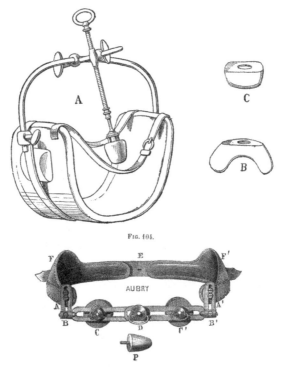

Fig. 105. — Ceinture compressive des ovaires.

FIGURE 12.4 Ovarian compression belt.
Private collection of the author.

of the periodic activity of the ovaries. In 1858, he wrote: *"In general, all of the conditions localized in the brain do not affect menstruation. On the contrary, the ovarian function has great influence on the diseases of the brain. . . . Ovulation noticeably worsens intellectual disturbances and frequently makes them hysterical in nature."*[46] As for Gilles de la Tourette, he included in his treatise this description by Albert Pitres (1848–1928):[47] *"The hysterogenic zones are circumscribed regions of the body, which may or may not be painful. During the prodromes, they are often the starting point of spontaneous attacks and special sensations that play a role in all phenomena of the hysterical aura. Pressure on these zones may either cause a convulsive attack, or part of the spasmodic phenomena of the attack, or put a sudden end to the convulsions. This definition can be completed by noting that pressure not only causes or stops the convulsive attack, but also any attacks of rhythmical chorea, coughing, yawning—in a word, all paroxysms."* Given their adherence to the concepts developed by Négrier, it is easy to understand why Charcot and Gilles de la Tourette attached essential importance to pain in the pelvic region. Today, women continue to consult their physicians for painful sensations during the menstrual cycle: premenstrual syndrome with mastodynia, pain during ovulation, and dysmenorrhea. They often find some relief from hot water bottles and other physiotherapies less brutal than those used at La Salpêtrière but nonetheless applied to the same "hysterogenic" or "hysterical hyperesthesia" zones.

The Hysterical Breast

"The hysterical breast" is another fascinating example. Gilles de la Tourette drew from the thesis of Brutus Connard (1853–1881),[48] defended in 1876: *"The breast swells, increasing in volume . . . . Palpation, which is difficult because of the horrible pain it causes, reveals small isolated nodules, which of course are only the more or less swollen divisions of the mammary gland."* For Gilles de la Tourette, vasomotor signs involving congestion and edema, according to his terminology, were sufficient to identify a manifestation of hysteria. His approach can be considered prudent, given that his main goal was to avoid the mammary amputations that certain surgeons practiced. These benign mastodynias, hormonal in origin, probably included premenstrual functional mastoses and the fibrocystic conditions described in 1829 by Astley Paston Cooper[49] (1768–1841) in England (Cooper's disease), and in 1883 by Paul Reclus[50] (1847–1914) in France (*La maladie de Reclus*).

Clou hystérique

Gilles de la Tourette listed all cutaneous and subcutaneous hysterogenic zones in his treatise. For example: *"Pains in the head, according to Briquet, are one of the perversions of sensitivity most often encountered in hysterical women."* Gilles de la Tourette then described tension headaches and what was known as the *"clou hystérique"* ("hysterical nail," an intense headache that seemed like a nail hammered into the vertex of the head). These headaches, frequently associated with vomiting, were part of a clinical picture called "pseudo-meningitis," the fear being misdiagnosis of tuberculous meningitis. Presenting the differential diagnosis, Gilles de la Tourette referred to the thesis of André Chantemesse (1851–1919), which described the initial symptoms of tuberculous meningitis as *"headache, vomiting, constipation, and fever, then convulsive movements and even delirium, frequently followed by a deceptive remission; then progression continues and worsens with a 'serious development,' the 'slowing of the pulse.' "*[51] In his transposition of Chantemesse, Gilles de la Tourette wrote: *"By their initial mode, by the successive evolution of symptoms that overall nearly characterizes tuberculous meningeal phlegmasia—violent headache, vomiting, diplopia, delirium, slowing of the pulse, meningitis rash, refractory constipation—these accidents simulate to a marvelous degree the disease we are interested in. It is only knowledge of the subject's antecedents, disturbances of sensitivity that can be attributed to hysteria, and a body temperature within normal range that make it possible to suspect the involvement of neurosis and to diagnose hysteria with a prudent margin of certitude."*

In a section on facial neuralgias, Gilles de la Tourette used the observations he provided to Jacques Artières (1863–1892)[52] for his thesis, defended in 1891 before Brouardel. All of these patients probably had organic trigeminal neuralgia, and the diagnosis of hysteria would not be considered today. The chapter on hysterical angina, hysterogenic zones of the mucosas, visceral hysterogenic zones, and dizziness is full of observations that seem confusing and vague to modern readers and are thus only of historical relevance. What does come across clearly is the difficulties faced by physicians who only had basic clinical knowledge with which to handle interlinked organic and functional pathologies, which in certain cases had not been fully described.

The conclusion to this chapter on hysterogenic zones leaves the reader perplexed: *"Quite often it is sufficient to bear in mind that they [hysterogenic zones] can exist or that they exist very frequently and in the most varied locations, in order to avoid causing and indefinitely perpetuating attacks. . . . There can be great advantages to provoking a convulsive paroxysm, which agitates the hysteric from top to bottom. . . . Causing a paroxysm can be, in certain cases at least, as useful as stopping one, as the attack may modify in all aspects the hysterical terrain and as a result, its current manifestations. . . . It may seem surprising that we have not put greater emphasis on the advantages of stopping an attack by pressure on these zones. In fact, this may be the least important element of their therapeutic action. Prolonged pressure may allow stopping an attack that occurs at an untimely moment, or in unfavorable conditions; this can help to calm the fears of a family frightened by the upheaval of hysterical convulsions . . . . But it must be understood that once the paroxysm starts, it must play out, and patients wearing a compressive ovarian belt are morally, if not physically under attack. At some point, many of them ask us to remove the compressor, preferring to struggle for an hour rather than to experience extremely uncomfortable sensations all over their bodies and locally, where compression is applied."*

Hysterical Disturbances of Vision

Hector Landouzy (1812–1864) wrote of hysteria during episodes of transitory amaurosis in his 1846 treatise.[53] Paul-Alfred Lebreton (1837–?), in his 1868 thesis[54] on hysterical paralyses, referred to the Englishman Edward Octavius Hocken (1820–1845)[55] as the first to have described, in 1842, a complete clinical picture associating rapidly progressive unilateral or bilateral amaurosis with corneal anesthesia.[56] The combination of anesthesia and amblyopia (hemianopsia), both reversible, seems to have been sufficient to posit hysteria as the cause. However, Xavier Galezowski (1832–1907) raised this question in his 1865 thesis: *"Are we to assume that hysterical conditions result in no material damage to the nervous substance? . . . There are other cases in which the disorders of the optical nerves are very pronounced in hysterics."*[57] Charcot[58] mentioned the thesis of Galezowski's Turkish student, Aristides Svynos (1848–?),[59] defended in 1873. Svynos's thesis included the description of one patient's fundus (eye): *"1) The blind spot is uniformly red throughout, following congestion in this area; 2) the contours of the blind spot are blurred, due to diffuse serous exudation that extends over the retina along the vessels; 3) the main branch of the central artery that supplies the lower part of the retina presents fusiform dilation, whereas it appears to be spasmodically contracted near the blind spot"* (Figure 12.5).[60] The diagnosis of hysteria was clearly erroneous given the appearance of the fundus, especially since Svynos added that *"optical atrophy will occur rapidly."* He did not hesitate, however, to proceed with *"faradization of the eye."* These descriptions may

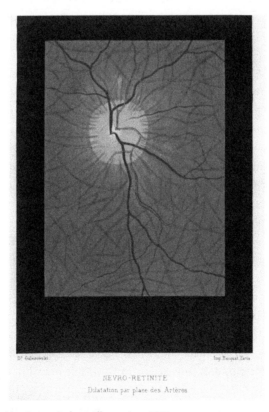

FIGURE 12.5 Aristides Svynos's thesis illustration, 1873.
Private collection of the author.

be referring to neuromyelitis optica, first described by Eugène Devic (1858–1930), who presented his findings at a French medical conference in Lyon in 1894.[61] Other observations reported by Gilles de la Tourette, in which facial anesthesia is combined with abolition of the eye-blink reflex, are undoubtedly indicative of multiple sclerosis. Victor Morax (1866–1935), then a student of Henri Parinaud (1844–1905), Charcot's ophthalmologist, provided detailed observations of ocular anomalies in hysterics based on the thirty examinations that he conducted: *"Eye examinations in hysterics take into account the visual field, dyschromatopsia, and the symptoms that almost always accompany this amblyopia: monocular polyopia and micromegalopsia. This is how Mr. Parinaud refers to the apparent shrinkage or enlargement of an object when it is brought near to, or far from the eye. Micromegalopsia, which is linked to reduced accommodation, exists almost constantly in hysterical amblyopia."* Parinaud also described hysterical ophthalmoplegia, during which voluntary eye movements are impossible while involuntary movements remain normal.[62] Another of Parinaud's students, Auguste François Hitier (1857–?), based his 1886 thesis on the study of the visual field in hysterics.[63] Gilles de la Tourette mentioned Hitier's thesis and described in detail his personal use of "Landolt's perimeter"[64] in order to assess the visual field. *"Disturbances of the visual field in hysteria cause concentric reduction."* Gilles de la Tourette then paid tribute to Galezowski for having identified dyschromatopsia, or color blindness, in hysterics. *"Unless it is complete, hysterical amblyopia, even in very severe cases, results in no serious inconvenience, probably owing, at least in part, to the fact that visual acuity is not modified. It is very rare that patients consult for this reason, and they are often quite surprised when shown how reduced their visual field has become."* Gilles de la Tourette briefly cited a few explanatory theories, but did not go into details. He listed the various conditions involved in differential diagnosis: amblyopia resulting from lead poisoning or alcoholism, locomotor ataxia, hemiplegia subsequent to hemorrhaging in the posterior limb of the internal capsule, and, last, multiple sclerosis. Allowing himself to drift off subject, he wrote at length about the visual field reduction diagnosed by Augustin Morvan (1819–1897)[65] who *"gave us the results of his specific investigations with the syndrome that, rightfully, bears his name and should be considered as syringomyelia, which he was thus one of the first to describe."*[66]

Gilles de la Tourette drew heavily from the thesis of Laurent Fink (1866–?), defended in 1891, to show that hysteria can trigger an ocular migraine: *"Certain ocular migraines are in fact manifestations of hysteria."*[67] Babiński had described with greater discernment and clarity the possible interlinking of the two pathologies in 1890.[68]

Finally, in a long chapter, Gilles de la Tourette discussed in great detail the *"hysterical affections of the ocular muscles,"* referring to the work of Georges

Borel (1860–1935)[69], an ophthalmologist in Neuchâtel, Switzerland: *"Although rarer than reduced accommodation, a particular sort of disturbance in the muscles of the eyelids and eyeballs is observed, resulting in some cases from contraction, in others from paralysis, and it is not always easy to determine which of these mechanisms predominates."*[70]

Contraction Diathesis

After covering the disturbances in sensitivity characteristic of *"interparoxysmic hysteria,"* Gilles de la Tourette went on to discuss *"the muscular disturbances that Charcot referred to as diathesis, or a state opportune for contraction,"* which Pierre Pomme (1735–1812) called in 1763 *"the hardening of the extremities."*[71] Gilles de la Tourette began by asserting: *"This is not specific to hysteria; it exists in all organic conditions that result in reflexive hyperexcitability of the pyramidal tract. Proceeding from this very fact, and reasoning by analogy, we have been able in hysteria, for which the lesions are still unknown, to interpret diathesis entirely based on anatomical control. But neurosis gives it such special traits that it must be studied on its own."* This chapter on contractions illustrates the progress in neurological knowledge made possible by hysteria. Obviously, Gilles de la Tourette lacked a semiology that would allow him to differentiate between organic contraction and functional contraction. Progress was gradual. In 1872, Désiré-Magloire Bourneville (1840–1909) and Paul Voulet (1842–1914) made a complete review of what was then known about contractions; however, the clinical aspects remained a source of confusion.[72] On March 15, 1875, Isidore Straus (1845–1896) spoke at length about "contractions" as the subject of his *agrégation* thesis,[73] in which he didactically summarized what was known at the time without contributing anything new. After the 1872–1873 lessons of Charcot, his *chef de clinique* Gilbert Ballet (1853–1916) and his *externe* Albert Delanef (1858–?) made a detailed account of *"the state of spinal reflectivity in diverse pathological situations,"* identifying the signature of hysteria only in the suddenness of onset and disappearance of contraction.[74] Edouard Brissaud (1852–1909), in his remarkable thesis defended before Charcot in 1880,[75] attributed to degeneration of the pyramidal tract the contraction of hemiplegics, characterized by exaggerated reflexes, "spinal tremor," and synkinesis, as Vulpian had described it on July 21, 1864.[76] At the December 15, 1883, session of the Société de Biologie,[77] Richer presented, on behalf of Charcot, a report on *"the contraction diathesis in hysterics,"* which he expanded into a book in 1892.[78] In addition to permanent fixed contraction, Richer characterized *"latent contraction, a state opportune for contraction that reveals itself by the simple exaggeration,*

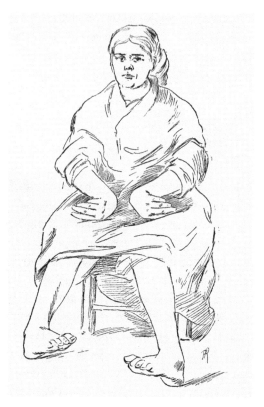

FIGURE 12.6 Hysterical prolonged contractions. Engraving by Paul Richer (1849–1933). Copyright Ecole Nationale des Beaux-arts, Paris. With kind permission.

more or less pronounced, of tendon reflexes." This sort of contraction could be triggered, among other things, by benign trauma, typically in hysterics. But there was still much confusion (Figure 12.6). Richer discussed the respective value of exaggerated tendon reflexes and *"triggered tremor": "these signs have the same significance but differ in value. Frequently, both can be observed at the same time in a given limb under special pathological conditions, but exaggeration of the patellar reflex usually appears at an early stage of the disease, when tremor in the limb cannot yet be provoked. On the other hand, the patellar reflex exists to a certain degree in the normal state, as a physiological fact, and only its exaggeration or its complete disappearance results from a pathological state. It is thus more difficult to assess than the phenomenon of triggered tremor, which is always pathological. Consequently, while the former has greater prognostic value than the latter due to its early appearance, it is far less valuable for diagnosis, since triggered tremor is never observed in the healthy state. The spasmodic character of hysterical paralysis can be more or less pronounced, from tendon reflexes that are simply heightened to extreme epileptoid shaking."* In his thesis defended before Charcot in 1888, Paul Blocq (1860–1896) attempted a pathophysiological theory, attributing permanent muscular contraction by *"lack of cerebral inhibition"* to *"a spontaneous strichnism* [strychnine poisoning]*"* of the cells in the anterior horn.[79] As for Gilles de la Tourette, he faithfully reported Richer's presentation, making no new contributions.

It was not until two years after Gilles de la Tourette's book was published, in 1893, that Babiński resolved the issue formally and established the differential diagnosis semiology: *"I accord great importance to the state of the tendon reflexes for differential diagnosis and, in my opinion, this is perhaps the sign with the greatest value. The clear exaggeration of tendon reflexes seems to me to be sufficient in the majority of contraction cases to confirm the existence of an organic affection of the nervous system, be it hemiplegia or paraplegia. . . . Hysterical contraction, on the contrary, is absolutely independent of exaggeration in these reflexes."* He was of the same opinion with regard to epileptoid tremor: *"This is not a true epileptoid tremor, but merely an imitation of the phenomenon, a shaking that differs significantly from spinal epilepsy."*[80] He also noted: *"I also maintain that the abolition of tendon reflexes is a phenomenon that hysteria is not liable to provoke."* It thus took twenty years before organic contractions could be distinguished from hysterical contractions. Gilles de la Tourette clearly lacked Babiński's perspicacity.

Hysterical Shaking

The chapter on shaking is not as indicative of the progress allowed by hysteria in neurological semiology. This is because Charcot, when he distinguished multiple sclerosis from paralysis agitans in 1868, opposed the shaking during intentional movement of the former to the shaking during rest of the latter.[81] The thesis of the German doctoral student Leopold Ordenstein (1835–1902), defended in 1867,[82] precisely explained how his teacher Charcot had differentiated the two diseases by describing the different types of shaking.[83] In 1869, Léon Guérard (1840–?) also prepared a thesis[84] that covered the different types of shaking. He published it shortly thereafter in book form, in collaboration with his teacher, Bourneville.[85] After presenting the various studies of Charcot and his students, Gilles de la Tourette did little more than copy, to a large extent, the thesis of Adolphe Dutil (1862–1929) on the clinical study of hysterical shaking,[86] which Dutil defended before Charcot on March 19, 1891. Dutil transcribed Charcot's teachings in stating that a differential diagnosis taking into account the various etiologies of shaking was based on rapid or slow onset, localized (head, hand) or generalized shaking, frequency, and regularity. Hysteria can closely simulate mercury or alcohol poisoning or Graves's disease,[87] but cases in which it resembles general paralysis, paralysis agitans, or multiple sclerosis are rarer. Louis Mugnerot (1862–?), in his thesis inspired by Maurice Letulle (1853–1929), argued that *"all shaking supposedly caused by mercury poisoning is hysterical in origin,"* based on the fact that he could bring about cessation with esthesiogenic agents or by suggestion.[88] But Charcot maintained: *"Until I have further information on the matter, I believe that true mercury-induced shaking exists independently of hysteria and results directly from hydrargyrism."*[89] Gilles de la Tourette aligned himself with Charcot, while Dutil remained doubtful.

Mental State of Hysterics

Gilles de la Tourette started this chapter with a quote: *"According to Mr. Charcot, hysteria must be taken for what it is—a psychic disease* par excellence.*"*[90] For him, understanding *"the hysterical mental state"* was important because it provided *"the key, the interpretation, for many phenomena that constitute the pathology of hysteria."* By and large, Gilles de la Tourette copied his own article published in 1890 in *Nouvelle Iconographie de La Salpêtrière*,[91] as well as that published in *Bulletin de la Société de Médecine Légale.*[92] He advised readers to consult an 1889 article[93] written by George Junkin Preston (1858–1908), who would become a neurology professor in Baltimore. Gilles de la Tourette presented Preston as his private student at La Salpêtrière, but, when Preston visited Paris, around 1884, Gilles de la Tourette was still an *interne* under Charcot. It seems more likely that Preston had come to hear the Master. In the book Preston wrote for American physicians in 1897, he noted that his data came from Charcot, Richer, and Gilles de la Tourette.[94] He even mentioned Loudun and Urbain Grandier. Gilles de la Tourette must have been pleased. In his book, Preston developed a theory of hysteria involving inhibition of cortical activity, less developed than that of Paul Sollier (1861–1933) but conceptually similar.

Gilles de la Tourette wanted to invalidate the clichés of the hysteric who simulates or concocts her condition, noting: *"What Charcot did for the physical phenomena of hysteria, he also did for the psychic phenomena."* The cause of the disease was heredity; hence this vivid expression: *"It is the most luxuriant heraldic tree that can be observed."* In his treatise, Gilles de la Tourette catalogued all mental pathologies, based on the work of Valentin Magnan (1835–1916), to show that the hysteric *"presents the most undeniable psychic stigmata of mental degeneration,"* the signature characteristic being *"suggestibility."* He described the hallucinations, sleeping problems, and anxieties of the patients hospitalized at La Salpêtrière, noting perfect similarity with *"possessed women"* such as Sœur Jeanne des Anges, Madeleine de la Palud, Loyse Capel, and Madeleine de Bavent.[95] Gilles de la Tourette did not fail to add that he had transcribed Charcot's lesson on *"spiritism and hysteria."*[96] He then included a long section on the suggestibility and self-suggestion of hysterics. This section is woven throughout with a historical theme he was particularly fond of, the life of religious women.

To complete his description of the mental state of hysterics, Gilles de la Tourette worked in several anecdotes gleaned from newspapers or from Pierre Janet (1859–1947).[97] Often, they provided him an opportunity to talk about himself. Gilles de la Tourette presented the observation of a patient suffering from obsessions, then added: *"Two weeks before her release from La Salpêtrière, she was placed next to a woman with convulsive tic disease, which we were the first to describe, under the direction of our Master. However, she seemed only moderately affected by seeing the convulsions and hearing the filthy words of her coprolalic neighbor. She then left the hospital, and one month later, she returned to us with the most perfect copy of convulsive tic disease that could possibly be imagined. The* delire du toucher *was even present, but the patient's suggestibility had not given way to it, and Mr. Charcot presented this woman to his audience as a remarkable example of hysterical simulation of convulsive tics, underscoring the coexistence of these two elements: hysterical suggestibility and stigmata of mental degeneration."*

Referring to descriptions which he qualified as *"most often those of alienists,"* Gilles de la Tourette noted: *"We can henceforth confirm it: there is no such thing as hysterical madness."* He argued against oft-repeated notions that the hysteric was *"a thief, beggar, adulteress, and murderess who no longer has the right to put an end to her life, as a simulator of suicide."* To support his arguments, he reported on several successful suicide attempts. He criticized Ambroise Tardieu (1816–1879),[98] Henri Legrand du Saulle (1830–1886),[99] Henri Taguet (1842–?),[100] Lasègue,[101] and others for having spread the idea, in particular in the literary world, that it was *"the need to simulate that pushed* [hysterics] *to stage their suicides."* The truth was that the risk of suicide was higher among hysterics and often led to real deaths.

Nutrition in "Normal Hysteria"

The first volume of Gilles de la Tourette's treatise ended with a study of the nutritional state of hysterics outside of hysteria major. Gilles de la Tourette needed the expertise of Henri Cathelineau (1861–?), a *"former clinical pharmacy intern for nervous system diseases and head of the chemistry laboratory at Hôpital*

Saint-Louis." Cathelineau measured urea and performed red blood cell counts, taking samples using a "suction cup," rather than by venipuncture. As elsewhere, Gilles de la Tourette simply copied, word for word, the first chapter of the book he had published with Cathelineau in 1890.[102] Regardless, the idea behind the study was truly novel. The only work on this theme was a thesis[103] by César-Constantin Empereur (1848–1929).[104] Gilles de la Tourette criticized Empereur's methodology because Empereur had not studied hysterics outside of attacks and thus could not credibly compare the two states. The notion of metabolism was not yet established, which led to the use of words such as "assimilation" and "disassimilation," for which the concepts were vague. Empereur concluded that *"certain hysterics maintained all of their nutritive functions,"* which was identical to the conclusion of Gilles de la Tourette and Cathelineau: *"In hysterics, aside from pathological manifestations of neurosis other than the permanent stigmata, nutrition occurs normally."*

End of Volume One

Charcot concluded his preface with these words: "[Gilles de la Tourette] *has presented us with a complete study, perfectly summarizing the current state of science in all matters, with the scrupulousness that characterizes his other works. I sincerely hope that my contribution will be advantageous to a work that represents considerable effort, sustained over a long period despite difficulties of every sort. Paris, October 15, 1891."*

In 1909, Henri Cesbron (1879–1952), the grandson of Lasègue, summed up in a few words the work's relevance: *"Gilles de la Tourette's treatise, published in 1891, can be considered the most faithful expression of Charcot's teaching. Everything the Master wrote in his articles, proffered in his lessons, or taught at his patients' bedsides is coordinated, explained, and amplified in this work. There are admittedly few new ideas, but it remains a marvelous presentation of the state of knowledge at that time."* And we share his opinion: *"Gilles de la Tourette never changed his conception of hysteria."*[105]

Notes

1. American Psychiatric Association. *Diagnostic and Statistical Manual of Mental Disorders*, Fifth Edition (DSM-5). Arlington: American Psychiatric Publishing. 2013.
2. Shorter Ed. Hysteria-psychosomatic-somatization. In Shorter (ed.), *A Historical Dictionary of Psychiatry*. New York: Oxford Press. 2005.
3. Spiegel D, Lewis-Fernández R, Lanius R, Vermetten E, Simeon D, Friedman M. Dissociative disorders in DSM-5. *Annu Rev Clin Psychol.* 2013;9:299–326.

4. Sonoo M. Neurology of hysteria (conversion disorder). *Brain Nerve.* 2014;66(7):863–871.
5. Miresco MJ, Kirmayer LJ. The persistence of mind-brain dualism in psychiatric reasoning about clinical scenarios. *Am J Psychiatry.* 2006;163(5):913–918.
6. Vuilleumier P. Hysterical conversion and brain function. *Prog Brain Res.* 2005;150: 309–329.
7. Luauté JP. 'Fin-de-Siècle' epidemiology of hysteria. *Front Neurol Neurosci.* 2014;35:20–27
8. LaFrance WC Jr. 'Hysteria' today and tomorrow. *Front Neurol Neurosci.* 2014;35:198–204.
9. Babiński J. Du phénomène des orteils et de sa valeur sémiologique. *La Semaine Médicale.* 1898;18:321–322.
10. Babiński J. *Diagnostic différentiel de l'hémiplégie organique et de l'hémiplégie hystérique. Extrait de La Gazette des Hôpitaux des 5 et 8 mai 1900.* Paris: Imprimerie F. Levé. 1900.
11. Claude H, Schnyder L. XVIIᵉ Congrès des médecins aliénistes et neurologistes de France et des pays de langue française. *La Presse Médicale.* 1907;15:532–534.
12. Le Gendre P. Gilles de la Tourette 1857–1904. *Bulletins et Mémoires de la Société Médicale des Hôpitaux de Paris.* 1905;21(3):1298–1311.
13. Gilles de la Tourette G. *Die Hysterie nach den Lehren der Salpêtrière. Normale oder interparoxysmale Hysterie.* Leipzig und Wien: Franz Deuticke. 1894.
14. Gilles de la Tourette G. *Traité clinique et thérapeutique de l'hystérie d'après l'enseignement de la Salpêtrière. (Préf. de M. le Dr J.-M. Charcot, 1°.)* Hystérie normale ou interparoxystique. Paris: Plon. 1891.
15. Gilles de la Tourette G. *Traité clinique et thérapeutique de l'hystérie, d'après l'enseignement de la Salpêtrière. 2°. Hystérie paroxystique.* Paris: E.Plon-Nourrit. 1895.
16. Richer P. *Étude descriptive de la grande attaque hystérique: ou attaque hystéro-épileptique et de ses principales variétés.* Thèse no. 179. Paris:. V. Adrien Delahaye. 1879.
17. Richer P. *Études cliniques sur l'hystéro-épilepsie, ou Grande hystérie; précédé d'une lettre-préface de M. le professeur J.-M. Charcot.* Paris: Delahaye et Lecrosnier. 1881.
18. Axenfeld H, Huchard H. *Traité des Névroses.* Paris: Germer Baillière. 1883.
19. Charcot JM, Richer P. *Les démoniaques dans l'art.* Paris: A. Delahaye et E. Lecrosnier. 1887.
20. Georget E. *De la physiologie du système nerveux et spécialement du cerveau: recherches sur les maladies nerveuses en général: et en particulier sur le siège, la nature et le traitement de l'hystérie, de l'hypochondrie, de l'épilepsie et de l'asthme convulsif.* Paris: JB. Baillière. 1821.
21. Brachet JL. *Recherches sur la nature et le siège de l'hystérie et de l'hypocondrie: et sur l'analogie et les différences de ces deux maladies.* Paris: Chez Gabon. 1832.
22. Briquet P. *Traité clinique et thérapeutique de l'hystérie.* Paris: JB. Baillière. 1859.
23. Charcot JM. *Leçons du Mardi à La Salpêtrière. Policlinique 1888–1889.* Paris: Aux Bureaux du Progrès Médical et E. Lecrosnier & Babé. 1889.
24. Féré Ch. *La famille névropathique.* Paris: Le Progrès médical et A Delahaye et E. Lecrosnier. 1884.
25. Dowbiggin I. Degeneration and hereditarianism in French mental medicine 1840–1890: psychiatric theory as ideological adaptation. In WF Bynum, R Porter, and M Shepherd (eds.), *The Anatomy of Madness*, vol. 1: People and Ideas. London and New York: Tavistock. 1985.
26. Lucas P. *Traité philosophique et physiologique de l'hérédité naturelle dans les états de santé et de maladie du système nerveux: avec l'application méthodique des lois de la procréation au traitement général des affections dont elle est le principe.* Paris: JB. Baillière. 1847–1850.
27. Morel BA. *Traité des dégénérescences physiques, intellectuelles et morales de l'espèce humaine et des causes qui produisent ces variétés maladives.* Paris: JB. Baillière. 1857.
28. Guinon G. *Les agents provocateurs de l'hystérie.* Thèse no. 140. Paris: Aux Bureaux du Progrès médical et A. Delahaye et Lecrosnier. 1889.
29. Lasègue Ch. De l'anesthésie et de l'ataxie hystériques. *Archives Générales de Médecine.* 1864;3(6°série):385–402.

30. Charcot JM, Richer P. De l'influence des agents æsthésiogènes sur l'hémianesthésie et l'achromatopsie cérébrales et particulièrement du phénomène des oscillations consécutives. *Le Progrès Médical*. 1879;7(46):893–894.

31. Haygarth J. *Of the Imagination, as a Cause and as a Cure of Disorders of the Body, Exemplified by Fictitious Tractors, and Epidemical Convulsions*. Bath: R. Crutwell. 1800.

32. Babiński J. Recherches servant à établir que certaines manifestations hystériques peuvent être transférées d'un sujet à un autre sous l'influence de l'aimant. *Le Progrès Médical*. 1886;14(47):1010–1011.

33. He reproduced the error of Axenfeld, whom he very likely copied.

34. John Hughes Bennett (1812–1875), not Bennet.

35. Daniel Hack Tuke (1827–1895).

36. Weber E. *De pulsu, resorptione, auditu et tactu: Annotationes anatomicae et physiologicae*. Lipsiae: Prostat Apud C.F. Koehler. 1834.

37. von Haller A. *Elemens de physiologie ou Traité de la structure et des usages des différentes parties du corps humain*. Paris: Chez Prault Fils. 1752.

38. Müller J. *Handbuch der Physiologie des Menschen für Vorlesungen*. Coblenz: J. Hölscher. 1838.

39. Landry O. Recherches physiologiques et pathologiques sur les sensations tactiles. *Archives Générales de Médecine*. 1852;4(29):257–275 et 1852;4(30):28–56.

40. Finger S. Origins of Neuroscience: A History of Explorations into Brain Function. New York and Oxford: Oxford University Press. 1994.

41. Sherrington Ch. Experiments in examination of the peripheral distribution of the fibres of the posterior roots of the spinal nerves. *Phil Trans R Soc (B)*. 1898;190:45–186.

42. Buet G. *Des zones hystérogènes*. Thèse no. 56. Paris: A. Parent. 1881.

43. Willis Th. Pathologiæ cerebri, et nervosi generis specimen. In *Quo agitur de morbis convulsivis et de scorbuto*. Londini: Apud Jacobum Allestry, Regalis Societatis Typographum. 1668.

44. Käbin L. Karl E. von Baer (1792–1876), le fondateur de l'embryologie contemporaine. *Histoire des Sciences Médicales*. 1998;32(1):57–62.

45. Négrier Ch. *Recherches anatomiques et physiologiques sur les ovaires dans l'espèce humaine: considérés spécialement sous le rapport de leur influence dans la menstruation*. Paris: Bechet Jeune et Labé. 1840.

46. Négrier Ch. *Recueil de faits pour servir à l'histoire des ovaires et des affections hystériques de la femme*. Angers: Imprimerie de Cosnier et Lachèse. 1858.

47. Pitres A. *Clinique médicale de l'hôpital Saint-André: Des zones hystérogènes et hypnogènes et des attaques de sommeil; leçons recueillies par M. le Dr Davezac*. Bordeaux: Imprimerie de G. Gounouilhou. 1885.

48. Connard B. *Du sein hystérique: étude sur le gonflement douloureux du sein chez les femmes hystériques*. Thèse no. 147. Paris: A. Parent. 1876.

49. Cooper AP. *Illustrations of the Diseases of the Breast*. London: Longman, Rees & Co. 1829.

50. Reclus P. La maladie kystique des mamelles. *Bulletin de la Société anatomique de Paris*. 1883;58:428–433.

51. Chantemesse A. *Étude sur la méningite tuberculeuse de l'adulte*. Les formes anormales en particulier. Thèse no. 124. Paris: V. Goupy et Jourdan. 1884.

52. Artières J. *Etude des névralgies hystériques en particulier de la névralgie faciale*. Thèse no. 335. Paris: Imprimerie H. Jouve. 1891.

53. Landouzy H. *Traité complet de l'hystérie*. Paris: JB. et G. Baillière. 1846.

54. Lebreton PA. *Des différentes variétés de la paralysie hystérique*. Thèse no. 111. Paris: A. Parent. 1868.

55. Hocken EO. *An Exposition of the Pathology of Hysteria: Elucidated by a Reference to the Origin, Diagnosis, Symptomatology, Pathology, and Treatment of Hysterical Amaurosis*. Philadelphia: Haswell and Johnson. 1842.

56. Jarius S, Wildemann B. "Spinal amaurosis" (1841). On the early contribution of Edward Hocken to the concept of neuromyelitis optica. *J Neurol.* 2014;261(2):400–404.

57. Galezowski X. *Etude ophtalmoscopique sur les altérations du nerf optique et sur les maladies cérébrales dont elles dépendent.* Thèse no. 239. Paris: Imprimerie Bonaventure et Ducessois. 1865.

58. Charcot JM. *Leçons sur les maladies du système nerveux faites à La Salpêtrière. Douzième leçon, de la contracture hystérique.* Paris: Adrien Delahaye. 1872–1873.

59. Aristide Svynos was born in Kalymnos (a Greek island in the Aegean Sea that was Turkish at the time; part of the Southern Sporades).

60. Svynos A. *Des amblyopies et des amauroses d'origine hystérique.* Thèse no. 253. Paris: A. Parent. 1873.

61. Devic E. *Myélite aiguë dorso-lombaire avec névrite optique. Autopsie. In Congrès français de médecine.* (Premiere Session; Lyon, 1894; procès-verbaux, mémoires et discussions; publiés par M. le Dr L. Bard.) Paris: Asselin et Houzeau & Lyon, Louis Savy. 1895:434–439.

62. Morax V. Compte rendu du service ophtalmologique de La Salpêtrière de M. Parrinaud pour l'année 1888 (hystérie, tabes, sclérose en plaques). *Archives de Neurologie.* 1889;27(51):436–469.

63. Hitier AF. *De l'amblyopie liée à l'hémianesthésie et spécialement de l'amblyopie hystérique.* Thèse no. 145. Paris: G. Steinheil. 1886.

64. Edmund Landolt (1846–1926), Swiss ophthalmologist.

65. Walusinski O, Honnorat J. Augustin Morvan (1819–1897), a little-known rural physician and neurologist. *Rev Neurol (Paris).* 2013;169(1):2–8.

66. Morvan A. Rétrécissement du champ visuel dans la paréso-analgésie (Maladie de Morvan). *Gazette Hebdomadaire de Médecine et de Chirurgie.* 1891;38(26):306–311.

67. Fink L. *Des rapports de la migraine ophtalmique avec l'hystérie.* Thèse no. 366. Paris: Henri Jouve. 1891.

68. Babiński J. De la migraine ophtalmique hystérique. *Archives de Neurologie.* 1890;20(60):305–335.

69. Even D. *Le Dr Georges Borel, le parcours d'un oculiste neuchâtelois.* Neuchâtel: Editions du Quadratin. 2007.

70. Borel G. Affections hystériques des muscles oculaires et leur reproduction artificielle par la suggestion hypnotique. *Annales d'oculistique.* 1887;48:nov-dec.

71. Pomme P. *Traité des affections vaporeuses des deux sexes.* Lyon: Benoit Duplain. 1763.

72. Bourneville DM, Voulet P. *De la contracture hystérique permanente.* Paris: Adrien Delahaye. 1872.

73. Straus I. *Des contractures.* Paris: JB. Baillière. 1875.

74. Ballet G, Delanef A. De l'état d'opportunité de contracture. *Gazette Médicale de Paris.* 1882;53(30):370–371.

75. Brissaud E. *Recherches anatomo-pathologiques et physiologiques sur la contracture permanente des hémiplégiques.* Thèse no. 38. Paris and Versailles: Imprimerie et Stéréotypie Cerf et fils. 1880.

76. Vulpian A. *Leçons sur la physiologie générale et comparée du système nerveux. Vingtième leçon du 21 juillet 1864: variations de l'action réflexe de la moelle (rédigée par Ernest Brémond).* Paris: Germer-Baillière. 1866

77. Richer P, Charcot JM. Diathèse de contracture chez les hystériques. *Le Progrès Médical.* 1883;11(51):1034–1035.

78. Richer P. *Paralysies et contractures hystériques.* Paris: Doin. 1892.

79. Blocq P. *Des contractures: Contracture en général.* La contracture spasmodique, les pseudo-contractures. Thèse no. 128. Paris and Chateauroux: Typographie et stéréotypie A. Majesté. 1888.

80. Babiński J. *Contractures organique et hystérique. Extrait des Bulletins et Mémoires de la Société médicale des Hôpitaux de Paris, séance du 5 mai 1893.* Paris: G Masson. 1893.

81. Charcot JM. *Leçons sur les maladies du système nerveux faites à La Salpêtrière. Cinquième leçon: de la paralysie agitante.* Paris: Adrien Delahaye. 1872–1873.

82. Ordenstein L. *Sur la paralysie agitante et la sclérose en plaques généralisée.* Thèse no. 234. Paris: Imprimerie E. Martinet. 1867.

83. Lehmann HC, Hartung HP, Kieseier BC. Leopold Ordenstein: on paralysis agitans and multiple sclerosis. *Mult Scler.* 2007;13(9):1195–1199.

84. Guérard L. *Essai sur la sclérose en plaques disséminées.* Thèse no. 95. Paris: Imprimerie Veuve Goupy. 1869.

85. Bourneville DM, Guérard L. *De la sclérose en plaques disséminées: suivi d'une nouvelle étude sur quelques points de la sclérose en plaques disséminées.* Paris: Delahaye. 1869.

86. Dutil A. *Contribution à l'étude clinique des tremblements hystériques.* Thèse no. 159. Paris: Lecrosnier et Babé. 1891.

87. Marie P. *Contribution à l'étude et au diagnostic des formes frustes de la maladie de Basedow.* Thèse no. 149. Paris: Goupy et Jourdan. 1883.

88. Mugnerot L. *Du tremblement mercuriel et de son traitement par les agents esthésiogènes.* Thèse no. 169. Paris: Imprimerie Henri Jouve. 1887.

89. Charcot JM. Des tremblements hystériques. *Le Progrès Médical.* 1890;18(36):179–182 / (37):195–197.

90. Charcot JM. *Leçons du Mardi à La Salpêtrière. Policliniques.* Paris: Bureaux du Progrès Médical & A. Delahaye et E. Lecrosnier. 1887.

91. Gilles de la Tourette G. Considérations sur les ecchymoses spontanées et sur l'état mental des hystériques. *Nouvelle Iconographie de La Salpêtrière.* 1890;3(2):49–72.

92. Gilles de la Tourette G. Ecchymoses spontanées, état mental des hystériques. Séance du 10 mars 1890. *Bulletin Société de Médecine Légale.* 1890;11:306–310.

93. Preston GJ. The mental condition in hysteria. *New York Medical Journal.* 1889;49:141–144.

94. Preston G. *Hysteria and Certain Allied Conditions: Their Nature and Treatment, with Special Reference to the Application of the Rest Cure, Massage, Electrotherapy, Hypnotism, etc.* Philadelphia: P. Blakiston, Son & Co. 1897.

95. Desmarets P. *Histoire de Madeleine Bavent: religieuse du monastère de Saint Louis de Louviers, avec sa confession générale et testamentaire, où elle déclare les abominations, impietez & sacrilèges qu'elle a pratiqué & veu pratiquer, tant dans ledit Monastere, qu'au sabat, & les personnes qu'elle y a remarquées. Ensemble l'interrogatoire de Madeleine Bavent. De plus, l'arrest donné contre Mathurin Picard; Thomas Boullé et ladite Bavent.* Paris, 1652.

96. Charcot JM. *Œuvres complètes. Leçons sur les maladies du système nerveux. Seizième leçon: spiritisme et hystérie.* Paris: Aux Bureaux du Progrès Médical & Lecrosnier et Babé. 1890.

97. Janet P. *L'automatisme psychologique: essai de psychologie expérimentale sur les formes inférieures de l'activité humaine.* Thèse d'État de Lettres. Paris: F Alcan. 1889.

98. Tardieu A. *Étude médico-légale sur la folie.* Paris: JB. Baillière. 1872.

99. Legrand du Saulle H. *Les hystériques: État physique et état mental: actes insolites, délictueux et criminels.* Paris: JB. Baillière. 1883.

100. Taguet H. *Du Suicide dans l'hystérie.* Paris: Impimerie de E. Donnaud. 1877.

101. Lasègue Ch. De l'anorexie hystérique. *Archives Générales de Médecine.* 1873;21(6ᵉ série):385–403.

102. Gilles de la Tourette G, Cathelineau H. *La nutrition dans l'hystérie.* Paris: Le Progrès Médical & Lecrosnier et Babé. 1890.

103. Empereur C. *Essai sur la nutrition dans l'hystérie.* Thèse no. 364. Paris: Pillet et Dumoulin. 1876.

104. He practiced medicine in Bourg-Saint-Maurice and would become a French Senator for Savoie under the Third Republic.

105. Cesbron H. *Histoire critique de l'Hystérie.* Thèse no. 133. Paris: Asselin et Houzeau. 1909.

13

Clinical and Therapeutic Treatise on Hysteria

Paroxysmic Hysteria

A FTER EXAMINING THE first volume of Gilles de la Tourette's *Traité de l'Hystérie*, on "normal hysteria," namely permanent hysterical stigmata, we survey the two remaining volumes, concerning "paroxysmic hysteria."

Paroxysmic Hysteria

In the face of the factual evidence, the supposed scientific skepticism that some still seem to adopt with regard to these studies will henceforth be recognized as purely arbitrary, barely masking the prejudice by which nothing new can be heard or seen.

—Jean-Martin Charcot (1825–1893)[1]

In his introduction, Gilles de la Tourette noted: *"Our aim is not to give a classification of hysterical paroxysms, which are too varied for the task."* Our aim here is similarly limited. The two volumes on paroxysmic hysteria are too vast to be analyzed in detail within the scope of a biography. Our goal, more modest, is to bring out a few specific points, especially those related to Gilles de la Tourette as physician.

Hysteria major, or *la grande hystérie*, is too well known to necessitate description, and Richer's drawings remain a magnificent reference.[1] As Gilles de la Tourette stated: *"The convulsive attack in hysteria is the traditional phenomenon par excellence."* It is the main subject of the second volume of his treatise, which covers its different phases: aura, epileptoid period, clownism period, and delusional period. Gilles de la Tourette drew largely and rather uncritically on the book of Paul Richer (1849–1933) but only referred to him with the few illustrative engravings he included. In general, he took it as established that hysteria was more frequent in women than in men and did not cover the social condition of patients.

Hysteria in Children

It was Jules Simon (1831–1899) at Hôpital des Enfants Malades who initiated the study of hysteria in children, starting at the end of the 1870s. The idea of hysteria in children seemed to come from the cerebralization of the disease, no longer associated solely with women. Two of Simon's students wrote a thesis on this subject in 1880, Henri Paris (1854–?)[2] and Georges Guiraud (1857–1942).[3] The cases observed, involving hemiplegia, ocular paralysis, choreas, and symptoms of meningitis, cast doubt on whether the young girls in question actually had hysteria. In 1885, the thesis that Paul Peugniez (1859–1943)[4] defended before Charcot, made a far-reaching survey of the various forms of hysteria in children, the first descriptions of which he dated back to Pierre Briquet (1796–1881). Peugniez noted: *"First and foremost, it is the disastrous law of nervous heredity that causes the development of hysteria in youngsters."* However, he did not fail to underscore such decisive causes as *"abuse, frightening experiences, moral emotions, and ceremonies."* It seems that many of these children suffered from what is currently known as attention deficit hyperactivity disorder. Others had authentic epilepsies or migraines, while still others had nascent psychoses. This study was used by Arthur Clopatt (1858–1933)[5] in Helsinki; he collected 270 observations for his book published in 1888.

Inspired by Bourneville, Hélène Goldspiegel (1865–?)[6] also focused her thesis on hysteria in children;[7] she defended it before Charcot on October 31, 1888. Among the observations, she included that of a fourteen-year-old boy, victim of anxiety-induced chest pain with throat tightening and the beginning of opisthotonos. Charcot had described this boy in his Tuesday lesson on February 21, 1888. He drew a parallel between this case and one of Richer's drawings in their book, *Les démoniaques dans l'art*: *"Here is a print reproduction of a fresco by Domenichino in Rome in which St. Nilus is curing a demonically possessed man. This man was certainly painted from nature and I have often shown him to the internes in this class."*[8] It was on this occasion that Charcot stated: *"Hysteria must be taken for what it is—a psychic disease par excellence."* Goldspiegel presented other cases of children from seven to fourteen years old, clearly anxious, perhaps the victims of abuse, subject to violent attacks of agitation, *"irritable and insubordinate,"* and suffering from anxiety-induced chest pain and hallucinations. Goldspiegel's thesis was one of the very first on child psychiatry in the contemporary sense of the term. Paul Blocq (1860–1896) provided a compelling explanation for these attacks of agitation, which seemed like temper tantrums and which he qualified as manic: *"Consciously,* [the child patient] *seeks to attract attention and is happy when someone notices him, exaggerating the signs of his condition accordingly; unconsciously, he is extremely impressionable and sensitive to everything he hears around him."*[9]

Ten years after the work of Jules Simon, perhaps due to the increase in studies on adult hysteria, the field of hysteria in children was boundless. Jules-François Burnet (1863–1937), in his 1891 thesis,[10] described pathologies that today appear completely unrelated to hysteria: actual hyperpyretic convulsions (meningitis?), fits of frustration associated with fainting and now known as sobbing spasms, night terrors, bedwetting, possible reactive depressions, and a host of other symptoms (abdominal pain, arthritis, hives, etc.) for which educational and moral hygiene measures were recommended, indicative of the mentalities of the time. Gilles de la Tourette strongly criticized Edmond Chaumier (1853–1931) for the opinion he presented to the Académie de Médecine in 1892, maintaining that Chaumier *"singularly exaggerated the frequency of convulsive accidents"* in newborns and children under the age of two.[11] In keeping with the views of his teacher Auguste Ollivier (1833–1894), a pediatrician at Hôpital des Enfants-Malades, Chaumier had indeed identified cases of hysteria in infants no more than a few weeks old.[12] As for Gilles de la Tourette, he only considered convulsive attacks as hysteria in children older than seven or eight, whose brains are *"so impressionable."* He helped one of his students, Arsène Bardol (1863–?),[13] prepare his thesis, which focused on children and aimed to parallel what Achille Souques (1860–1944)[14] had done two years earlier in his thesis on adults, the idea being that infantile hysteria simulated neurological pathologies. But could cases of hemiplegia accompanied by epileptic seizures, blepharospasms, hemichorea, unilateral amaurosis, and meningitis syndromes in children under ten be the result of hysteria? A tuberculous etiology probably explained some of these clinical pictures. Psychiatric causes only seem possible in the case of isolated transitory mutism.

Cultural Hysteria

Gilles de la Tourette was quite sensitive about criticisms of Charcot. When Hippolyte Bernheim (1840–1919) in Nancy contested the regularity of hysteria major as Charcot had established it, Gilles de la Tourette's response was, oddly enough, to turn to observations from military medicine. Bernheim wrote: *"I have not observed this regularity of successive phases, and I don't think it has been observed outside of La Salpêtrière. In light of how suggestible hysterics are, even during their attacks, how easily they manifest the phenomena expected of them or that they have seen in others, it is difficult not to conclude that imitation, based on self-suggestion, plays a major role in these manifestations. . . . I therefore believe that hysteria major, which La Salpêtrière considers the classical attack, occurring in clear, precise stages like beads on a rosary, is an example of cultural hysteria."*[15] Bernheim's criticism was severe and direct. Gilles de la Tourette retorted in his treatise: *"Mr. Bernheim is suggesting that Mr. Charcot, from the beginning of his research, artificially created a type of attack that he went on to cultivate in his department. The patients, men and women from around the world, supposedly did their utmost, acting on unconscious suggestion or self-suggestion, to copy the various phases of the attack and reproduce them in the same regular order. And this gave rise to the 'Salpêtrière attack, or cultural hysteria.' Quite a singular notion."* For Bernheim's edification, Gilles de la Tourette strongly advised him to read foreign authors and, rather comically, those who had described hysteria in armies. He specifically suggested the article[16] of August Knoblauch (1863–1919) and Ferdinand Andrée,[17] which he had translated for *Nouvelle Iconographie de La Salpêtrière*.[18] Charcot had used this article in his Tuesday lesson on March 19, 1889.[19] Its unsigned drawings with *"their excellent figures"* were not by Paul Richer, even though the style is similar. *"In minute detail, they describe, one by one, the periods that succeed each other with the regularity indicated by Charcot. Note that here we see a Prussian grenadier in his barracks, showing clear signs of hysteria major and very likely thinking of something entirely different than the cultural hysteria dear to Mr. Bernheim."* Gilles de la Tourette completed his demonstration by advising Bernheim to study the seventy photographs of Annita B., taken in Siena, Italy, by Gaetano Rummo (1853–1917),[20] who, it should be noted, was Charcot's translator. These pictures are very similar to the photos taken at La Salpêtrière by Albert Londe (1858–1917).[21] Gilles de la Tourette listed other works on hysteria in armies. Edouard Lanoaille de Lachèse (1839–1914) studied *"troubles of the soul"* in French army soldiers.[22] Emile Duponchel (1850–1891), professor at the Faculté de Médecine in Toulouse and author of a thesis on "hysterical madness,"[23] noted the following: *"In the general nosology of the army, hysteria holds an important place that has gone unnoticed until now and could not have been suspected prior to the latest research on male hysteria. In numerous cases, this ignorance led patients suffering from very real hysterical convulsions to be considered simulators, or epileptics."*[24] Regarding the Dutch army, Gilles de la Tourette referred to an article by H. A. Janssen de Helder.[25]

Biological Analyses Used for Diagnosing Hysteria

Gilles de la Tourette pointed out that *"authors of the past, and those writing today, have made the purely clinical observation that once the attack is over, hysterics spontaneously secrete a relatively large quantity of urine which, compared to the normal liquid, has special characteristics."* Hence his interest in the variations in concentration of several urine components, outside of and immediately after a hysteria major attack. Gilles de la Tourette selected a sample of ten patients hospitalized at La Salpêtrière and performed daily urine analyses while monitoring body weight. *"The convulsive attack was most often followed by immediate polyuria. Normal miction generally varies between 150 and 200 grams; we noted a quantity sometimes reaching 700 grams."* He observed that urine secreted immediately after the attack was of low density, low acidity, and contained half of the urea of that secreted during calm periods. *"The analysis of phosphates is as instructive as that of urea. It enabled us to identify special characteristics in urine from the attack period, which we were the first to highlight, along with the other characteristics mentioned above."*

In 1884, Albert Mairet (1852–1935),[26] *"professor of clinical medicine for mental and nervous diseases"* in Montpellier, published a report on his research into elimination of phosphoric acid in healthy men and in lunatics.[27] *"From a biological point of view, it is indispensable to comparatively study phosphoric acid bound to rare earths and phosphoric acid bound to alkalis, and we shall see that this study enables distinguishing, for a given case, between what results from muscular work and what results from intellectual work, in the elimination of phosphates."* Was it possible that biological measurement could certify the diagnosis of a mental illness? Gilles de la Tourette, inspired by Mairet's publication, studied *"the elimination of phosphates in a hysterical attack,"* as well as chlorides and sulfates. He arrived at the following result: *"The constant residue of urea, phosphates, chlorides, and sulfates is reduced by a third, relative to the normal state. The ratio of rare earth phosphate to alkaline phosphate (which together form total phosphate), which in the normal state consists of whole numbers such as 1/3, tends to become 2/3 or greater."* Diet did not modify the results, and Gilles de la Tourette was categorical: *"We repeated our experiments too many times to leave any room for doubt: the chemical formula discovered for the first time with Mr. Cathelineau in Mr. Charcot's department is directly dependent on the hysterical attack."* Gilles de la Tourette noted that, for Mairet, *"alkaline phosphate was a product of muscular activity, whereas rare earth phosphate was a product of intellectual activity. Based on our differential analyses of the two phosphates, does the hysterical attack, with is dreaming and its passionate attitudes, involve an activity that is more intellectual than muscular? . . . The chemical formula we discovered in studying the convulsive attack is applicable to other hysterical paroxysms occurring as simple or prolonged attacks or as status epilepticus; this is as we expected. . . . The formula is unchanged for attacks limited to the epileptoid period, attacks resembling partial epilepsy, and attacks of coughing, yawning, shaking, or rhythmical chorea."* Armed with this diagnostic tool, Gilles de la Tourette did not hesitate to use it to distinguish *"pseudo-angina, pseudo-meningitis, and hysterical facial neuralgias"* from organic forms. Although he was careful not to use the term "hystero-epilepsy," he was confronted with cases where differential diagnosis between hysteria and epilepsy remained quite difficult. But with his new tool, he was confident: *"Based on our research, we have chemically established—that is, independently of all objective interpretation—a means for differential diagnosis between convulsive attacks of hysteria and epileptic seizures"*; he probably meant to write *"subjective interpretation."*

After noting that his results corroborated Mairet's, he validated his own work by referring to Raphaël Lépine (1840–1919)[28] in Lyon, who claimed to be the first to have demonstrated that, in epileptics, *"rare earth phosphates, rather than alkaline phosphates, increase significantly relative to nitrogen immediately after an attack."*[29] Following publication of these results, Grasset in Montpellier[30] and Pitres in Bordeaux agreed that *"the findings of the analyses performed at La Salpêtrière by Gilles de la Tourette seem sufficiently accurate to allow, in almost all cases, diagnosis of hysteria and epilepsy by the simple comparison of urine secreted by the patients in the twenty-four hours that precede, and the twenty-four hours that follow the convulsive paroxysms."*[31] Gilles de la Tourette must have been quite proud that Grasset used "his" biological test to differentiate a case of convulsive tic disorder from hysteria.

Gilles de la Tourette noted that *"it would have been quite unusual if the results of Mr. Cathelineau and myself, and our conclusions, had gone uncontested."* He proceeded to list those who challenged him and their arguments, including Joseph Denis Voulgre (1868–1963).[32] In his 1892 thesis defended in Lyon, Voulgre wrote: *"We found ratio changes that were absolutely identical or even more exaggerated in other pathological states that have nothing in common with hysteria, for example in cases of ataxia, trauma-induced paraplegia, neurasthenia, and phosphate diabetes."*[33] But, in response, Gilles de la Tourette rejected the soundness of the challenge with an argument based on methodology—*"it was the entire chemical formula including the inversion of phosphates that we found pathognomonic for hysteria attacks"*—and with a disingenuousness that comes as no surprise: *"That phosphate inversion exists in locomotor ataxia or phosphate diabetes, conditions for which differential diagnosis with epilepsy is not called for, is of little import to us."* On January 7, 1893, a student of Féré, M. F. Royer, presented results to the Société de Biologie confirming those that his teacher presented in 1892. Royer stated bluntly: *"The supposed inversion for establishing a differential diagnosis between hysteria and epilepsy cannot be used to draw any conclusions because it may be missing in hysteria and present in epilepsy."*[34] Féré had concluded: *"This formula is not a law."*[35]

What Gilles de la Tourette took for a significant advance, despite the criticism, would have no future. It was roundly ignored by Joseph Babiński (1857-1932), Paul Sollier (1861-1933), Pierre Janet (1859-1947), and Sigmund Freud (1856-1939).

Status Epilepticus

Gilles de la Tourette paid tribute to Charcot and Bourneville for identifying cases of *"prolonged hysterical paroxysms,"* which they differentiated for the first time from status epilepticus owing to epilepsy. In a lesson, Charcot noted: *"Our dear patient, Cotte, was subject to attacks with such a predominant and pronounced epileptoid character that status epilepticus persisted for more than two months and at times reached the highest degree of intensity. For example, on January 22, a succession of epileptoid convulsions took place without interruption from nine o'clock in the morning, until eight o'clock at night. From eight to nine o'clock, there was a period of respite, then the attacks started again with renewed intensity and no recovery of lucidity; they persisted for about the same length of time. It would be no exaggeration to say that during this period, she had approximately 150 to 200 epileptoid attacks in the space of a day."*[36] Long before Gilles de la Tourette's attempts to find a biological measurement for distinguishing epilepsy and hysteria, Bourneville had tried to refine diagnosis by comparing body temperature changes during attacks. His thesis on this subject, relative to nervous system diseases, defended in 1870,[37] mainly examined *"hemorrhages and softening of the brain."* He completed his study in 1872[38] and 1873[39] with the addition of uremia, *"puerperal eclampsia,"* epilepsy, and hysteria. Charcot reported on Bourneville's results: *"When a number of true epileptic seizures are repeated in a short space of time, core temperature increases very remarkably. . . . In the common clonic hysterical attack, whatever the intensity of the convulsions, there is no significant change in core temperature."* Charcot would return several times to this method of diagnosing hysterical status epilepticus and to the possibility of differential diagnosis through temperature measurements: first, when he helped Ernest Dieu with his 1876 thesis,[40] then in 1884 during a lesson[41] transcribed by Pierre Marie (1853–1940) and an *externe* from Brazil, José-Dantas de Souza Leite (1857–1904?),[42] and finally, in his Tuesday lesson on June 26, 1888, during which he noted that *"Bl."* (i.e., Blanche Wittmann) had three hundred attacks in two days without an increase in her temperature.[43] Gilbert Ballet (1853–1916) and Gaston Crespin (1858–?) published an observation of hysterical status epilepticus simulating Bravais-Jackson epilepsy; the patient reportedly had more than 20,000 attacks in one month—without an increase in her temperature.[44] In his treatise, Gilles de la Tourette indicated that if body temperature continued *"to rise with prolongation of status epilepticus, reaching 40, 41, 42.2, and even 42.4, this was an unmistakable sign of imminent death."* And death did occur in this way for epileptics. Gilles de la Tourette's conclusion is unequivocal: *"Similarly, Mr. Bourneville demonstrated that the hysterical status epilepticus was never accompanied by an increase in temperature, which always remained below 37.8 or 38.2. Today, these facts have the force of a law."* But he did not fail to add: *"To the very important sign based on temperature observed comparatively between hysterical status epilepticus, and status epilepticus in epilepsy, discovered by Mr. Bourneville, we have added other elements of assessment by studying the nutritive exchanges in the two states."* A patient suffering from status epilepticus loses up to five hundred grams per day: *"hysterical status epilepticus is, from a chemical point of view, a prolonged attack of hysteria characterized, like the attack itself, by a reduction in volume, constant residue, urea, and phosphates, with the characteristic inversion of the phosphate formula."*

Hysterical Hypersomnia

"Hypersomnia has always attracted attention from observers, and it is to this phenomenon that we must look to explain the apparent deaths and miraculous resurrections, which are only so numerous in the literature because their undeniable singularity." After surveying a few historical examples of prolonged lethargic states followed by inexplicable awakenings and perfectly restored health, Gilles de la Tourette explained these episodes as *"ordinary attacks"* of hysteria major ending with *"interference of lethargic phenomena,"* as Charcot and Richer had described them. To illustrate the regrettable confusions of the past, he cited the thesis defended in 1872 by Louis Boutges, a student of Lasègue, in which the diagnosis of comatose hysteria was applied to clinical symptoms of hemiplegia, very likely brought on *"by apoplexy."*[45] For Gilles de la Tourette, representative cases of *"hysterical hypersomnia"* were best described by Bourneville in the 1880 *Iconographie Photographique de La Salpêtrière*. The observation of Hel– Eudoxie was used by Charles Hyvernaud (1866–1948)[46] in his thesis.[47]

Bourneville had known this twenty-seven-year-old woman in the department of Louis Delasiauve (1804–1893) before she was moved to Charcot's department, then that of Auguste Voisin (1829–1898). Tall and obese, bedridden due to paraplegia, her belly massively deformed by a pelvic tumor, Eudoxie had undoubtedly had attacks of hysteria major followed by lethargic states, but her *"wheezing inhalation with heavy exhalation"* and her *"frequent yawning"* are evocative of an obstructive sleep apnea syndrome, resulting in diurnal episodes of somnolence (Figure 13.1). Her moments of delirium, hallucination, and catatonia suggest schizophrenic psychosis or a manic-depressive state due to the alternating paradoxical euphorias and lethargic slumps.

Gilles de la Tourette can be credited with clearly stating that *"establishing a differential diagnosis between narcolepsy (without any premature judgments about this syndrome) and hysterical lethargy should not entail much hesitation,"* especially given that confusion had reigned on this matter since the descriptions—by Carl Westphal (1833–1880)[48] in Germany and Edouard Gélineau (1828–1906)[49] in France in 1880—of sudden attacks of narcoleptic sleep. In 1890, Emile

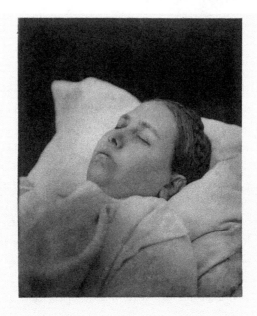

Planche XII.

HYSTÉRO-ÉPILEPSIE

ATTAQUE DE SOMMEIL

FIGURE 13.1   Hel– Eudoxie, a clinical case of hysterical sleep. *Iconographie de La Salpêtrière,* 1879.
Private collection of the author.

Parmentier (1860–1940), a former Charcot *interne*, attributed typical cases of narcolepsy[50] to hysteria: *"What are the common symptoms? Sudden onset, rapid awakening, yawning, closure of the eyelids, lack of bodily awareness, and the need to lie down out of a fear of falling."* Ballet and Gustave Samain (1869–1937)[51] did not see *"the sleeping disease as anything other than a symptom that indeed entails a special physiognomy, but does not constitute in and of itself a morbid entity."*[52]

The absence of any knowledge on sleep physiology, along with the reigning confusion between "lethargy" and coma at the end of the nineteenth century, shed light on Gilles de la Tourette's long discussions of "melancholic stupor," "apoplectoid attacks of general paralysis," hemorrhaging and brain softening, "simulated lethargy," and other brain conditions (meningitis, poisoning), but what is most apparent is how difficult and dangerous differential diagnosis was at that time. Nonetheless, hysteria was always, as if by principle, among the first of the diagnoses mentioned.

In the following chapter, Gilles de la Tourette copied long passages from his book *L'hypnotisme et les états analogues* to deal with somnambulism during hysteria and *"ambulatory automatisms."*

Trophic Dysfunction in Hysteria

Although Gilles de la Tourette claimed that *"hysteria in women wears a much more luxuriant mask than in men,"* in the second part of his treatise on pathological hysteria, he described a significant number of pathologies, found in both genders and often unpleasant, that have no link with hysteria. Readers are left with the impression that any illness deemed incomprehensible, either by its form or its cause, was considered a manifestation of hysteria. We can only feel empathy for the poor patients. To the much repeated dictum, *"the hysteric suffers because she goes onstage in the wrong theater,"* one can reply: the doctor is mistaken when he sees hysteria everywhere. As early as 1886, Babiński saw things clearly: *"All possible manifestations of hysteria seem to have been identified already and even their number has been exaggerated, since there is perhaps not a single functional disturbance that has not in certain cases, correctly or incorrectly, been linked to this neurosis."*[53]

Unfortunately, Charcot himself initiated most of the errors committed in the name of hysteria. In his preface for the commercial edition of the thesis of Alexandre Athanassio (1863–?), a native of Bucharest and former La Salpêtrière *externe*, he wrote: *"The vast domain of hysteria seemed for a long time to only accommodate those phenomena I would readily qualify as psychic, in opposition to organic phenomena resulting from damage to tissues and known in neuropathology under the general term of trophic dysfunction. The work of Mr. Athanassio strikes at the very foundations of this immaterial notion, which for too long has been applied to neuroses, and to hysteria in particular. It is important to realize that hysteria absolutely has its laws and its determinism, as a nervous affection with material lesions. The anatomical location of these lesions is still beyond our means of investigation, but they are undeniably perceptible to attentive observers in the form of trophic dysfunction, similar to what is seen in cases of organic lesions of the central nervous system or the peripheral nerves. Along this same line of reasoning, the humors are also profoundly modified, as shown recently by two of my students, Mr. Gilles de la Tourette and Mr. Cathelineau, who studied urinary dysfunction in hysteria. Now the way is open wide, and I dare hope that some days, the anatomical-clinical method will triumph once again, this time for hysteria, finally identifying the primordial impairment, the anatomical cause for what is known today to have so many material effects."*[54]

In his thesis, Athanassio thanked Gilles de la Tourette *"for amiably helping us to complete our work, and for his example and his wise advice as* chef de clinique*"* (during 1888–1889).

And now, a few examples of dysfunctions abusively attributed to hysteria. Gilles de la Tourette coined the expression *"vasomotor diathesis"* to designate dermographism, hives, and *"local asphyxia of the extremities."* This last term refers to Raynaud's disease,[55] covered in detail by Auguste Martin (1852–?), along with erythrocyanosis, in his 1876 thesis.[56] Dramatic progression to *"gangrene in the extremities"* probably illustrates cases of scleroderma and thromboangiitis obliterans, or Buerger's disease.[57] In 1881, Jules Comby (1853–1974)[58] published observations of patients suffering from *"localized sweating"* (currently known as hyperhidrosis), or who perhaps simply had increased anxiety levels.

"Hysterical Edema"

The term "hysterical edema" appeared for the first time in France[59] in the writings of François Damaschino (1840–1889)[60] and was used by Charcot in his Tuesday lesson on June 28, 1889, in the description of a case of syringomyelia, or Morvan's disease:[61] *"You can see singular tumefaction in all parts of the right hand, especially the dorsal region. This is caused by a hard edema, not indented by a touch of the finger. The tumefied parts are purplish in color and the temperature is lower than the corresponding parts of the left hand."*[62] Charcot devoted a specific lesson to this topic on May 6, 1890,[63] during which he presented the patient observation that Paul Trintignan (1863–?)[64] had based his thesis on. Charcot noted how to establish a differential diagnosis with Raynaud's disease. The symptom he focused on, occurring unilaterally, at the end of a limb, and resulting in a sheath around one or more joints that rapidly stiffen, corresponds to algodystrophy, currently referred to as complex regional pain syndrome type I by rheumatologists and orthopedic surgeons. Gilles de la Tourette indicated in his treatise the very long progression, over two to five years, with good functional recovery. During his lesson, Charcot related the history of Pauline Schey–, aged twenty-three: *"On April 26, 1890, with the patient hypnotized in the somnambulistic stage, it was suggested to her that her right wrist and hand would swell and turn purple. In the days that followed, this gradually occurred and on April 30, the right hand was swollen to a volume much greater than the left. The fingers, the dorsal side of the hand, and the wrist were purplish in color, with scattered patches of bright red. The fingers appeared blocked at the joints."* Then the seemingly miraculous resolution: *"What one suggestion had brought about, another undid."* After massage of the hand, it regained its normal appearance in about fifteen minutes. The possibility of a factitious disorder was not mentioned, only the diagnosis of hysteria.

The list of skin diseases attributed to hysteria is long in Gilles de la Tourette's treatise, which often merely copies from other authors: pemphigus, eczema, vitiligo, prurigo, zona, canities, alopecia areata, telogen effluvium, ereuthophobia, leg ulcers, lichen planus, erythromelalgia, and so forth. Gilles de la Tourette's sources include Ferdinand Hebra (1816–1880, Brno, Moravia); Moriz Kaposi (1837–1902)[65] in Vienna; Louis-Gabriel Mermet (1850–1900)[66] in Lyon; Henri Leloir (1855–1896),[67] former *interne* under Vulpian and first to hold the Chair of Cutaneous and Syphilitic Diseases in Lille; Charles Féré (1852–1907)[68]; Adrien Veillon (1864–1931), one of Fournier's students at Hôpital Saint-Louis[69]; Aristide Lebrun (1860–?) in Lille[70]; and Maurice Lannois (1856–1942).[71] Thus many of the most famous authors of his day, some of whom are cited earlier, held similar nosographical views and attributed to hysteria the etiology of numerous symptoms.

"Hysterical Sweating of Blood"

The chapter dealing with *"hemorrhages of the skin, mucous membranes, and sense organs caused by hysteria"* is not only surprising today; it also reveals the suffering inflicted on patients in the name of treatment. The poor understanding of physiological blood coagulation mechanisms led Gilles de la Tourette to consider various interpretations, some from theses without any scientific basis, such as the works of Georges Froidefond (1854–?)[72] and Virgile Mora (1841–1883).[73] *"Hysterical sweating of blood"*[74] and spontaneous bruising may have involved several pathologies such as thrombocytopenia and hemophilia. *"What we have reported above might be subject to discussion, but it is impossible to remain unconvinced by the facts we shall now analyze."* Thereby ruling out any contradiction, Gilles de la Tourette presented cases of cutaneous hemorrhaging, where letters had been traced on a limb and then appeared when the hysteric awoke, after this phenomenon had been predicted during a session of hypnotic suggestion. He supported his position by citing a similar case reported by Henry Mabille (1852–1918), head physician at an asylum in La Rochelle: *"This hemorrhage occurred during somnambulism, without any intermediary and at the point of old stigmata; I propose that its cause was self-suggestion. And this self-suggestion was cortical in origin, given that the starting point of the peripheral impressions was eliminated. It was similar to awakening and exteriorization of previously stored sensations."*[75] It is quite possible to remain unconvinced despite Gilles de la Tourette's certitudes!

Gilles de la Tourette did not hesitate to attribute hemorrhages in the eye or ear to hysteria: *"Hemorrhaging may occur in the conjunctiva, and when the blood mixes with lachrymal fluid, "tears of blood" or hematidrosis may result. However, hemorrhaging may be more frequent at the base of the lashes, occurring more rarely at the eyebrows."* As an example, he cited the case of a female hysteric with conjunctival hemorrhaging, an observation he had found in the *agrégation* thesis of Xavier Arnozan (1852–1928), a professor of therapeutics in Bordeaux.[76] These were probably subconjunctival hemorrhages, a common phenomenon most often caused by capillary fragility related to age or to violent efforts with glottis obstruction that increase pressure in the superior vena cava (refractory constipation, childbirth, coughing fits).

Even more extraordinary is what Gilles de la Tourette had to say about the ears: *"Hysterical auricular hemorrhaging is very rarely isolated; the patient, while bleeding from the ear, generally has similar blood flow from the skin, the pituitary, the conjunctiva, the gastric mucosa, and so forth."* Today's physicians would not think to ascribe to hysteria such serious coagulative dysfunction, which would clearly indicate a vital danger. Jean Baratoux (1855–?) studied bleeding from the ear that occurred periodically in hysterics[77] and which, as Gilles de la Tourette noted, *"was in addition to, or totally replaced menstrual flow. In the particular case of these patients, there was a pre-existing lesion in the middle ear with perforation of the eardrum, whereas the characteristic of hysterical hemorrhages is that they generally take place in the healthy outer ear canal, without perforation of the tympanic membrane. Or, if hysterical hemorrhaging of the inner ear does exist, it has not yet been reported."* In 1882, in *Le Progrès Médical*, Gilles de la Tourette translated and provided commentary on an article by a Dr. Field, published on February 8, 1882, in the American journal, *Medical Press*. Its title—evoking compensatory menstruation via the outer ear canal—was as enigmatic as it was surprising.[78] It should be noted, however, that Gilles de la Tourette hypothesized a fall during a lethargic state resulting in a fracture of the petrous part of the temporal bone, while pointing out that *"we know of no example for this hypothesis."* We can surmise, as an assumption underlying Gilles de la Tourette's thinking, that menstruation was still viewed as having the age-old virtue of purification, the same virtue associated with bleeding to remove contaminated humors, whatever the location of the bleeding.

Hysterical Fever

Gilles de la Tourette was clearly uncomfortable writing about "hysterical fevers": *"Their inner workings are still almost completely unknown to us, and until recently their reality was still contested."* Since the discoveries of Louis Pasteur (1822–1895), infection was considered the main cause of fevers. The thesis of Jules Gagey (1844–1905)[79] and Henri Briand (1854–?),[80] based on short-term fevers without any specific diagnosis did not escape criticism from Gilles de la Tourette: *"The research of Mr. Gagey and Mr. Briand, not supported by any conclusive observations, must be viewed as highly questionable."* As to the hysterical cause posited by the authors, Gilles de la Tourette wrote: *"The diagnosis is very debatable and we deny its existence."* He gave a list of fifteen articles from different countries on the subject of hysterical fevers but concluded: *"Among these studies, not one came directly from La Salpêtrière. To our knowledge, an authentic case of hysterical fever has never been observed in Mr. Charcot's department, probably a sign that this manifestation is not frequent. But we shall see once again that, in most cases, hysterical fever wears the mask of an acute illness: typhoid fever, malarial fever, pulmonary tuberculosis."* The one explanation he did consider plausible for hysteric fever, although his reasons are unclear, is that given by Marcel Vérette (1848–?): *"The common etiology of hysterical accidents is strong emotions and sudden cessation of menstruation."*[81] According to Henri Fabre (1858–?), hysterical fevers differed by their progression and their pseudo-meningitic, pseudo-typhoidal, and dyspneic aspects, among others,[82] but there was no demonstrated proof. Georges Debove (1845–1920) reported on a case of fever at the February 13, 1885, session of the Société Médicale des Hôpitaux:[83] *"This fever, essentially continuous, involved intermittent attacks."* The hysterical etiology of such prolonged fevers left Gilles de la Tourette perplexed; they were probably due to chronic inflammatory diseases (connective tissue diseases). Gilles de la Tourette concluded by citing Eugène Chauveau (1862–1900), who *"admitted a direct action of neurosis on the thermal centers of the cerebral cortex,*

the excitation or inhibition of which could produce hysterical fever and perhaps hypo-
thermia. These are mere hypotheses that should be mentioned, but we shall not delve
into them further."[84]

Muscular Atrophy Caused by Hysteria

"It was in 1886 that Babiński established, in Mr. Charcot's department, the reality
of muscular atrophy as a trophic dysfunction caused by hysteria." Babiński based
his work on six cases, in male patients.[85] His aim was to show that hysterical paralyses could be complicated by muscular atrophy. The atrophy set in
rapidly, affected all muscles, and stopped progressing after a time without
arriving at complete atrophy despite the persistence of complete paralysis
or of contraction. It should be noted that examining the reflexes provided
contradictory information because they were sometimes exaggerated or,
on the contrary, very weak. Gilles de la Tourette's discussion, based on
the observations of other authors and Charcot's Tuesday lesson on March
12, 1889,[86] is quite confusing in contrast to Babiński's clear deductions.
Whereas Babiński did not note any fibrillation, Gilles de la Tourette indicated *"muscular tremors"* in certain cases. Babiński specified that all muscles
of a limb were impaired, but Gilles de la Tourette maintained that sometimes atrophy *"can limit itself to certain muscular territories."* The drawings
of Paul Richer illustrating his text show typical aspects of monkey's hand,
which in his thesis, Jean-Baptiste Charcot (1867–1936)[87] referred to as
Duchenne-Aran hand, as a tribute to Guillaume Duchenne de Boulogne
(1806–1875). What this suggests is that these patients actually had organic
impairment from syringomyelia, amyotrophic lateral sclerosis, or brachial
plexus injury, for example.

At Gilles de la Tourette's request, Romain Vigouroux (1831–1911), head
of the electrotherapy department at La Salpêtrière, examined a patient in
1889 and found *"a reaction of degeneration."* This went against the opinion of
Babiński, who maintained the absence of electrical anomalies during hysterical muscular atrophy. Gilles de la Tourette re-examined the same patient
in 1893, then again in 1894, with the help of Jules-Louis Larat (1857–?), *"an*
expert in electricity," who found *"considerable reduction in faradic and galvanic*
contractilities. No trace of a reaction of degeneration." Even though the atrophy
persisted for more than five years, Gilles de la Tourette maintained his diagnosis of hysteria. He concluded: *"The positive diagnosis of hysterical mus-*
cular atrophy is easy to establish, if those characteristics specific to it, and rarely
absent, are considered: superposition on a paralysis or contraction, disturbances

of sensitivity, and coexistence of other hysterical manifestations." The prognosis was extremely variable and *"the atrophy [could] persist for months or even years."* Once again, hysteria was probably masking other unrecognized organic pathologies.

Muscular Contractions of the Head and Neck

In 1821, Etienne-Jean Georget (1795–1828) introduced the notion of sequelae, *"in cases where spasmodic cerebropathy resists."* One of the possible outcomes is that *"the patients become sensory paralytics, or suffer total or partial motor paralysis, while others have convulsive tics, dancing manias, or spasmodic retractions of the limbs."* Richer would later add that *"like the muscles of the limbs, the muscles of the face are also subject to contraction. . . . Cases of contraction limited to the face and parts of the face have been observed in which all other parts of the body remain unaffected."* For example, in blepharospasms, *"the contraction of the face may be tonic or clonic. In the first case, the deformation is permanent and persists to the same degree. In the second, it results in involuntary movements that are sudden and often repeated. The clonic form is not rare; it constitutes a variety of non-painful facial tics."*[88] As for the second form of contraction localized in the face and neck: *"Glossolabial hemispasm is not at all a rare symptom in hysteria. . . . The permanent deformation it gives the face in the resting state is generally not very pronounced, and initially has the appearance of a paralysis on the opposite side. But when movement occurs, the damage to the features is accentuated, and one sees the grimace captured in stone by the sculptor of Sancta Maria Formosa."*[89] Gilles de la Tourette illustrated his treatise with drawings by Richer (Figure 13.2) and discussed differential diagnoses for *"hysterical facial paralysis,"*[90] adding: *"In November 1887, when I became chef de clinique at La Salpêtrière, I proceeded to study glossolabial spasms in hysterics, as well as ten cases of spasms in the tongue and the muscles of the face and neck, including the orbicularis oculi. We came to the important finding that disturbances of sensitivity—anesthesia or hyperesthesia—were always superposed on these various spasms. By carefully studying these disturbances of sensitivity, we showed that what is known as glossolabial spasm frequently extended to the platysma muscle; hence the name glossolabial platysmal spasm, which should be attributed in most cases."* The history of neurology has not retained this modest discovery. In his thesis defended before Charcot, René Belin (1863–?) included thirty-six observations and, among them, the complete observation of Lelog–, a kitchen hand, depicted by Richer. Belin added commentary provided by his *chef de clinique,* Gilles de la Tourette: *"In attentively exploring the sensitivity of the tongue in several*

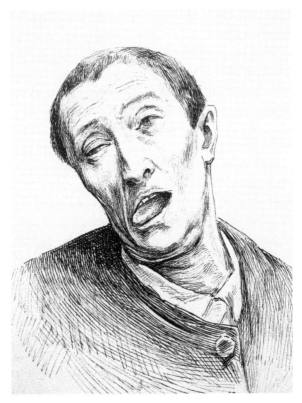

FIGURE 13.2 Hysterical (psychogenic) hemifacial spasm. Engraving by Paul Richer (1849–1933), ref 196.
Private collection of the author.

cases of hysterical glossolabial spasm, we constantly observed that the tongue was to-
tally anesthetized, even though the subjects suffered from general hemianesthesia."[91]

Gilles de la Tourette continued his chapter with hysterical torticollis, *"an*
abnormal position of the head maintained by contraction of the neck muscles."
The attribution of a psychopathological cause to these twisting movements,
introduced by the Salpêtrière School among others then perpetuated by
psychoanalysts, persisted into the 1970s. Currently, these symptoms are referred to as dystonia—that is, a muscle tone dysfunction characterized by
inappropriate muscular activity involving co-contraction of agonist and antagonist muscles at rest and when a position is held. Dystonias can exist alone
or in association with other abnormal movements. Today they are considered
the result of basal ganglia dysfunction.[92] Although their identification is complex, psychogenic dystonias, like other abnormal psychogenic movements, are
still diagnosed.[93]

Louis Hallion (1862–1940) defended his thesis before Charcot in 1892, after serving as his *interne* in 1891. Hallion's thesis addressed neuropathic vertebral deviations but contained no descriptions of scoliosis with hysterical etiology.[94] Hallion even criticized the 1889 thesis of Eugène Landois for not providing sufficient and valid proof for its claim of a possible hysterical etiology in scoliosis.[95] That did not prevent Gilles de la Tourette from accepting its existence, based on several publications, including that of Henry Duret (1849–1921), then a professor of surgery at the Université Catholique de Lille.[96] For Duret, *"hysterical contraction involved the deep muscles of the posterior abdominal region— that is, the quadratus lumborum and the iliopsoas."*[97]

As usual, Gilles de la Tourette cited himself on paralysis and contraction in the limbs: *"As I established in my inaugural thesis, during the first phase of organic hemiplegia, the lower limb is limp and sweeps against the ground as in hysterical hemiplegia."* Gilles de la Tourette then reviewed all forms of paralysis—hemiplegias, monoplegias, and paraplegias—acknowledging that *"in hysterical paralyses, tendon reflexes are generally not impaired."* It was the sensory deficits, considered very rare in organic paralysis, that allowed him to confirm a hysterical etiology.

Next, Gilles de la Tourette described in detail those contractions affecting only one limb, as illustrated by the fine drawings of Richer: *"Diagnosis* [of hysterical etiology] *generally presents no difficulties: the often rapid onset, the observation of hysterical phenomena, and the complete resolution under chloroform is nearly sufficient to settle any remaining doubts."*

Astasia-Abasia

In 1883, Charcot and Richer published an article in Italian in the journal, *A Medicina Contemporanea*, *"on a special form of motor impairment in the lower limbs involving lack of coordination."*[98] Richer qualified the article as *"the first consistent publication, supported by observations, on this bizarre form of paralysis of the lower limbs, in which muscular power is preserved for all movements other than those necessary for standing upright or walking. This form of paralysis has been given the name astasia-abasia."*[99] In fact, Sigismond Jaccoud (1830–1913) had already described the illness as an atypical form of ataxia in 1864, entitling a chapter of his book: *"Ataxia due to a lack of automatic coordination."* Jaccoud wrote: *"Until now, this very rare form has only been seen in hysterics. . . . Movements are normal when executed in a lying or sitting position. They only become ataxic in the standing position and during walking, at which time involuntary contractions interfere with balance, or disrupt the harmony of the functional act, every time the sole of the foot strikes the ground—that is, when the centripetal forces resulting from contact engage the morbid hyperkinesis of the spinal cord.*"[100] In 1888, Paul Blocq (1860–1896) returned to this description in an article in *Les Archives de Neurologie* entitled *"On a condition characterized by astasia and abasia."*[101] Blocq's coinage comes from the Greek terms for instability[102] and walking, respectively. Paul Berbez (1859–?), Charcot's *interne* in 1886, just before Blocq, used a musical metaphor to explain the syndrome: *"Most of the functional centers in the brain and spinal cord are organized like musical pieces notated on special rolls and enclosed in a barrel organ."* When *"spikes or cleats"* are missing from the organ roll, the melody is lost, as walking is impaired if coordination is no longer established.[103] Blocq noted that *"in 1884, Mr. Charcot covered this subject in several lessons published by Dr. Miliotti."*[104] The lessons in question took place on successive Tuesdays, March 5 and 12, 1889. To describe the various movements performed by the patients as they tried to raise themselves, he used the expressions *"paralytic abasia," "choreic abasia,"* and *"trembling abasia."* The last of these resembled a case described by Grasset, who used Charcot's lesson as an opportunity to present a panorama of hysteria and Gilles de la Tourette convulsive tic disorder in *Le Montpellier Médical* of March 1889.[105] Abasia generally occurs after emotional shock, especially when accompanied by a fall. One of Charcot's patients was recovering from carbon monoxide poisoning, making the diagnosis of pure hysteria unlikely. Charcot referred to Blocq's article, in which his own thinking *"was skillfully elaborated upon."* Blocq presented eleven observations, including eight of his own, compiled during his year as an *interne* under Charcot, in 1887; two of the observations were from Babiński. Gilles de la Tourette noted: *"This new syndrome will lead to numerous publications."* For example, the Brazilian physician Augusto Duprat Mazeron (1865–1940)[106] wrote his thesis on it in 1892,[107] at the end of his *internat* in Paris. He underscored that Jaccoud had been the first to describe the condition, even though Blocq had not failed to cite him. In 1892, Edmond Weill (1858–1924), working in Lyon, published a case in *Les Archives de Neurologie*; the woman, twenty-eight years of age, regained normal walking while pressure was maintained from behind on both shoulders.[108] In his 1890 thesis, Georges Cahen (1865–?) included among his thirty-seven observations three that concerned children aged eight to eleven.[109] Gilles de la Tourette in his treatise copied nearly in their entirety the lessons of Charcot and, like the Master, advised readers to consult Brissaud for *"the interesting study in his* agrégation *thesis"*[110] as well as Hippolyte Bourdon (1814–1892) for his 1843 thesis on *"paralyses following asphyxia induced by coal steam."*[111] Gilles de la Tourette recommended looking for *"stigmata of hysteria"* in atypical forms, for example those that mimed chorea, as in the observation reported by Pierre Jolly.[112] Paul Maigre (1863–1927), in his 1892 thesis, described the case of

Font– Astride, twenty-one years old and *"profoundly anemic."* Upon standing, the patient *"is overcome with trembling at a high rate of oscillation, generalized to her entire body. Her facial trembling is characterized by a rapid succession of alternating movements involving abduction and adduction of the lower jaw. In her forearms, there is rapidly alternating pronation and supination. Her lower limbs undergo successive flexing and extension of the foot on the leg, and of the lower leg on the thigh. . . . The attack lasts 4 to 5 minutes and usually ends in tears."*[113]

Like Charcot, Gilles de la Tourette pointed out *"that it could be difficult to differentiate certain cases of paralytic astasia-abasia from phenomena arising from an organic lesion of the cerebellum, known as ataxia or cerebellar incoordination."* He described in detail the difficulties of establishing an exact diagnosis, especially when several neurological pathologies were interlinked. As an example, he cited Babiński's observation of a case of astasia-abasia in a woman suffering from general paralysis.[114] He also summarized a pathophysiological hypothesis formulated by Sollier based on a case of amnesia: *"Organic memory can undergo dissociation in hysteria. The explanation for astasia-abasia can only be found in the disappearance of elements, relative to walking and standing upright, from the organic memory."*[115] Sollier successfully treated the patient by means of *"reviviscence of memories,"* first using associated sensorial images presented repeatedly, *"always giving priority to vision."* This can be considered an early form of cognitive-behavioral therapy.[116]

Hysterical Yawning

"We shall briefly cover yawning, which Mr. Huet[117] *and Mr. Georges Guinon detailed in a specific study based on five observations."*[118] Charcot dedicated his Tuesday lesson on October 23, 1888, to this subject[119] (Figure 13.3). As Gilles de la Tourette noted, the first patient presented by Charcot *"yawned around eight times per minute, 480 times per hour, or 7200 times in fifteen waking hours."* Interrupted by sleep, this yawning returned when the patient awoke *"and [could persist] for weeks and months without any noticeable deterioration of general health."* Gilles de la Tourette developed detailed arguments to convince his readers of the hysterical etiology: premonitory urges, contraction of the limbs, anesthesia of the right arm, dyschromatopsia in the right eye only, *"pain elicited by pressure on the left ovary,"* yawning attacks alternating with *"convulsive attacks"*—all examples of *"stigmata that, aside from the yawning itself, do not permit the observer to doubt."* The urinary test invented with Cathelineau supported his demonstration: *"While doubt may subsist between hysterical yawning attacks and epileptic yawning, urine analysis will quickly resolve*

the matter." Gilles de la Tourette drew a parallel between these yawning salvos and sneezing fits, which were also qualified as hysterical and observed in other patients. In reality, this sneezing was probably secondary to vasomotor rhinitis or allergies. In his lesson, Charcot added to the observation of Ler–Augustine, seventeen years old, a maid with exceptional yawning; he noted bitemporal amputation of her visual field, amenorrhea, and complete loss of taste and smell. He considered all of these symptoms as *"permanent stigmata of hysteria,"* especially since they were associated with convulsive attacks. Gilles de la Tourette evoked the notion of anorexia and reported recurrent episodes of vomiting. Although galactorrhea is not indicated, this patient probably suffered from a large adenoma in the pituitary gland (prolactinoma?) with possible intracranial hypertension. Today, a patient with these symptoms would not be diagnosed with hysteria. However, Charcot concluded: *"There is no point in further discussion; all of the various accidents in our patient are clearly hysterical—everything here is due to hysteria. What is the prognosis in this case? There are positive points: pronounced hysteria in older women is much more tenacious and persistent, sometimes incurable."* Unfortunately, the outcome of this case is not documented anywhere.

The other observations are not as exaggerated, and it is difficult to make diagnoses based solely on clinical descriptions expressly used to demonstrate that repeated yawning had to be hysterical in nature, whereas the possible causes are numerous and varied.[120]

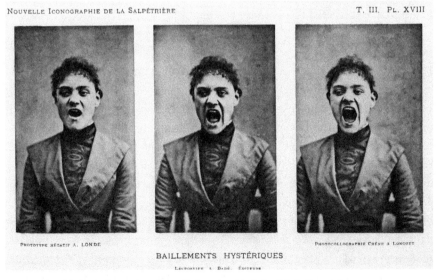

FIGURE 13.3　Hysterical yawning. *Nouvelle Iconographie de La Salpêtrière,* 1889.
Private collection of the author.

Hysterical Hemoptysis

We will only briefly mention the chapter on hysterical hemoptysis as such a diagnosis seems wholly inconceivable. Gilles de la Tourette reported that auscultation may be abnormal and coughing is constant. In the epidemic context of his day, tuberculosis must have been responsible for nearly all of these cases. He cited the thesis of A. Tostivint (1860–?), for whom *"hysterical hemoptyses appear to be more abundant than in tuberculous. The blood is crimson, like current jelly."*[121] Gilles de la Tourette took an optimistic view: *"Overall, the prognosis of hysterical hemoptysis is not serious. . . . There is always either direct cessation, or transformation into another manifestation. While hemorrhaging can be so abundant as to cause death directly, hemoptysis, like other visceral hemorrhaging linked to neurosis, does not seem likely to provoke such an outcome."* He did not adhere to the theory developed by one of Grasset's students, François Largaud (1855–?), which was *"an often impassioned argument in favor of the inhibitory influence of hysteria on pulmonary tuberculosis,"* the corollary of this argument being *"that hysteria in phthisics should not be treated."*[122] Gilles de la Tourette defended the opposing opinion: *"Based on what we have seen at La Salpêtrière, hysteria singularly favors the growth of tubercles; in this facility, where the sanitary conditions are generally very good, we have often noted that hysterics were particularly vulnerable."* Gilles de la Tourette could have cited Charcot, who stated on Tuesday, March 12, 1889: *"In addition to the agents that trigger hysteria, aside from major moral disturbances, trauma, detoxification, and so forth, poverty can be cited, with all its hardships and cruelties. In the etiological domain, one cannot overemphasize the significance of poverty, and this is what I wish to highlight."*[123]

Hysterical Anorexia

Hysterical anorexia or "hysterical inanition" is masterfully described, with an exceptional literary style evoking Victor Hugo, by Charles Lasègue (1816-1883) in 1873, who focused on *"bizarre perversions of appetite."* Here is a brief example: *"The family had only two methods at its disposal—begging or threatening—and always exhausted them. Both served as touchstones. Great efforts were made in food presentation and selection in the hopes of stimulating the patient's appetite. The greater the solicitude, the more her appetite diminished. She tasted new foods with disdain, and having made this show of willingness, she did not consider herself obliged to do more. Her family begged her, as a favor, as a sovereign proof of her affection, to resign herself to ingesting just one more mouthful of a meal she had declared finished. Their excessive insistence met with excessive resistance. The well-known rule among hysterics, roundly confirmed by experience, is that the best way to redouble their stubbornness is to implicitly or explicitly suggest that if they wished, they could control their unhealthy impulses. Having to make the slightest concession turns them from patients into capricious children, and they will never consent to such concessions, partly from instinct and partly from resolve.*"[124] Gilles de la Tourette recognized that *"Lasègue's clinical picture of this mental perversion is excellent."* His very long treatment of this subject does not make any new contributions. He remarked on insensitivity in the epigastric region, one of the hysterical stigmata, and did not hesitate to mention several times his work with Cathelineau, which he claimed made it possible to flawlessly distinguish real primitive anorexia, as described by Lasègue, from other etiologies, such as *"gastric anorexia."* Gilles de la Tourette also cited *"several important texts"* by Sollier, who used the term *"mental anorexia."* Sollier wrote: *"There is only one sort of nervous anorexia—mental anorexia—as the psychic element is really the essential one. But the term 'mental anorexia' is misleading. Etymologically, it simply means 'a loss of appetite or feeling of hunger,' whereas in reality, for anorexia to be pronounced clinically, something further is required: the systematic refusal of food, which is comparable to sitophobia in lunatics, but stems from a different motivation in the patient."*[125] His coinage of *"sitieirgia"* ("food" + "I refuse"), which he admitted was *"a little barbaric and given here for whatever it is worth,"* was not to have any lasting usage.

Effects of Hysteria on the Digestive System

"Studying the effects of hysteria on the digestive system is difficult, as they are so varied and often complex." We might add that many aspects of the physiology of digestion were still unknown in Gilles de la Tourette's day. An 1880 reference treatise on the diseases of the digestive tracts written by his teacher and friend, Damaschino, indicates that infectious pathologies were dominant, including membranous tonsillitis, typhoid fever, ulcerative-membranous stomatitis, constipation, and dysentery.[126] Intestinal worms were very frequent, and this was the usual explanation for stomach pain. Since hysteria was *"mobile in its gastric manifestations,"* Gilles de la Tourette included a vast catalogue in this chapter: gout, gastralgia, gastrodynia, anorexia, vomiting, pain, and so forth. The following paragraphs describe a few examples.

What was meant by "nervous dyspepsia"? *"Real change in gastric acid, at least according to our current knowledge, would not explain the clinical modalities of interest."* In sum: *"The influence of neurosis dominates all of these disturbances."* This turned out to be prophetic since we now know that the digestive tube contains as many, if not more neurons than the brain and that the two structures communicate closely.[127] Gilles de la Tourette described a psycho-somatic theory of digestive problems that stood in contrast to other theories, such as that of Maurice Soupault (1864–1905), who would become a hospital physician. In his thesis, Soupault examined his patients using gastric intubation and believed he could classify digestive troubles based on changes in gastric chemistry. He employed the terms "hyperchlorhydria" and "anachlorhydria" and based therapies on these concepts.[128] This type of controversy, on whether dyspeptic disturbances were psychic or gastric in origin, had existed for a long time. It is reflected in numerous theses, such as that of Lucien Deniau (1852–?), ten years before Gilles de la Tourette's treatise, in 1883.[129]

Gilles de la Tourette found himself enmeshed in the debate when he presented hematemesis: "*Strictly speaking, hematemesis is never in addition to menstruation; it sometimes modifies the quality and regularity of catamenial flow. . . . Blood in the vomit is observed in men as well as women. . . . Hematemesis, like a number of other trophic disturbances in the mucosas, hemoptysis in partic-ular, is generally part of a paroxysm easily recognizable by the aura common to all attacks, whether entailing convulsive, vasomotor, or other phenomena.*" Gilles de la Tourette recommended Louis Ferran's thesis[130] as "*excellent*"; it summed up "*several studies conducted in 1874 at La Salpêtrière*" on vomiting blood in hys-teria "*which led to later research.*" In the absence of endoscopic examination to find the cause of digestive bleeding, physicians at that time could only make guesses based on related symptoms: location of pain, burning, anorexia, and so forth. "*Syncope or fainting subsequent to hematemesis is found in many of the observations. As it is indicated even in cases where very little blood was vomited, we believe that in most cases, it cannot be attributed to true syncope due to blood loss, but rather to a demi-syncopal or lethargic state owing to hysteria.*" It is impossible to ig-nore the main flaw in this discursive sequence intended to persuade—namely, its erroneous premises.

To resolve the mystery of pathogenesis in the case of the round stomach ulcer as described by Jean Cruveilhier (1791–1874)[131] in 1830, Gilles de la Tourette, with his expertise in anatomical pathology,[132] referred to the thesis of Henri Bruchon (1868–?):[133] "*We know that hysteria is liable to produce many local circulatory disturbances, in particular spontaneous bruising, which, if located on the stomach, can initiate ulcerous lesions.*"[134] To facilitate diagnosis, Gilles de la Tourette proposed a sign for clinical examinations: "*Are cases of round ulcer attributed to hysteria often accompanied by a phenomenon of clinical importance? We are referring to acute cutaneous hyperesthesia in the epigastric region and, when it exists, a driving, rod-like pain in the lower back.*" While the first part of the assertion is false, the second is relevant, and many gastric ulcers involve pain that occurs essentially in the back, like pancreatic pain, the source of much confusion in the diagnosis of the various types of lumbagos due to joint and connective tissue problems.

Gilles de la Tourette included a long chapter on "hysterical tympanites," causing abdominal pain and bloating, sometimes to a significant degree. These were clearly cases of spastic colon, Crohn's disease and other chronic intestinal inflammations, cancer, or ovarian tumor, but, at that time, differential diagnosis focused on chronic tuberculous peritonitis. With his usual assurance, perhaps a sign of megalomania from his general paralysis, Gilles de la Tourette wrote: *"In an eighteen-year-old woman, we ourselves were able to confirm hysterical tympanites, where tuberculous peritonitis had been previously suspected. This diagnosis seemed corroborated by hemoptysis, which was in fact due to hysterical hemorrhaging."* He did not give any information on what became of this tubercular woman.

"Vomiting is so dominant that it is currently used as a general qualifier for almost all manifestations of gastric hysteria." Gilles de la Tourette referred to the observations in the thesis of Honoré Basset (1862–?)[135] to explain chronic vomiting. Excluding pregnancy, hysterical anorexia should be the primordial diagnosis before uremia or peritonitis are considered, according to Basset. Aside from migraines, also considered hysterical, there is no mention of intracranial hypertension, unknown in Gilles de la Tourette's day. Also beyond the knowledge of the time was the possibility of hypercalcemia.

Hysteria Treatments

"As the medical art is now a science increasingly committed to finding the direct causes of morbid phenomena, it is only natural that before presenting the rules of rational treatment of hysteria, we explain the nature of the neurosis. If we knew exactly which organ was the substratum of the hysterical process, and the damage it underwent, clearly our therapies would aim to eliminate the anatomical lesion, thereby abolishing the effects by destroying the cause. Unfortunately, in this regard hysteria is still within the domain of neurosis—this disease sine materia, or at least whose substance has yet to be identified." After this introduction, Gilles de la Tourette traced the history of the theories proposed since the beginning of the nineteenth century and leading up to the psychic theory: *"While there is little doubt that hysteria proceeds from the nervous system and particularly the ideational, psychic part of the brain, it is no less certain that the anatomical nature of the process escapes us completely."* Gilles de la Tourette then described advances made through the innovative work of his contemporaries Janet[136] and Sollier.[137] This final chapter starts with an overview of childrearing advice for mothers to prevent the development of

neurosis, advice that can seem quite severe to modern readers. Then Gilles de la Tourette reviewed Charcot's recommendations for treating hysterics. As Charcot explained in a lesson transcribed by Gilles de la Tourette,[138] the first measure was isolation and rest, far removed from any sources of excitation. The choice of a hydrotherapy facility was a difficult one: *"Many of them are excellent in terms of comfort, for example, but have radical shortcomings because their directors are not sufficiently qualified for their complex task."* The question of treatment cost was never addressed; most of the patients belonged to the poorest sectors of society. This may explain hospitalizations that lasted months and even years, at La Salpêtrière in particular. *"Hydrotherapy is frequently used"*; *"the physician will work with cold water."* More specifically: *"Experience has shown that the most satisfactory results have been obtained with short, cold showers using a jet shower head."* Next, Gilles de la Tourette covered the use of *"electricity in its various forms"* and advised readers to consult the work of Larat.[139] He rightfully criticized surgery practices that had come into fashion beginning in the 1870s: *"Despite its lack of success, oophorectomy quickly became known as a radical cure for neurosis. . . . It is difficult to say how many women have been castrated in this way, but in any case, the number is considerable."* He cited extracts from the thesis of Léon Tissier (1856–1948): *"Castration was proposed to all women lunatics. Goodell*[140] *seriously proposed removal of the ovaries as a remedy for masturbatory habits and dysmenorrhea."*[141] Gilles de la Tourette noted that, in France, *"Péan*[142] *was one of the first to use castration to treat pelvic manifestations caused by hysteria. And to justify his surgical operations, he did not hesitate in the least to create surgical hysteria."* Surgical excesses were such that Roland Pichevin (1857–1914) wrote his 1889 thesis on them: *"What was so unfortunate in this castration applied to nervous affections is that although the surgeons were skilled, they had little knowledge of nervous system diseases."* Pichevin also underscored the fact that compression of the ovaries is mostly a compression of the muscular wall: *"Stopping attacks of hysteria by ovarian compression is not significant. One can stop certain hysterical fits by pinching the larynx with the fingers. No one has ever used this clinical observation to prove that hysteria proceeds from the larynx."* Highlighting the frequency of deaths secondary to the operation, Pichevin concluded: *"one has no right to test a remedy that is worse than the disease, as the disease does not endanger the patient's life."*[143]

Key Points from Gilles de la Tourette's Hysteria Treatise

Such a voluminous treatise represents an enormous amount of work. Aside from a few flamboyant moments, the style is often flat and monotonous, with numerous repetitions and some unnecessary digressions. Gilles de la Tourette successfully compiled the work of a vast number of authors across three centuries of medicine. Most of them were French, but his fluency in English allowed him to translate from publications originating in Great Britain or the United States. And he did not neglect schools whose writings were in German, Italian, or Spanish. Unfortunately, the bibliographic references are often approximate or incomplete, with frequent errors in the dates. As was still tolerated at the time, he copied several of his own previously published texts, drawing on articles in *Archives de Neurologie, La Pratique Médicale, Nouvelle Iconographie de La Salpêtrière,* and *La Semaine Médicale.* He also copied passages of his previous books, notably *Sœur Jeanne des Anges* and *Hypnotisme et les états analogues.*

The treatise clearly breaks down into two parts—not along the lines he proposed, distinguishing hysterical attacks from what occurred outside the attacks—but rather hysteria related to actual neurological symptoms, on one hand, and everything that is not neurological, on the other. The first part is the perfect illustration of the lessons and works of Charcot and the School he formed at La Salpêtrière, with a key role played by Paul Richer, from whom Gilles de la Tourette borrowed heavily, to the point of plagiarism. This first part has maintained its value, both in its content and as a historical record of the concepts associated with hysteria. The second part strikes twenty-first-century readers as preposterous due to the lack of scientific proof for claims that depart radically from the rigor of the anatomical-clinical method, which had given rise to so many of Charcot's discoveries at La Salpêtrière. The Master apparently had the time to read the entire work shortly before his death, but he was already seriously ill. Had he lost his critical edge? The praise he showered on Gilles de la Tourette in his preface was flattering and ensured the commercial success of the book when it was published. But was it justified?

The reality of the work's content presaged rapid obsolescence, which did indeed occur. Only the first volume was translated into German.[144] Did the excessive content prevent translation of the other two volumes? *"Hysteria, which simulates all of the organic diseases of the nervous system, can also wear the mask of almost any visceral disease."* This maxim, which Gilles de la Tourette originated, was reflected in an 1883 book on heart failure and other subjects[145] by Augustin Fabre (1836–1884), professor of clinical medicine at the medical school in Marseille. This belief drove Gilles de la Tourette onward in his uncritical elaboration of extravagant concepts in all branches of medicine. The most extraordinary of these may have been his concept of compensatory hysterical hemorrhages in amenorrheic women, from the ear, eye, or as hematemesis or hemoptysis. This very likely played a significant role in discrediting Charcot's work on hysteria, which fell into disfavor shortly after his death. Several passages in the treatise can be seen as the product of megalomania, a symptom of Gilles de la Tourette's insidious disease. Or are they simply the expression of his relentless need for recognition, apparent from his earliest days as a medical student? *"Like everyone, hysterics ask for love, but with them, it's harder to give."* Jacques Lacan (1901–1981) could very well have written these words about Gilles de la Tourette.[146]

Notes

1. Lettre-préface de M. le professeur J.-M. Charcot. In Richer P. *Études cliniques sur l'hystéro-épilepsie, ou Grande hystérie.* Paris: Delahaye et Lecrosnier. 1881.

2. Paris H. *De l'hystérie chez les petites filles, considérée dans ses causes, ses caractères, son traitement.* Thèse no. 82. Paris: A. Parent. 1880.

3. Guiraud G. *Essai sur l'hystérie précoce se développant chez les jeunes filles avant la puberté.* Thèse no. 138. Paris: A. Parent. 1880.

4. Peugniez P. *De l'hystérie chez les enfants.* Thèse no. 307. Paris: Camille Lebas. 1885.

5. Clopatt A. *Eudes sur l'hystérie infantile.* Helsingfors: Frenckell. 1888.

6. Born in Warsaw, also known by her married name (Goldspiegel-Sosnowska). She thanked Babiński, Blocq, and M. Brzeziński.

7. Goldspiegel H. *Contribution à l'étude de l'hystérie chez les enfants.* Thèse no. 3. Paris: Henri Jouve. 1888.

8. Charcot JM. *Leçons du Mardi à La Salpêtrière. Policliniques.* Paris: Aux Bureaux du Progrès Médical & A. Delahaye et E. Lecrosnier. 1887–1888.

9. Blocq P. *Hystérie maniaque infantile.* Paris: Librairie de M. Décembre. 1890.

10. Burnet JF. *Contribution à l'étude de l'hystérie infantile: son existence au-dessous de l'âge de 5 ans.* Thèse no. 131. Paris: Henri Jouve. 1891.

11. Chaumier E. L'hystérie chez les nouveau-nés et chez les enfants au dessous de deux ans. A. Ollivier rapporteur. Séance du 28 juin 1892. *Bulletin de l'Académie de Médecine.* 1892;27(3) série):883–897.

12. Ollivier A. *Leçons cliniques sur les maladies des enfants.* Paris: Steinheil. 1889.

13. Bardol A. *De l'hystérie simulatrice des maladies organiques de l'encéphale chez les enfants.* Thèse no. 82. Paris: L. Bataille et Cie. 1893.

14. Souques A. *Contribution à l'étude des syndromes hystériques "simulateurs" des maladies organiques de la moelle épinière.* Thèse no. 158. Paris: Lecrosnier et Babé. 1891.

15. Bernheim H. *Hypnotisme & suggestion, psychothérapie.* Paris: Octave Doin. 1891.

16. Andrée F, Knoblauch A. Über enein Fall von Hystero-Katalepsie bei einem Manne. *Berliner klinische Wochenschrift.* 1889;10(26):204–207.

17. Dr. Oberstabsarzt Andrée, Chef Arzt des Garnisonlazaretts in Karlsruhe.

18. Gilles de la Tourette G. L'hystérie dans l'armée allemande. *Nouvelle Iconographie de La Salpêtrière.* 1889;2(7):318–326.

19. Charcot JM. *Leçons du Mardi à La Salpêtrière. Policliniques.* Paris: Bureaux du Progrès Médical & A. Delahaye et E. Lecrosnier. 1889.

20. Rummo G. *Iconografia fotografica del grande isterismo (Istero-Epilessia).* Napoli: Tipografia Angelo Trani. 1890.

21. Walusinski O. The girls of La Salpêtrière. *Front Neurol Neurosci.* 2014;35:65–77.

22. Lanoaille de Lachèse E. *"Tarassis," troubles de l'âme et du corps chez l'homme dans les temps modernes et dans l'histoire.* Paris: JB. Baillière. 1886.

23. Duponchel E. *De la folie hystérique.* Thèse no. 1. Paris: F. Pichon, 1874.

24. Duponchel E. L'Hystérie dans l'armée. *Revue de Médecine.* 1886;6:517–542.

25. Janssen HA. Over Hysterie bij soldaten. *Nederlands Tijdschrift voor Geneeskunde.* 1887;30(13):321–334.

26. Professor Albert Mairet. Orbituary. *Br Med J.* 1935;2(3908):1078.

27. Mairet A. *Recherches sur l'élimination de l'acide phosphorique chez l'homme sain, l'aliéné, l'épileptique et l'hystérique.* Paris: G Masson. 1884.

28. Raphaël Lépine was Charcot's *interne* in 1867.

29. Lépine R. *Titres et Travaux scientifiques.* Lyon: A Stock. 1887.

30. Grasset J. Leçons sur un cas de maladie des tics et un cas de tremblement singulier de la tête et des membres gauches. *Archives de Neurologie.* 1890;20(58):27–45 / (59):187-211

31. Pitres A. *Leçons cliniques sur l'hystérie et l'hypnotisme: faites à l'Hôpital Saint-André de Bordeaux, précédé d'une lettre-préface de M. le professeur J.-M. Charcot.* Paris: O. Doin. 1891.

32. Joseph Denis Voulgre would practice medicine in Congo, then at Val-de-Grâce military hospital during World War I.

33. Voulgre JD. *De l'élimination des phosphates dans les maladies du système nerveux et de l'inversion de leur formule dans l'hystérie.* Thèse no. 640. Lyon: Rey. 1892.

34. Royer MF Note sur la soi-disant formule urinaire de l'hystérie. *Comptes Rendus hebdomadaires des Séances et Mémoires de la Société de Biologie.* 1893;45:2–4.

35. Féré Ch. A propos de la soi-disant formule urinaire de l'hystérie. *Comptes Rendu hebdomadaires des Séances et Mémoires de la Société de Biologie.* 1893;45:151–153.

36. Charcot JM. De l'hystéro-épilepsie. Leçon faite à La Salpêtrière en juin 1872, recueillie par Bourneville. *Revue Photographique des Hôpitaux de Paris.* 1872;4(9):273–286.

37. Bourneville DM. *Etudes de thermométrie clinique dans l'hémorrhagie cérébrale et dans quelques autres maladies de l'encéphale.* Thèse no. 213. Paris: Victor Goupy. 1870.

38. Bourneville DM. *Etudes de thermométrie clinique dans l'hémorrhagie cérébrale et dans quelques autres maladies de l'encéphale. Premier fascicule: hémorrhagie et ramollissement du cerveau.* Paris: Adrien Delahaye. 1872.

39. Bourneville DM. *Etudes de thermométrie clinique dans l'hémorrhagie cérébrale et dans quelques autres maladies de l'encéphale.* Deuxième fascicule: urémie et éclampsie puerpérale; épilepsie et hystérie. Paris: Adrien Delahaye. 1873.

40. Dieu E. *De l'état du mal hystérique.* Thèse no. 332. Paris: Typographie Malverge et Dubourg. 1876.

41. Charcot JM. Attaques hystériques ayant, par leur nombre er leur durée simulée l'état de mal épileptique. Leçon recueillie par P. Marie et Souza-leite. *Le Progrès Médical.* 1884;12(38):755–757.

42. José-Dantas de Souza Leite (1857–1904?) would serve as an *interne* at the Aliénés de la Seine asylums and defended his thesis in 1890: de Souza-Leite JD. De l'acromégalie: maladie de P. Marie. Thèse no. 136. Paris: Lecrosnier et Babé, Libraires-Éditeurs. 1890.

43. Charcot JM. *Leçons du Mardi à La Salpêtrière. Policliniques.* Paris: Aux Bureaux du Progrès Médical & A. Delahaye et E. Lecrosnier. 1887–1888.

44. Ballet G, Crespin G. Des attaques d'hystérie à forme d'épilepsie partielle (étude d'une nouvelle variété d'état de mal épileptiforme). *Archives de Neurologie.* 1884;8(23):129–151 / (24):277-295.

45. Boutges L. *De la forme comateuse de l'hystérie.* Thèse no. 51. Paris: A Parent. 1875.

46. Charles Hyvernaud would be elected as mayor and regional administrator in Beaugency (Loiret), from 1906 to 1940.

47. Hyvernaud Ch. *Quelques recherches sur les attaques de sommeil hystérique.* Thèse no. 206. Paris: Henri Jouve. 1892.

48. Westphal C. Eigenthümliche mit Einschläfen verbundene Anfälle. *Archiv. Psychiatr. Nervenkr.* 1877;7:631635.

49. Gélineau JBE. De la narcolepsie. *Gazette des Hôpitaux civils et militaires.* 1880;53:626–628.

50. Parmentier E. De la forme narcoleptique de l'attaque de sommeil hystérqiue (pseudo-narcolepsie hystérique). *Archives Générales de Médecine.* 1891–2;28(7ᵉ série):528–548; 662–685.

51. Samain G. *Contribution à l'étude de la narcolepsie: ses rapports avec l'hystérie et l'épilepsie.* Thèse no. 496. Paris: Ollier-Henry. 1894.

52. Ballet G. Contribution à l'étude du sommeil pathologique. Quelques cas de narcolepsie. *Revue de Médecine.* 1882;2:945–956.

53. Babiński J. De l'atrophie musculaire dans les paralysies hystériques. *Archives de Neurologie.* 1886;12(34):1–27

54. Athanassio A. *Des troubles trophiques dans l'hystérie.* Thèse no. 162. Paris: Henri Jouve. 1890.

55. Maurice Raynaud (1834–1881) described this syndrome, which was named for him, in his 1862 thesis. Gangrene is a final stage in the progression of scleroderma. See Raynaud AGM. *De l'asphyxie locale et de la gangrène symétrique des extrémités.* Thèse no. 36. Paris: Rignoux. 1862. Charles-Victor Racle (1819–1867) had already described, in 1849, "stupor of the extremities" and gangrene. See Racle Ch. Mémoire sur de nouveaux caractères de la gangrène et sur l'existence de cette lésion dans les maladies où elle n'a pas encore été décrite. *Gazette médicale de Paris.* 1849;193(4):958–963.

56. Martin A. *Des troubles vaso-moteurs dans l'hystérie.* Thèse no. 136. Paris: A Parent. 1876.

57. http://www.orpha.net/consor/cgi-bin/OC_Exp.php?Lng=FR&Expert=36258

58. Comby J. Hystérie larvée, sueurs profuses des extrémités. *Journal de médecine et de chirurgie pratiques.* 1881;51:344–347.

59. The Englishman Thomas Laycock (1812–1876) is credited with the first description of this type of "*hysterical edema,*" for example that in "*hysterical ischuria,*" two concepts that were adopted by Charcot. See Laycock T. On anomalous forms of hysteria containing analysis of new phenomena. *Edinburgh Med J Psychiatry.* 1838;163:394–402].

60. Damaschino F. Des troubles trophiques dans l'hystérie. Leçon recueillie par Revillout. *Gazette des Hôpitaux civils et militaires.* 1888;60(3ᵉ série):561–563.

61. Walusinski O, Honnorat J. Augustin Morvan (1819–1897), a little-known rural physician and neurologist. *Rev Neurol (Paris).* 2013;169(1):2–8.

62. Charcot JM. *Leçons du Mardi à La Salpêtrière. Policliniques.* Paris: Bureaux du Progrès Médical & A. Delahaye et E. Lecrosnier. 1889.

63. Charcot JM. *L'œdème bleu des hystériques. Clinique des maladies du système nerveux. Leçons recueillies par G. Guinon.* Tome 1. Paris: Bureaux du Progrès Médical & A. Delahaye et E. Lecrosnier. 1892.

64. Trintignan P. *De l'œdème hystérique.* Thèse no. 186. Paris: Henri Jouve. 1890.

65. Hebra F, Kaposi M. *Traité des maladies de la peau comprenant les exanthèmes; traduit et annoté par A. Doyon.* Paris: G. Masson. 1872–1878.

66. Mermet LG. *Du pemphigus dans les névroses.* Thèse no. 345. Paris: A Parent. 1877.

67. Leloir H. *Recherches cliniques et anatomopathologiques sur les affections cutanées d'origine nerveuse.* Thèse no. 11. Paris: A. Delahaye. 1882.

68. Féré Ch. Notes pour servir à l'histoire de l'hystéro-épilepsie: le zona hystérique. *Archives de Neurologie.* 1882;3(8):160–175 / (9):281–309.

69. Veillon A. Troubles trophiques symétriques des mains et des avant-bras d'origine probablement hystérique. *Nouvelle Iconographie de La Salpêtrière.* 1892;5(4):201–203.

70. Lebrun A. *Du vitiligo d'origine nerveuse.* Thèse. Lille: Le Bigot frères. 1886.

71. Lannois M. *Paralysie vaso-motrice des extrémités ou érythromélalgie.* Thèse no. 166. Paris: A. Parent. 1880.

72. Froidefond G. *Contribution à l'étude de quelques hémorrhagies névropathiques.* Thèse no. 28. Paris: A. Parent. 1879.

73. Mora V. *Des hémorrhagies dans l'hystérie.* Thèse no. 192. Paris: A Parent. 1880.

74. Parrot J. Etude sur la sueur de sang et les hémorragies névropathiques. *Gazette Hebdomadaire de Médecine et de Chirurgie.* 1859;6(40):633–635; (41):644–647; (43):678–681; (45):713–715; (47):743–748.

75. Mabille H. Note sur les hémorragies cutanées par auto-suggestion, dans le somnambulisme provoqué. *Le Progrès Médical.* 1885;13(35):155–156.

76. Arnozan X. *Des lésions trophiques consécutives aux maladies du système nerveux.* Thèse d'agrégation. Paris: Adrien Delahaye. 1880.

77. Baratoux J. *Des affections auriculaires et de leurs rapports avec celles de l'utérus.* Paris: Goupy et Jourdan. 1880.

78. Gilles de la Tourette G. De la menstruation compensatrice par le conduit auditif externe. *Le Progrès Médical.* 1882;10(35):668.

79. Gagey J. *Des accidents fébriles qu'on remarque chez les hystériques.* Thèse no. 4. Paris: Lefrançois. 1869.

80. Briand H. *De la fièvre hystérique.* Thèse no. 515. Paris: A. Parent. 1877.

81. Vérette M. *De l'hystérie aiguë conséquence de l'arrêt subit de la menstruation.* Thèse no. 334. Paris: A. Parent. 1875.

83. Debove G. De la fièvre hystérique. Séance du 13 février 1885. *Bulletin de la Société médicale des hôpitaux de Paris.* 1885;2(3ᵉ série):43–46; 1886;3(3e série):209–211.

82. Fabre H. *Contribution à l'étude de la fièvre hystérique.* Thèse no. 99. Paris: Davy. 1888.

84. Chauveau E. *Formes cliniques et pathogénie de la fièvre hystérique.* Thèse no. 145. Paris: Steinhel. 1888.

85. Babiński J. De l'atrophie musculaire dans les paralysies hystériques. *Archives de Neurologie.* 1886;12(34):1–27; (35):154–196.

86. Charcot JM. *Leçons du Mardi à La Salpêtrière.* Paris: Policliniques. Bureaux du Progrès Médical & A. Delahaye et E. Lecrosnier. 1889.

87. Charcot JB. *Contribution à l'étude de l'atrophie musculaire progressive type Duchenne-Aran.* Thèse no. 313. Paris: Alcan. 1895.

88. Richer P. *Paralysies et contractures hystériques.* Paris: Octave Doin. 1892.

89. Charcot JM, Richer P. Le mascaron grotesque de l'église Santa Maria Formosa, à Venise, et l'hémispasme glosso-labié hystérique. *Nouvelle Iconographie de la Salpêtrière.* 1888;1(2):87–92.

90. Holland NJ, Bernstein JM. Bell's palsy. *BMJ Clin Evid.* 2014. pii:1204.

91. Belin R. Déviation de la face dans l'hémiplégie hystérique et dans l'hémiplégie organique: Hémispasme glosso-labié des hystériques. Thèse no. 37. Paris: Henri Jouve. 1888.

92. Ranoux D. Mouvements anormaux. In J Bogousslavsky, JM Léger, JL Mas (eds.), *Interprétation des troubles neurologiques.* Paris: Doin, 2002.

93. Schrag A. Psychogenic dystonia and reflex sympathetic dystrophy. In M Hallett, S Fahn. J Jankovic et al. (eds.), *Psychogenic Movement Disorders, Neurology and Neuropsychiatry (AAN).* Philadelphia: Lippincott Williams & Wilkins. 2006.

94. Hallion L. *Des déviations vertébrales névropathiques.* Thèse no. 349. Paris: Louis Battaille. 1892.

95. Landois E. *Des déviations du rachis dans leurs rapports avec la névropathie héréditaire.* Thèse no. 25. Paris: Henri Jouve. 1889.

96. Walusinski O, Courrivaud P. Henry Duret (1849–1921): a surgeon and forgotten neurologist. *Eur Neurol.* 2014;72(3-4):193–202.

97. Duret H. Déformation de la région lombaire de nature neuro-musculaire (cypho-scoliose hystérique). *Nouvelle Iconographie de La Salpêtrière.* 1888;1(5):191–195.

98. Charcot JM, Richer P. Su di una forma speciale d'impotenza motrice degli orti inferiori per diffetto di coordinazione. *A Medicina Contemporânea.* 1883;1(1):6–10.

99. Richer P. *Notice sur les titres et travaux scientifiques.* Paris: L Battaille et Cie. 1896.

100. Jaccoud S. *Etudes de pathogénie et de sémiotique.* Les paraplégies et l'ataxie du mouvement. Paris: Adrien Delahaye. 1864.

101. Blocq P. Sur une affection caractérisée par de l'astasie et de l'abasie. *Archives de Neurologie.* 1888;15(43):24–51; (44):187–211.

102. In physics, astatine is an instable element (atomic number 85), a radioactive halogen discovered by bombarding bismuth with accelerated helions.

103. Berbez P. Du syndrome astasie-abasie. *Gazette Hebdomadaire de Médecine et de Chirurgie.* 1888;35(8):754–757.

104. Charcot JM. *Lezioni cliniche dell'anno scolastico 1883–1884 sulle malattie del sistema nervoso, redatte dal dottore Domenico Miliotti.* Milan: Dottor Francesco Vallardi. 1885.

105. Grasset J. *Leçons sur un cas d'hystérie male avec astasie abasie, recueillies par L. Bourguet.* Montpellier: Camille Coulet. 1889.

106. Born in Recife (Brazil) on May 14, 1865, Duprat worked at the hospital in Rio Grande Do Sul and died on September 10, 1940, in Porto Alegre.

107. Duprat A. *Contribution à l'étude des troubles moteurs psychiques. Syndrome de Jaccoud (Astasie-Abasie).* Thèse no. 329. Paris: A. Lanier et ses fils. 1892.

108. Weill E. Astasie-abasie à type choréique. Arrêt instantané de l'astasie abasie par la pression de certaines régions. *Archives de Neurologie.* 1892;23(67):88–92.

109. Cahen G. *Contribution à l'étude de l'astasie-abasie.* Thèse no. 63. Paris: Ollier-Henry. 1890.

110. Brissaud E. *Des paralysies toxiques.* Paris: Asselin & Houzeau. 1886.

111. Bourdon H. *Des paralysies consécutives à l'asphyxie par la vapeur de charbon.* Thèse no. 137. Paris: Rignoux. 1847.

112. Jolly P. *Contribution à l'étude de l'astasie-abasie.* Thèse no. 769. Lyon: Alexandre Rey. 1892.

113. Maigre P. *Quelques considérations sur l'astasie-abasie.* Thèse no. 277. Paris: Henri Jouve. 1892.

114. Babiński J. *Association de l'hystérie avec les maladies organiques du systèmes nerveux, névroses et diverses affections. Bulletins et Mémoires de la Société Médicale des Hôpitaux (séance du 11 novembre 1892).* Paris: Masson. 1892

115. Séglas J, Sollier P. Folie puerpuérale, amnésie, astasie et abasie. Idées délirantes communiquées. *Archives de Neurologie.* 1890;20(60):386–404.

116. Walusinski O. Paul Sollier, Pierre Janet, and their vicinity. *Front Neurol Neurosci.* 2014;35:126–138.

117. Ernest Huet (1858–1917).

118. Gilles de la Tourette G., Huet E, Guinon G, Contribution à l'étude des bâillements hystériques. *Nouvelle Iconographie de La Salpêtrière.* 1890;3(2):97–119.

119. Charcot JM. *Leçons du Mardi à La Salpêtrière. Policlinique 1888–1889.* Paris: Aux Bureaux du Progrès Médical et E. Lecrosnier & Babé. 1889.

120. Walusinski O. Yawning in diseases. *Eur Neurol.* 2009;62(3):180–187.

121. Tostivint A. *Contribution à l'étude de l'hystérie pulmonaire (pseudo-phthisie hystérique).* Thèse no. 268. Paris: Henri Jouve. 1888.

122. Largaud F. *De l'influence de l'hystérie sur la phthisie pulmonaire.* Thèse no. 23. Montpellier: S. N. 1882.

123. Charcot JM. *Leçons du Mardi à La Salpêtrière. Policliniques.* Paris: Bureaux du Progrès Médical & A. Delahaye et E. Lecrosnier. 1889.

124. Lasègue Ch. Anorexie hystérique. *Archives Générales de Médecine.* 1873;21(6e série):385–403.

125. Sollier P. Anorexie Hystérique (Sitieirgie hystérique). *Revue de Médecine.* 1891;11:625–650.

126. Damaschino F. *Maladies des voies digestives.* Paris: Germer Baillière. 1880.

127. Mayer EA. Gut feelings: the emerging biology of gut–brain communication. *Nature Rev Neurosci.* 2011;12(8):453–466.

128. Soupault M. *Les dyspepsies nerveuses.* Thèse no. 126. Paris: Steinheil. 1893.

129. Deniau L. *De l'hystérie gastrique.* Thèse no. 119. Paris: A. Davy. 1883.

130. Ferran L. *Du vomissement de sang dans l'hystérie.* Thèse no. 368. Paris: A. Parent. 1874.

131. Vayre P. Jean Cruveilhier (1791–1874), chirurgien promoteur de la preuve par les faits à la médecine fondée sur la preuve. *E-mémoires de l'Académie Nationale de Chirurgie.* 2008;7(2):1–12. (disponible sur www.bium.univ-paris5.fr/acad-chirurgie)

132. Frexinos J. L'ulcère de Cruveilhier. In F Vicari and A Papazian. *De Barrett à Zollinger-Ellison. Quelques cas historiques en gastroentérologie.* Paris, Berlin, and Heidelberg: Springer, ALN éditions. 2007.

133. Bruchon H. *Considérations sur l'étiologie et la pathogénie de l'ulcère rond de l'estomac, sa statistique dans les Hôpitaux de Paris.* Thèse Paris no. 486. Besançon: Jacquin. 1894.

134. Gilles de la Tourette G. L'ulcère rond de l'estomac dans les Hôpitaux de Paris. Pathogénie et statistique. Séance du 15 juin 1894. *Bulletins et Mémoires Société Médicale des Hôpitaux de Paris.* 1894;11(13ᵉ série):393–408.

135. Basset H. *Des vomissements incoercibles chez les hystériques.* Thèse no. 164. Paris: Librairie Ollier-Henry, 1888.

136. Janet P. Quelques définitions récentes de l'hystérie. *Archives de Neurologie.* 1893;25(76):417–438.

137. P. Sollier, Faits nouveaux relatifs ci la nature de l'hystérie. *La Semaine Médicale.* 1894;13(22):178–181.

138. Charcot JM. De l'isolement dans le traitement de l'hystérie. *Leçon recueillie par Gilles de la Tourette. Le Progrès Médical.* 1885;13(9):161–164.

139. Larat J. *Précis d'électrothérapie. Préface de Cl. Gariel.* Paris: Lecrosnier et Babé. 1890.

140. William Goodell (1829–1894). *Goodell W. Lessons in Gynecology.* Philadelphia: DG Brinton. 1880.

141. Tissier L. *De la castration de la femme en chirurgie (opération d'Hégar ou de Battey).* Thèse Paris no. 208. Le Mans: A. Drouin. 1885.

142. Jules Emile Péan (1830–1898). "A decent man, simple and gruff, capable of goodness and generosity, extremely light on his feet, there being no equivalent for the hands. As jovial as a butcher in his slaughterhouse, he cut into the living as one cuts into wood." See Daudet L. *Devant la douleur: souvenirs des milieux littéraires, politiques, artistiques et médicaux de 1880 à 1905.* Paris: Nouvelle librairie nationale. 1915.

143. Pichevin R. *Des abus de la castration chez la femme.* Thèse no. 271. Paris: Typographie G. Chamerot. 1889.

144. Gilles de la Tourette G. *Die Hysterie nach den Lehren der Salpêtrière. Normale oder interparoxysmale Hysterie.* Leipzig and Wien: Franz Deuticke. 1894.

145. Fabre A. *Nouveaux fragments de clinique médicale. L'hystérie viscérale: les dilatations du cœur droit.* Paris: A. Delahaye et E. Lecrosnier. 1883.

146. Lacan J. *Le séminaire Livre V. Les formations de l'inconscient 1957–1958. Texte établi par Jacques-Alain Miller.* Paris: Éditions du Seuil. 1998.

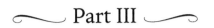

Part III

Writer and Polemicist

14

Sœur Jeanne des Anges, supérieure des Ursulines de Loudun

A Book by Gabriel Legué and Georges Gilles de la Tourette

Bibliothèque Diabolique

In 1886, Désiré–Magloire Bourneville (1840–1909) added a fifth book, suggested by Gabriel Legué (1847–1913) and Gilles de la Tourette, to his "Bibliothèque diabolique" collection. The book was entitled: *Sœur Jeanne des Anges, supérieure des Ursulines de Loudun (XVII* siècle), autobiographie d'une hystérique possédée, d'après un manuscrit inédit de la bibliothèque de Tours, annoté et publié par les docteurs Gabriel Legué et Gilles de la Tourette, préface de M. le Professeur Charcot, membre de l'Institut* (Sister Jeanne of the Angels, Superior of the Ursuline Convent in Loudun [seventeenth century], autobiography of a possessed hysteric based on an unpublished manuscript at the library in Tours, annotated and published by Doctor Gabriel Legué and Doctor Gilles de la Tourette, preface by Professor Charcot, member of the Académie des sciences). The editorial concept behind this collection, which included a total of nine books, was based on Bourneville's secular republican views. He chose books that would advance his efforts to demystify superstitious beliefs through scientific demonstration. Despite the controversy surrounding Charcot's experiments on hysteria at Hôpital La Salpêtrière, this pathology, though steeped in centuries-old beliefs in the supernatural, was in line with the anti-clerical ideals that, albeit unofficially, united all of the Master's disciples. The timeless pantomime of the possessed—witch or saint, depending on the place, era, and mindset—was precisely reflected in the three phases of *grande hystérie*, or hysteria major. The secular mind saw such states as illness and proposed medical treatment, without seeking a cause—at least at first.[1] Medical thinking at the time did not encompass the possibility that the spectacular, dramatic aspects of hysteria could be caused by emotional trauma or that patients were expressing suffering through the body and movement when words failed. With its gallery of historical portraits, the "Bibliothèque diabolique" collection provided the elements for a demonstration that sought to convince and then urged readers to adopt its forthright proselytizing.[2]

Role of Alexandre Axenfeld

A now-forgotten teacher and peer of Charcot, Auguste Alexandre Axenfeld (Aksenfeld, 1825–1876) (Figure 14.1), influenced several generations of

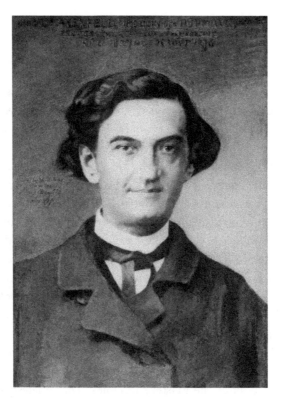

FIGURE 14.1 Auguste Alexandre Axenfeld (1825–1876), painted by his brother, Henry Axenfeld (1824–1892).
Postcard, private collection of the author.

medical students between 1857 and 1872. Son of Israel Axenfeld (1787–1866), a Yiddish lawyer and writer, Axenfeld, born in Odessa, came to Paris to study medicine after completing his secondary education in his native city. He was an *interne* (house officer or resident) in 1848, and, in 1853, he wrote his thesis on the consequences of tracheotomies performed on children with croup.[3] For his service during the cholera epidemics in Paris in 1849 and 1854, he was awarded two medals. He obtained naturalization in 1856, then passed the exams to become a professor and a hospital physician in 1857, the year Charcot failed. Axenfeld wrote a remarkable *agrégation* thesis on a subject that remains highly relevant: nosocomial diseases.[4] He was appointed *chef de service* first at Hôpital Beaujon, later replacing Léon Rostan (1790–1866) at Hôtel-Dieu. He succeeded Professor Gabriel Andral (1797–1876) at the Faculté de Médecine, occupying the Chair of General Pathology. Axenfeld spoke Hebrew, Russian, German, and French fluently, and his contemporaries wrote of his prodigious memory, his eloquent diction, his distinguished elegance, and his handsome appearance. Due perhaps in part to his book entitled *Des névroses*, Victor Hugo (1802–1885) called upon Axenfeld to treat Adèle Hugo (1830–1915) in 1872, shortly before she was committed to an asylum. In his journal, Edmond de Goncourt (1822–1896) left a poignant description of an after-dinner discussion on February 22, 1878: *"The evening's libations had begun to go to our heads, and the overall mood was colored by the uncertainty of death that each of us faced. Axenfeld, who was feeling unwell that night, was silent at first, then rose suddenly and spoke above the din: 'My brain is what will kill me,' he said loudly, and began describing how his death would occur. Then turning to the person on his right, and looking intently at him with the deep, piercing gaze of great diagnosticians, he told him how and of what he would die, and went on at length, in almost cruel detail, about the suffering that would accompany his death. Then, turning to the person on his left, he predicted his death and gave a horrific account of the details . . . all of the diners were utterly sober by this time."*[5] In 1872, Axenfeld indeed had a stroke that ruined his splendid intelligence. He began a slow, gradual decline that ended in death four years later.[6] Some documents suggest general paralysis.

Unaware of the consequences of his decision, the new dean of the Faculté de Médecine, Eugène Tardieu (1818–1879), authorized historical lectures to be held on school premises in 1865, lectures that Albert Regnard (1836–1903) transcribed and left to posterity. Regnard wrote the following preface: *"These lectures had the great merit of bringing major questions—questions of doctrine—back to the table, and of reviving the conflict between past and future, routine and method, to achieve faster resolution. I have always thought that the triumph of the science of materialism was related not only to progress in biology, but to humanity's progress as well. Therefore, in these critical essays, I made every effort to connect the field of medicine over the course of history to the great doctrine of social progress—that is, to socialism.*"[7] After thirteen lectures, the very spirit of what was being presented led the government of Napoleon III to ban the initiative.

Aimé-Philippe Tartivel (1829–1890) reported on the June 1865 lecture in *L'Union Médicale*: "*The appeal of the lecture's intriguing title was enhanced by the highly esteemed talent of the speaker, who far exceeded the promise of his reputation and his program. In elevated, often witty, even eloquent language, Mr. Axenfeld presented a historical overview of sixteenth-century witchcraft and witches and also spoke of their advocate, Jean de Wier.*"[8] Inspired by the doctrine of positivism developed by Auguste Comte (1798–1857), Axenfeld galvanized his young audience and did not hesitate to say that *"witches were the crime of the Church."* As if he could step into Wier's shoes and lend him a pathologist's point of view, Axenfeld stated that witches would have *"appeared to all as what they really were: suffering from illness. Their crimes would have taken the name of symptoms and the court records would have been nothing more than vast collections of clinical data."*[9] Regnard's praise was far-reaching: "*It was already quite daring of the young* agrégé *to have chosen such a subject from the prestigious position of his chair. And we must praise him all the more for being up to the task. Speaking with conviction and flair, he denounced the ignominious beliefs of the Middle Ages and what still remains of them today. He continually emphasized the constant connection between the state of science, the state of medicine, and that of society as a whole.*" In 1855, Bourneville, who presented himself as a disciple of Axenfeld, published writings attributed to Jean de Wier, or Johann Weyer (1515–1588), in the third volume of his "Bibliothèque diabolique."[10] The text written by Wier[11] was preceded by a biography, which was in fact an excerpt from Axenfeld's lecture. Axenfeld had pointed out that Wier was a contemporary of André Vésale (1514–1564) and had written several medical books, including one in which he described scurvy. Wier wisely recommended eating "cochlearia," a plant rich in vitamin C, something Axenfeld had not known himself. The following is Axenfeld's homage to the work undertaken by Wier: "*Let us celebrate him as the elder brother of Pinel, who freed lunatics from their chains, and the precursor of Pinel's students, who saved many of their patients from the guillotine and helped the insane in general by working to ensure their legal right to assistance. And now, is this sufficient? On the question of crime and punishment, on the most solemn of social issues, all of which are rooted in the physiological and deserving of our examination, are we to believe that science no longer has anything to say? Far from it. There is the final step to be taken, the most decisive step, and indeed the hardest to take. Today we no longer put people to death for fantastical crimes such as magic. Nor do we put people to death for an avowed crime if madness accounts for this act, and this is a sign of immense progress. However, we do continue to put non-insane criminals to death, with perfect peace of mind. For outside of madness, moral freedom seems unquestionable, and insanity is only recognized when thinking is disordered. Free will exists, such is the dogma."* Axenfeld then vehemently argued against capital punishment, stating: *"These arguments may appear rash. They aim for nothing less than this: to remove from any judicial consideration the delicate, complex, and often unsolvable problems of responsibility, and to replace public vengeance with society's sole obligation: to defend itself from any threats or dangers. Though my thinking may appear too bold, I wanted to express it in its entirety."*

Gabriel Legué

We have few biographical sources[12] for Gabriel Legué (18?–1913), born in Bonnétable in the Sarthe (northwestern France). Legué very likely attended Axenfeld's lecture; on the subject of hysteria in nuns, he wrote in his thesis: *"Agrippa, Paracelsus, and especially Jean de Wier, whose greatness Professor Axenfeld so eloquently recalled, were the first to courageously maintain that these women were sick, that we needed to save them from the devil whose plaything they had become, and heal them, not burn them."*[13] Inspired by Axenfeld's example, Legué turned his attention to the turbulent history of the convents in Loudun, the subject of his thesis. In a short footnote on page 23, he states that, in Doctor de la Tourette's office in Loudun, he had read of a nun who had admitted to having *"a pact with the devil."* Legué had thus obtained documents from Léon Gilles de la Tourette (1828–1882), Marie Gilles de la Tourette's uncle. It is our opinion that Legué, without acknowledging his sources, considerably extended and developed the thesis defended in 1839 by Jean-Charles Sauzé de Lhoumeau (1815–1889) on demonic possession in Loudun.[14] Legué's thesis was published as a book in 1874,[15] followed by two editions (1880[16] and 1884[17]) of his voluminous masterpiece, *Urbain Grandier et les possédées de Loudun*, the scrupulously researched and erudite work of a true historian. Building on the success of its second edition, Legué published *Médecins et empoisonneurs au XVIIᵉ siècle*[18] in 1896, then *La messe noire*[19] in 1903. Charles Richet (1850–1935), another actor in the demystification movement, turned frequently to Legué's thesis to prepare the three consecutive articles he published in the acclaimed *Revue des Deux Mondes* in 1880.[20] At the time, Richet was Secretary General of the Société de Psychologie Physiologique. He won the Nobel Prize for medicine "in recognition of his work on anaphylaxis" in 1913.

Urbain Grandier and the Mother Superior of the Ursuline Convent in Loudun

Included here is a brief historical summary on the protagonists of the political-religious events that disrupted life in Loudun in the era of Richelieu (1585–1652) and that re-emerged after 1870 as a political-medical ferment driving republican positivism.

In the seventeenth century, Gilles de la Tourette's beloved town of Loudun was primarily Catholic and home to many different orders of nuns and priests who unanimously spoke and preached against a Protestant minority that was, fortunately, protected by the Edict of Nantes. The Jesuits had appointed a priest from their ranks, Urbain Grandier (1590–1634) (Figure 14.2), to the parish of Saint-Pierre du Marché. Urbain Grandier rapidly came into conflict with the orders living in convents throughout Loudun and made numerous enemies. However, the tall, elegant, charming, and compassionate Grandier quickly won the sympathy of Loudun's inhabitants, especially the ladies. The governor, the King's *procureur*, and Théophraste Renaudot (1586 –1653) also came under his sway. But not everyone was charmed. *"He was an intelligent and haughty man whose provocative appearance and scorn for lowly opinion, more than his overly gallant ways, stirred part of the city up against him. As for the nuns, there is no doubt that this highly intelligent, widely-acclaimed man had made a strong impression on their imagination."*[21] Unfortunately, Grandier seduced the daughter of the *procureur*, and, when the young woman became pregnant, his one-time ally turned on him, vowing to avenge himself. *"As if this misdeed were not enough, he soon added to his list of conquests the good and kind Madeleine de Brou, for whom he had written a treatise on priestly celibacy. Based on logic worthy of his Jesuit training, his treatise demonstrated that the priest's vow of celibacy did not proceed from his own volition, but was dictated by the Church, which imposed this difficult condition on the priest whether he liked it or not, a condition without which he could not perform the duties of the priesthood."*[22]

Shortly thereafter, in 1626, the nuns in the order of Saint Ursula settled in Loudun under their twenty-five-year-old Mother Superior, Jeanne des Anges, a beautiful and proud young woman subject to convulsions that always culminated in erotic delirium. Sister Jeanne des Anges failed in her attempt to seduce Grandier and joined the ranks of those seeking his demise. Shortly

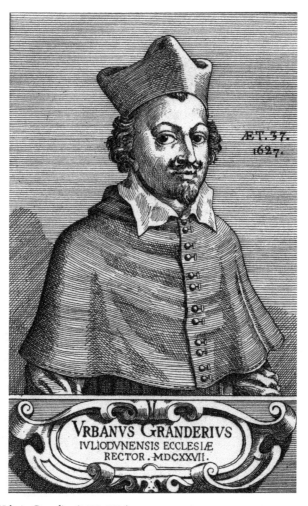

FIGURE 14.2 Urbain Grandier (1590–1634).
Private collection of the author.

thereafter, Grandier was condemned for *"sacrilegious indecency,"* but was later absolved. Despite this and other signs that it would be prudent to leave the city where he was so despised, *"attachments of the heart"* kept him from fleeing. Grandier later showed great courage in combating a terrible outbreak of plague in Loudun. Nonetheless, when the hysterical fits of Sister Jeanne des Anges began to occur daily and then spread to all of the nuns in the convent, Grandier was accused of instigating this evil possession. *"The convulsions were so horrible, the postures so terrifying that this assembly could be taken for a Sabbat."* After a biased investigation and a trial that was obviously rigged (Figure 14.3), Grandier was found guilty: *"Duly convicted of the crime of magic, enchantment,*

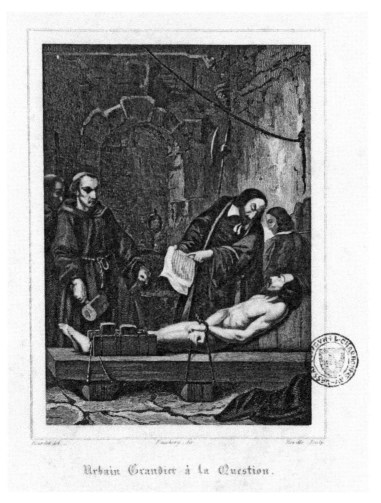

Urbain Grandier à la Question.

FIGURE 14.3 Grandier interrogated. The mode of torture employed at Loudun was a variety of the boot and one of the most painful of all. Engraving by Auguste Fauchery (1798–1843). Copyright Musée Charbonneau-Lassay, Ville de Loudun, with kind permission.

and possession as perpetrated against several Ursuline nuns in Loudun, and other secular persons, as stated during the trial. " Grandier was sentenced to be burned at the stake and underwent horrible torture beforehand. The fire was lit by the monks themselves.

Book by Legué and Gilles de la Tourette

During Legué's research in the city archives of Tours for his *"Urbain Grandier,"* he came upon an intriguing manuscript, the autobiography of a possessed hysteric. Legué wanted to publish the text with all of the necessary medical and psychological explanations but realized his own expertise on hysteria was insufficient. The year was 1885; Gilles de la Tourette had just completed part of his *internat* under Charcot. Legué, who knew the Gilles de la Tourette family in Loudun, saw Georges as the perfect partner for his project. Gilles de la Tourette's diary for the year 1886 was found in the Loudun archives and shows repeated meetings between the two men. In May 1886, they dined together twice a week. One Sunday, Bourneville joined them for dinner. The following letter from a youthful Jean-Baptiste Charcot (1867–1936), dating from 1885 or 1886 and addressed to his father, attests to how hard the two men worked:

Dear Father, I have just dined at Hôpital de la Charité with Gilles de la Tourette and Doctor Leguay.[23] After dinner, I accompanied them to Rue de Beaune where Gilles resides. The two of them are collaborating on a long work concerning possession. They have already written 551 pages, *grand aigle* or *petit aigle*; I am not sure, perhaps *moyen aigle*[24]. . . . Dr. Leguay discovered the authentic manuscript of the Ursuline Mother Superior. This precious book is at the library in Tours, under the protection of Mr. Dubost. Nothing is more touching than sentiment to Dubost (a weak-minded man). Mr. Leguay approaches literature like Pathouter [?—difficult to decipher] approaches china and he is a wonder with dates, knows all of the holy and profane scriptures, knows Albert Wolff and Lambardemont, along with Father Mignon and Baschet.[25]

Legué's find included not only the hysteric's autobiography, but also *"a digest of the most significant events during the possession of the nuns in Loudun"* and other letters and documents. These enabled Legué and Gilles de la Tourette to deepen their critical discussion: *"It was by availing ourselves of the original documents, the manuscripts from that time, that we were able, as we went along, to note the errors and make sense of the interpretations. Our medical work had to be done in the context of the manuscript, and not with historical remove. We made every effort to interpret each symptom experienced by the sister herself, based on the knowledge of the most authoritative masters on the subject. We were very sparing in our use of citations, as the way in which this work was devised does not allow for a luxuriant bibliography. However, relevant resources were not overlooked. We took special care to familiarize ourselves with the latest research of the most respected authors. Above all others, we must cite the work of our eminent Master, Professor Charcot, and his associate, our knowledgeable friend Dr. Paul Richer. Their studies on hysteria, like those of Briquet, are among the most brilliant medical works of our century."*

Paul Richer (1843–1933) defended his doctoral thesis in 1879, entitled *Etude descriptive de la grande attaque hystérique,*[26] to which he added magnificent

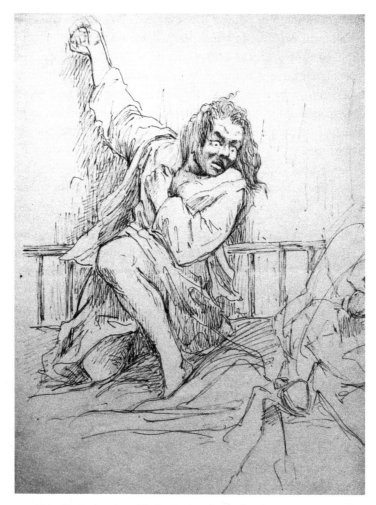

FIGURE 14.4 Magnificent drawing of hallucinations by Paul Richer (1849–1933).
Private collection of Philippe Richer, with kind permission.

drawings (Figure 14.4) and engravings for his 1881 book, *Etudes cliniques sur l'hystéro-épilepsie ou grande hystérie.*[27] In this way, our two authors aligned themselves with the opinion of Jacques Boutreux, sieur d'Estiau (15?–1639), who had witnessed comparable events in other places: *"Reasons for all of these symptoms and accidents must be given through the rules and maxims of medicine such that the signs and proof of illness seem fairly obvious."*[28]

There are three parts to the book by Legué and Gilles de la Tourette. The first is a deftly written chapter that reads like a novel and tells the story of Sister Jeanne des Anges. The second is the literal transcription of her autobiography. Gilles de la Tourette added footnotes to draw attention to the pathological nature of the content: *"Because Sister Jeanne admitted herself in this manuscript that she had never even seen Grandier prior to her illness, this is clearly a case of the hallucinations so frequent in hysterics"*; or, *"During exorcisms, the devil was thought to speak, when questioned, through the mouth of the possessed person. Note that at such a time, the victim was suffering an attack, or was even subject to somnambulic phenomena combined with the convulsive phenomena that occur during ordinary attacks."* In other cases, he provided a medical explanation for the signs described: *"Like all hysterical phenomena, the abdominal tympanites vanished as suddenly as it had appeared, whatever the cause, which in most cases is emotional in nature. The suddenness with which hysterical accidents appear and disappear should be noted, whatever the accident may involve: paralysis, cramps, and so forth"*; and, later in the text: *"This set of symptoms has been called 'status hysteroepilepticus' by Mr. Charcot, as compared with status epilepticus, with which it could be confused."* He sometimes cited other authors such as Alexandre Brierre de Boismont (1797–1881): *"Most of those who experienced cataleptic ecstasy, once the attack was over, spoke of the overwhelming joy they had felt, the terrifying phantoms they had seen, the divine visions, the angelic unions they had been privy to."*

In his preface, Charcot summarized perfectly what the text of Legué and Gilles de la Tourette illustrated about hysteria, the disease he had done so much to elucidate: *"In the Ursuline superior, we see hysterical passion develop with the entire cortege of nervous accidents characteristic of the major types of the disease. Somatic phenomena—such as hysteria major, sensory and sensorial anesthesia, vasomotor disturbances leading to the vomiting of blood, and stigmata—are present, along with phenomena that are specifically psychic in nature—such as visual and auditory hallucinations, and also suggestibility, heightened to such a degree that the mind dominates the body and brings about a false pregnancy and a false pleurisy, as well as having a marked influence on various secretions."*

The third part of the book includes *"excerpts from letters that Jeanne des Anges, Mother Superior of the Ursuline convent in Loudun, wrote to Reverend Father Saint Jure, of the Society of Jesus, her Director."* Most of these letters attest to hallucinatory delirium, though some reveal a state of great mental clarity, such as the June 2, 1645, letter: *"My interior languor and weakness still continue with these pains, which sometimes cause me to faint. I would be most grateful if Our Lord could remove these exterior manifestations. I beg you, my dearest Father, if you deem it fitting, to ask that He grant me this grace. You cannot know the sorrow this causes me. Everyone is always wanting to turn me over to the physicians. Up till now, I have resisted, using my weakness as an excuse, and I shall continue to do so until I receive your instructions."* At the end of the book, Legué and Gilles de la Tourette included reproductions of two of the letters written by Jeanne des Anges.

Douglas Aigre (1851–1932) concluded his summary of the book in *Le Progrès Médical* as follows: *"Thanks to the annotations by these two distinguished associates, this manuscript is more than just a find; it is a complete restitution."*[29] *Les démoniaques dans l'art*, published by Charcot and Richer one year after the book by Legué and Gilles de la Tourette, was similar in its approach: *"Our sole aim is to reveal the role that external attacks of hysterical neurosis have had in art, at moments in history when they were considered not as an illness, but as a perversion of the soul, due to demonic machinations. . . . It is not difficult to find traces of the disease we are studying in the demonic possessions that caused such havoc during the Middle Ages. The reports that eyewitnesses, most certainly reliable, have left us about the speech and actions of the possessed leave no room for doubt in this regard. Their contemporaries could not help but view these extraordinary phenomena as supernatural, but this interpretation disappeared as scientific investigation spread and modern science extended the territory of its conquests. . . . Demonic possession, of which history has left us long and meticulous descriptions, is illustrated with no less force and veracity in works of art. Miniatures, ivory carvings, tapestries, bronze bas-reliefs, frescoes, paintings, and engravings have all depicted scenes of exorcism as well as the attitudes and contortions of 'the possessed,' in which science now finds the exact rendering of a purely pathological condition."*[30] In its mission to demystify superstitions, the Salpêtrière School took a somewhat paradoxical approach. That is, they fought against these false notions by bringing them to the attention of the public at large.

Beyond its historical value, how was the work of Legué and Gilles de la Tourette relevant? It examined a context in which religion was the only acknowledged and accepted means to express and personify psychological suffering, for example through possession and ecstasy. To do away with references to the supernatural, Charcot and his students replaced religion with medical symptomatology to describe the same afflictions. Nevertheless, this laudable change did very little to improve management of the social, economic, and psychological causes of the disorders in the late 1800s. The drama that had unfolded in Loudun was now playing out on the stage of Charcot's lecture hall and would be followed by other metamorphoses. Each era has its own language and explanations. In the historical relationship Legué and Gilles de la Tourette established between mystical delirium and hysteria, we see the invention of a new paradigm. This paradigm, dominated by visual images—so important to Charcot—created a special link between femininity and trance states, which would lead to many regrettable developments in psychoanalysis. Jacques Lacan (1901-1981) went so far as to say: *"What so many of the good people in Charcot's entourage were seeking to do was to reduce mysticism to mere sex."*[31] It took a certain degree of effrontery to distort hysteria major and the neurological knowledge that had developed around it by equating it with female orgasm, and Lacan was not the only one to do so.[32]

There is considerable literature on the subject of the Ursulines in Loudun. The recent book by Michel Carmona, *Sœur Jeanne des Anges, diabolique ou sainte au temps de Richelieu,* can be commended for presenting the historical facts in their political and religious context.[33] *Mère Jeanne des Anges,* a 1961 film by Polish director Jerzy Kawalerowicz (1922–2007), is a cinematographic version of what happened in Loudun.

Michel de Certeau (1925–1986) beautifully describes modern-day Loudun, a city that remembers the tragic events of the seventeenth century but has largely forgotten Legué and Gilles de la Tourette, despite their instrumental role in perpetuating the memory of these events. *"Even though it has lost two-thirds of its population and huddles, shrunken, around its narrow streets filled with too many ghosts, Loudun is worth visiting. From the Courthouse to the Church of Sainte-Croix, you will be led along the ultimate path of the Hero, as if the city had reorganized its architecture into a Way of the Cross. The scattered venues, brought together by the guides' explanations, recreate a lost tale."*[34]

In his recent thesis, Nils Froment builds on the findings of Victor Ségalen (1878–1919) in his 1902 thesis.[35] Froment examined the emergence and development of "nervous diseases" in literature during the second half of the nineteenth century. Not only did Gustave Flaubert (1821–1880), the Goncourt brothers Edmond (1822–1896) and Jules (1830–1870), Emile Zola (1840–1902), Joris-Karl Huysmans (1848–1907), Jules Lermina (1839–1915), Octave Mirbeau (1848–1917), and Jules Claretie (1840–1913) draw from medical treatises to endow their neurotic protagonists with sufficiently morbid traits and flaws; physicians such as Legué and Gilles de la Tourette also took an interest in the "nervous" troubles of characters described in fiction. According to Nils Froment, the objective of these writers and physicians—which, unknown to them, aligned them with certain conservative politicians at the time—was to eradicate "nervous diseases" through exaggerated descriptions and to criticize religion for its role in the emergence of these diseases. For Froment, their books called for women's return to the home, especially working-class women, so that they could raise large families and instill bourgeois social values. This was in opposition to the initial goal of emancipation put forward by progressive republican thinkers such as Bourneville.[36] Froment's reasoning should be considered alongside Nicole Edelman's research on the sociological and economic foundations of hysteria in the nineteenth century,[37] which has led her to similar conclusions.[38]

Notes

1. Goldstein J. The hysteria diagnosis and the politics of anticlericalism in late nineteenth-century France. *J Mod Hist*. 1982;54(2):209–239.

2. Galanopoulos Ph. La bibliothèque diabolique du docteur Bourneville (1882–1902). *Vesalius*. 2001;17(2):89–98.

3. Axenfeld A. *Des principaux accidents que l'on observe après la trachéotomie chez les enfants atteints du croup*. Thèse no. 264. Paris: Rignoux. 1853.

4. Axenfeld A. *Les influences nosocomiales. Thèse pour le concours d'agrégation*. Paris: Félix Malteste. 1857.

5. Goncourt (de) J, de Goncourt (de) E. *Journal, Mémoires de la vie littéraire. postf. de M. Lucien Descaves. Édition définitive publiée par l'Académie Goncourt*. Paris: E. Flammarion Fasquelle. 1936.

6. Nécrologie. Professeur A. *Axenfeld. L'Union Médicale*. 1876;22(102):320.

7. Regnard A. *Essais d'histoire et de critiques scientifiques à propos des conférences de la Faculté de Médecine*. Paris: Chez l'Auteur. 1865.

8. Tartivel AP. Conférences historiques de médecine et de chirurgie. M. Axenfeld.—Jean de Wier et les Sorciers. *L'Union Médicale*. 1865;26(74):577–585.

9. Axenfeld A. *Jean Wier et la sorcellerie*. Paris: Germer-Baillière. 1866.

10. Bourneville DM, Axenfeld A. *Histoires, disputes et discours: des illusions et impostures, des diables, des magiciens infâmes, sorcières et empoisonneurs: des ensorcelez et démoniaques et de la guérison d'iceux: item de la punition que méritent les magiciens, les empoisonneurs et les sorcières. Le tout compris en six livres / par Iean Wier, Médecin du Duc de Clèves. Deux dialogues touchant le pouvoir des sorcières et de la punition qu'elles méritent / par Thomas Erastus, Professeur en médecine à Heidelberg*. Paris: Aux Bureaux du Progrès médical, A. Delahaye et E. Lecrosnier. 1885.

11. Jean Wier, Johann Weyer, or Johannes Weier; in Latin, Joannes Wierus, or by the pseudonym Piscinarius.

12. Couvreur A. Gabriel Legué. *La Chronique Médicale*. 1913;20(23):716.

13. Legué G. *Documents pour servir à l'histoire médicale des possédées de Loudun*. Thèse no. 63. Paris: A. Parent. 1874.

14. Sauzé JC. *Essai médico-historique sur les possédées de Loudun*. Thèse no. 353. Paris: Rignoux 1839.

15. Legué G. *Documents pour servir à l'histoire médicale des possédées de Loudun*. Paris: A. Delahaye. 1874.

16. Legué G. *Urbain Grandier and les possédées de Loudun, documents inédits de M. Charles Barbier*. Paris: L. Baschet. 1880.

17. Legué G. *Urbain Grandier and les possédées de Loudun, documents inédits de M. Charles Barbier*. Paris: Charpentier. 1884.

18. Legué G. *Médecins and empoisonneurs au XVIIᵉ siècle*. Paris: G. Charpentier and E. Fasquelle. 1896.

19. Legué G. *La messe noire*. Paris: E. Fasquelle. 1903.

20. Richet Ch. Les démoniaques d'autrefois. Les procès de sorcières and les épidémies démoniaques. *Revue des Deux Mondes*. 1880;37(4):828–863.

21. Richet Ch. Les démoniaques d'autrefois. *Revue des Deux Mondes*. 1880;37(2): 340–372 / (3):552–583 / (4):828–863.

22. Gilles de la Tourette G. Urbain Grandier and les Possédées de Loudun par le dr G. Legué, Charpentier 1884. *Le Progrès Médical*. 1886;14.1(11):231–232.

23. In fact Gabriel Legué, whom J-B. Charcot most likely did not know at the time and whose name he misspelled.

24. *Petit aigle* and *grand aigle* are two sizes of paper used for large-format drawings. J-B. Charcot's use of the term *"moyen aigle"* is incongruous, as this size does not exist.

25. Albert Wolff (1835–1891) was a writer and journalist. The clergymen Mignon and Lambardemont were involved in the Grandier trial, and Ludovic Baschet (1834–1909) was the publisher of Legué's book.

26. Richer P. *Étude descriptive de la grande attaque hystérique: ou attaque hystéro-épileptique and de ses principales variétés*. Thèse no. 179. Paris: Adrien Delahaye. 1879.

27. Richer P. *Etudes cliniques sur l'hystéro-épilepsie ou Grande Hystérie*. Paris: A. Delahaye and E. Lecrosnier. 1881.

28. Boutreux J. *(ou Syette, Pierre)*. *De la Puissance roialle, sur la police de l'Eglise*. Paris: De l'Imprimerie de Pierre Durand. 1625.

29. Aigre D. Sœur Jeanne des Anges, supérieure des Ursulines de Loudun par G. Legué and G. Gilles de la Tourette. Aux bureaux du Progrès médical, 1886. *Le Progrès Médical*. 1887;15-1(6):118–119.

30. Charcot JM, Richer P. Les Démoniaques dans l'art. Paris: A. Delahaye and E. Lecrosnier. 1887.

31. Lacan J, Miller JA. *Encore: Le séminaire, livre XX*. Paris: Le Seuil. 1975.

32. Israël L. *La jouissance de l'hystérique, séminaire 1974*. Paris: Seuil. 1996.

33. Carmona M. *Sœur Jeanne des Anges, diabolique ou sainte au temps de Richelieu*. Waterloo (Belgique): A. Versaille Ed. 2011.

34. de Certeau. *La possession de Loudun*. Paris: Gallimard-Julliard, Collection Archives. 1980.

35. Ségalen V. *L'observation médicale chez les écrivains naturalistes*. Thèse. Bordeaux: Cadoret. 1902.

36. Froment N. *Mots pour Maux: maladies nerveuses and écrits contagieux sous le Second Empire and la Troisième République*. Sarrebruck: Presses Académiques Francophones. 2014.

37. Edelman N. *Les métamorphoses de l'hystérie, du début du XIXe siècle à la Grande Guerre*. Paris: La Découverte. 2003.

38. Edelman N, Walusinski O. Socioeconomic background of hysteria's metamorphosis from the 18th century to World War I. *Front Neurol Neurosci*. 2014;35:11–19.

15

Théophraste Renaudot (1586–1653)

Gilles de la Tourette's Hero

History is the account of things that have occurred; the gazette carries only the rumors they give rise to.

—Théophraste Renaudot

GILLES DE LA Tourette always showed strong attachment to the town of Loudun where many members of his family lived. Loudun's long and rich history is due partly to its geographical location on the borders of three provinces: Poitou, Anjou, and Touraine. This border region was involved in the Hundred Years War, the conflict between the French and the English, and Loudun, built on top of a hill, was a strategic observation point. Later, during the Wars of Religion, Loudun was the scene of brutal battles between Catholics and Protestants. The city is home to vestiges of a fortress and to the beautiful city mansions built after the fortress's fall. In short, Loudun's rich past played an important role in stimulating Gilles de la Tourette's early interest in history. As his friend Paul Le Gendre (1854–1936) wrote: *"With his taste for history and literature, he might have been tempted to abandon his classes at the Faculté de Médecine and the hospitals for the classes at the Sorbonne and the Collège de France. Or he may have slipped into one of the literary or mainstream newspapers and ended up exclusively a journalist, rather than finding in journalism a pastime that provided diversion from his medical career."*[1] Gilles de la Tourette considered writing a biography of Théophraste Renaudot (1586–1653) in 1882 (Figure 15.1), then began the project in 1883 while an *interne* (house officer or resident) under Professor François Damaschino (1840–1889): *"We undertook to*

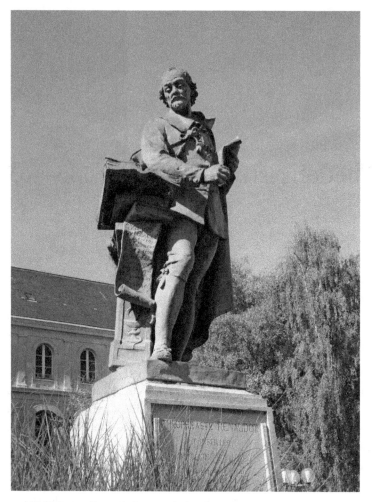

FIGURE 15.1 Théophraste Renaudot's statue in Loudun.
Photographed by the author.

highlight on this unfortunate philanthropist, dispelling the obscurity that had settled all too soon on a great figure. The fact that Renaudot, a contemporary of Urbain Grandier, was born in Loudun gave us yet another reason to honor his memory. We drew on family archives, historical manuscripts, and other documents that we hope will cast new light on this little-known figure." [2]

Théophraste Renaudot, the Man

Achille Chéreau (1817–1885), a physician and librarian at the Faculté de Médecine, left us this portrait: *"In 1612, a physician who was later to create quite an uproar came from the Montpellier School to settle in Paris. He combined a singularly inventive genius with profound loathing for his colleagues in the capital city. This character went by the name of Théophraste Renaudot. The ingenious, courageous Renaudot, founder of* La Gazette, Le Bureau d'adresses, Le Mont-de-piété, *and initiator of free medical consultations for the indigent, did much to merit recognition. In a dazzling, colossal demonstration of thanks, posterity has adopted all of the fertile, useful ideas in his work and avenged him for the outrage he suffered during his lifetime, the countless difficulties he had to overcome, one step at a time, and the scornful opposition he encountered in the premier medical corps in the Kingdom of France. Nothing deterred this extraordinary personage, not lawsuits, defamation, mockery, or any of the other machinations that targeted him. The Gazeteer, as he was called, the sneak, the extortionist, the charlatan, broker of love and advertisements, withstood it all with unshakeable courage, certain, as he was for over twenty-five years, that his efforts were valiant. Despite his enemies, his work took root and thrived to the point of making periodicals one of the most influential forces in the world. Renaudot was born in a Protestant family in Loudun in 1586, and received his doctoral cap in Montpellier in 1606. Having completed his medical studies at a provincial university, he professed doctrines that were contrary to those upheld at the school in Paris. Any one of his titles—head of the antimony party, friend of apothecaries, favorite of those in power—would have sufficed to make him offensive to the physicians on Rue de la Bûcherie. Things took a turn for the worse when our physician, influenced by an alliance judged highly unseemly, became a journalist, a pawnbroker, opening a shop and trafficking in valets, land, houses, and nurses. He also organized charitable medical care on a large scale and for this, he was accused of deal-making and being in cahoots with apothecaries and sellers of drugs."[3]*

Biography by Gilles de la Tourette

As a young man, Gilles de la Tourette identified with Renaudot and looked to him as a role model. Renaudot was a physician and a scientist, the inventor of a new remedy (Polychreston),[4] and a benefactor of the poor who helped them find jobs, fought mendacity and thievery (*Bureau d'adresses*), and sought to improve their medical care (*Consultations charitables*). He was also a philanthropist who introduced a new system of loans that countered usurers (*Mont-de-piété*, based on an idea that originated in Italy), and a journalist and writer who disseminated information and invented advertising (*La Gazette*, said to be the first weekly newspaper). Renaudot also conceived of a new way of teaching medicine. His Faculté libre, or Free School, accepted, for example, the discovery of circulation by William Harvey (1578–1657) and refused the scholastic method, limited to Hippocrates and Galen and used at the medical school under Guy Patin (1601–1672). *"He dreamed of nothing less than introducing experimental method into medical science."* In 1620, he published an anatomical work on the human skeleton, *Discours sur le scelet, c'est a dire sur les os de l'homme. Avec une leçon anatomique faicte en suitte sur le mesme scelet.*[5]

Gilles de la Tourette emphasized that he had attempted to situate Renaudot *"in the context of his era, by focusing on the history of his time and on his relations."* He had also attempted to account for *"an enigma and a major error. It is, indeed, difficult to understand why the name of Théophraste Renaudot is practically unknown today, given that he founded journalism in France, if not in all of Europe, with his Gazette, as well as commercial advertising with his Bureau d'adresse, not to mention the fact that as a disciple of Bacon and Pierre Ramus, he defied the scholastic tradition by seeking free and experimental teaching."* Gilles de la Tourette described Renaudot as follows: *"He was a robust man with a wiry build, of average height, severe in dress with a black pourpoint buttoned to the top. His face was thin and bony, his features unsightly and ravaged by smallpox. His nose was broad and short, a perpetual target for sarcastic comments from Guy Patin and other enemies. However, his forehead was clear and wide, his eyes set well apart. His entire face conveyed compassion and kindness, driven by tenacious intelligence and an untamed spirit that would be sorely tried but never defeated."*

The goal here is not to provide a complete summary of Gilles de la Tourette's book, nor a biography of Théophraste Renaudot. But it should be noted that Gilles de la Tourette carried out the work of a true historian in exhuming a forgotten text by Renaudot: *"We discovered the existence of this little book, of which there is, to the best of our knowledge, only a single copy that no one has ever analyzed. For its time, it was a nearly complete treatise on diagnostics. The work is entitled:* La présence de abscens, ou facile moyen de rendre présent au médecin l'estat d'un malade absent, dressé par les docteurs médecins consultant charitablement à Paris pour les pauvres malades [The presence of absence, or an easy way to present a physician with the condition of an absent patient, established by the physicians consulting for free in Paris for poor patients]." Gilles de la Tourette noted: *"Some will undoubtedly criticize consultations by correspondence that entail filling out a form. At the very least, they were handled by competent men and created with a humanitarian objective; above all, in contrast to current practices, they were absolutely free."*[6]

Gilles de la Tourette set an example with his efforts at rehabilitation that others followed, such as Michel Emery (1855–1896), who wrote his 1888 thesis *"in order to glorify the Montpellier medical school and prove its role in the introduction of therapeutic chemical remedies."* Introducing such remedies was a task that Renaudot considered crucial in his fight against Patin.[7]

In his biography of Gilles de la Tourette, Le Gendre devoted considerable attention to the Théophraste Renaudot book and paid Gilles de la Tourette this compliment: *"For a young interne whose studies had not prepared him for scholarly research or historical criticism, this book is truly very honorable."*

Praise from His Correspondents

Gilles de la Tourette sent his book to friends and to notables in Loudun. Some of the letters he received in return can be found in the archives at the Charbonneau-Lassay Museum. Of the dozen letters, we have selected three that indicate the esteem with which Gilles de la Tourette's work was met, a work that that continues to be of interest today. Though the cover page of his book indicates 1884 as the date of publication, he most likely obtained several copies in advance since he began receiving praise from his correspondents in the fall of 1883.

Poitiers, December 12, 1883, Léopold Thépard:

Dear Sir, I wanted to finish your book before I thanked you for sending it, but various obligations have kept me from completing it as quickly as I planned. I have now finished reading it and can tell you how much it interested me. Not only have you brought an important figure back to life; you have also honored his sense of truth and his moral example. Your book, with its accuracy and detail, is a chapter that had been missing in the history of the seventeenth century. Have no doubt that it will find great success among readers interested in historical studies. In Paris, there is talk just now about holding literary conferences and it would be easy to reserve a place of honor for you. With haste I shall inform you about the most conducive circumstances for you and your hero. Yours most sincerely."

This invitation must have been deeply gratifying for Gilles de la Tourette.

Paul Girard replied on January 22, 1884:

I feel very remiss for not having thanked you sooner for your book, which I read with great interest. You have successfully revived an inspiring figure, who definitely deserves to be better known. I, myself, was totally unaware of your subject, but have learned quite a bit from your detailed descriptions of Renaudot's various philanthropic undertakings. I believe you did well, as you state in your preface, not to limit yourself solely to your hero. It is easier to grasp his influence within the historical context in which he lived. This gives greater depth to your study, and greater appeal. Once again, please forgive my negligence. Yours most sincerely.

Paris, May 31, 1884:

"My dear friend, . . . *Théophraste Renaudot*, my dear friend, is quite simply a master-piece. Being the persnickety fellow that I am, I shall come immediately to my one criticism: some passages could have been more highly polished, but I find nothing else to reproach. Your style is clear and correct and very attractive; your serious study of language is apparent, as are the workings of your mind. The subject matter is solid, and the book is substantial, full of facts and new insights on the customs and quarrels of the intellectual world at that time. Lastly, the personality of Renaudot, extremely appealing, captivates the reader. In short, you have written a book that distinguishes you, setting you apart from the crowd. I heartily congratulate you. We no longer see you at the lodge. Do you intend to leave us like your friend, Dr. Blanchard, who has just sent us his resignation? He will be receiving the visit that is dictated in such cases, but will the three visitors, of which I may be one, succeed in bringing him back? I hardly dare allow myself such hope. Please tell him, if you see him, how much I miss him. Devotedly yours, Charles Beaumont."

In addition to warmly praising Gilles de la Tourette, this letter also confirms that he had been inducted into a Masonic lodge.[8]

An Aborted Plan

Pierre Mainguet (1855–1926), one of directors at the Plon-Nourrit publishing firm, informed Gilles de la Tourette of important news on January 31, 1884: "*Sir, A person has written us from England requesting authorization to translate your book,* Théophraste Renaudot, *into English. We can scarcely ask for more than 300 francs and even if we were offered only 200, we should perhaps accept it.*" Louis-Robert Nourrit (1833–1894) provided the translator's name: "*Sir, The person who requested authorization to translate your book is Mr. Darragh Mahony. Here is his address that we found in his letter: Culleria, Killarney, Ireland. We have sent him our answer, in keeping with our conversation with you during your last visit. Yours sincerely.*" Apparently, nothing came of this project, as no English translation of the book was ever published.

Unacknowledged Debt to Eugène Hatin

In contrast to these accolades were the words written by Eugène Hatin (1809–1893) (Figure 15.2), a journalist and historian who gained fame in 1846 with his *Histoire du journal en France*,[9] followed by his monumental *Histoire politique et littéraire de la presse en France*,[10] published in 1859. In a pamphlet whose aims were ambivalent, Hatin[11] described his contact with Gilles de la Tourette: "*Naturally I had never heard of this apprentice physician, when one fine*

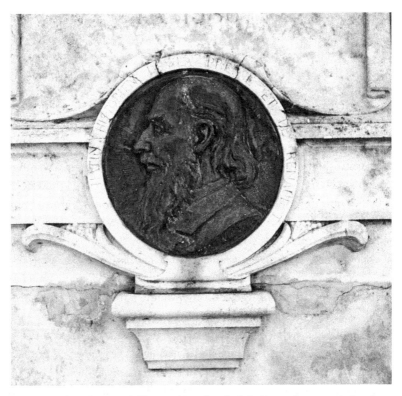

FIGURE 15.2 Eugène Hatin medallion on the pedestal of the Renaudot statue in Loudun.
Photographed by the author.

morning he visited me, after—he made a point to say—much effort to find my refuge;
I had long since passed into the nether world. Reading my works, he told me, had
inspired in him the ambition to write the life story of Renaudot. He was already in
the process of translating the registers of the medical school. Furthermore, he had
unpublished documents at his disposal and unfettered access to a library open to him
alone. And yet, with all of that, it was to me that he owed the idea of the work he was
preparing. It was from me that he had borrowed the essential materials and content—
in short, he had 'pillaged me to death.' Those were his first words when he approached
me, and he sought to ensure he would have neither claims nor competition from me. He
came back to this time and time again. He would acknowledge me in his preface, he
said, and even spoke of dedicating his book to me."

"We had fairly frequent discussions. He knew he could find me when I was out
walking, and he would approach me and ask endless questions in the Luxembourg
Gardens. In short, I left him free to do as he pleased, and he took full advantage of it,
but was perhaps overly hasty, eager as he was to be published, and especially to surpass
me. So much so that he forgot his debt to me, perhaps thinking he had done enough by

mentioning my name here and there, in a footnote or two. He hid as best he could all that he had borrowed from me, and this preoccupation was not only superfluous, it was puerile and ridiculous. I am anything but demanding, but really, my own goodness toward him deserved better than that, and the limits of gratitude would not have been exceeded had he offered me a copy of his book. When he had gotten everything he could from me, he took his leave, always with a show of politeness. After a final, three-hour meeting in the Luxembourg Gardens, I never saw him again."

Hatin was clearly resentful, and there is every reason to believe that Gilles de la Tourette had generously helped himself to the former's writings. In his pamphlet, Hatin went on to meticulously list the errors he had noted in Gilles de la Tourette's book, such as the latter's failure to distinguish between Renaudot father and son, both physicians and both with the first name of Théophraste. He judged the young author severely: *"His Renaudot is, as I have amply demonstrated, a confusing compilation put together at his desk at the medical school; both form and content are mostly, if not entirely, what one would expect from a student."* And yet, strangely enough, Hatin's tone softened in his conclusion: *"To sum up, the book by de la Tourette is actually nothing more than the amplification of my own. He took from me all of the content, everything that made up Renaudot's life. The heretofore-unpublished documents he so pompously touted are nothing more than the registers from the Paris medical school—which, while never before published in full, are familiar to many and have been widely used, particularly, as concerns Renaudot and his era, by the erudite librarian at the school.[12] I, myself, summed up the spirit of these registers insofar as I considered it relevant; what I overlooked had much more to do with the history of the medical school than it did with Renaudot. That said, it does not cost me to acknowledge that parts of de la Tourette's book left me surprised that such a young writer could have written them. Overall, the book attests to considerable and skillful work that I would not have thought possible from a young hospital interne with little literary experience. I remain convinced that, despite its weaknesses, it has largely contributed and will continue to contribute to rehabilitating Renaudot's reputation, a task I have devoted myself to for some time now. May this young author be successful in this endeavor; no one will applaud more warmly than I."*

A letter, kept in the archives, compares the two books. Charles Barbier, Poitiers, November 30, 1883:

"Dear Sir, I would like to thank you for the beautiful book you so kindly sent me. I have begun to read it and am extremely interested, as everything about this man from Loudun intrigues me. I know the book by Monsieur Hatin, which Mr. Odin, the printer, gave me, and I do not hesitate to predict that yours will be more successful. Mr. Hatin's borrows somewhat heavily from his book on the press, whereas yours, full of unpublished and unknown documents, sheds entirely new light on Renaudot. I was pained to see, in Mr. Hatin's preface, the attacks against Mr. de la Tourette, whose memory I cherish. Rest assured that I shall do my utmost, should the occasion arise, to present the facts as they actually occurred. The city of Poitiers showed greater respect for Renaudot than did Loudun. In the ceremonial staircase of the Poitiers Town Hall hangs a portrait of Renaudot, alongside three other famous persons from the region. Thank you once again for sending me the book. Sincerely yours."

Campaign to Erect a Statue

When Hatin published this pamphlet, Gilles de la Tourette was conducting his campaign to erect a statue of Renaudot in Paris. He turned to his friend Georges Montorgueil (1857–1933) and Montorgueil's paper, *L'Eclair,* for lobbying purposes, and he relied on Jules Claretie (1840–1913) for intellectual and moral support. Hatin wrote ironically about the terms used by Montorgueil in *L'Eclair* to describe Gilles de la Tourette: *"The distinguished practitioner, former chef de clinique at La Salpêtrière, devoted his leisure time, seven years ago, to writing such a complete biography of the founder of journalism that one wonders what more could be added."* Then he railed: *"The manner in which this campaign has been conducted would suggest that patriotism, or to put it more accurately, Renaudotism, is not the sole, nor even the main purpose of its leaders. How else to explain, for example, that Poitiers has been left by the wayside; or that it was—in the words of a local paper as recently as January 15—'through the Paris dailies' that we learned of plans to raise a statue of Renaudot on one of the public squares in Loudun! And it is through these Paris newspapers that I and everyone else have learned many other things, one after the other. A public square in Loudun is no longer the issue; the matter is out of the hands of the local committee—perfectly honorable, of course, but lacking the necessary prestige. Now the focus is on a major pubic square in Paris and on a grand committee, both literary and medical, which has yet to be organized, but already has a secretary general. It is easy to imagine what is being said and thought about all of this in and around Poitou."*

The mayor of Loudun, Alphonse Dumereau (1834–1897), and the Loudun town council deliberated on January 11, 1892, in order keep pace with Paris. Their decision was unanimous: *"Responding to the wishes of the district's Senators but without consulting an unauthorized committee formed in our town on this matter, we have decided to support the project to erect a statue of the illustrious Théophraste Renaudot, born in Loudun."* It was also declared that *"the names of Mr. Hatin and Mr. Gilles de la Tourette, the two biographers of Renaudot, and who have both graciously provided the municipality with a copy of their respective books, shall be inscribed on the pedestal of the statue."* The first statue of Renaudot in Loudun was a simple bust, which is now displayed in front of his birthplace. The statue that replaced it was inaugurated on May 12, 1894 (Figure 15.1). Located on the square in front of the Town Hall, it showed a larger-than-life Renaudot standing tall, holding notes for the articles of his *Gazette* in his left hand. In his right hand was a pen, and a cloak was slung casually over his shoulders. His registry of addresses was shown lying open on a platform from that period, embellished with the symbolic serpent and cup. The inscriptions on the pedestal stated his titles: *"Counselor to the King, Ordinary Physician, Historiographer of Louis XIII, Minister of Public Charity, born in Loudun in 1586."* The bronze statue, the work of Alfred-Joseph Charron (1863–1955), a sculptor from the region, was melted down in 1942 during the German occupation. The current statue, an identical replica of the original, is a bronze-coated plaster work that Charron had originally given to the museum in Poitiers in 1895, and which was moved to the public square in 1950. On the pedestal of the replacement statue is a medallion dedicated to *"Eugène Hatin, historian of the press and of Renaudot"* (Figure 15.2). There is no reference to Gilles de la Tourette.

By the time the Loudun town council announced its plans, Gilles de la Tourette had already leveraged his relations in Paris and founded, in December 1891, *"a committee for the erection in Paris of a statue to Théophraste Renaudot, founder of journalism and of charitable consultations."* He did not fail to point out that *"unlike Paris, Loudun, where Renaudot was born, still has done nothing for the most illustrious of its native sons. There is no street that bears his name, nothing at all that identifies the home where he lived, which still stands on the corner of Rue Centrale and Rue du Jeu de Paume. In 1884, when we published our book on Renaudot, we wrote to the mayor of Loudun, Mr. Duméreau, to inform him of our intention to organize a lecture that would overcome the indifference of his fellow townsmen and lay the ground for Mr. Renaudot's rehabilitation, which was our goal. Mr. Duméreau did not even deign to answer. In 1891, a second letter also went unanswered."*[13] Gilles de la Tourette, who knew how to hold a grudge, wrote to Montorgueil on May 15, 1894: *"The old mayor of Loudun, the one who disparaged me, wanted the red ribbon; he is still chasing after it."* This undoubtedly explains why only Hatin's name is inscribed on the medallion in Loudun, instead of both Hatin and Gilles de la Tourette, as the town council had decided in 1892.

Among the correspondence discovered in the Loudun archives was a letter dated November 26, 1883, to an unknown addressee; it may be the unanswered letter to Duméreau:

Sir, In recognition of the warm welcome you extended to me when I was a student in Poitiers, I have enclosed my book on Théophraste Renaudot, Loudun's illustrious native son who has nearly been forgotten. I thought several of the points covered in this book might be of interest to you, particularly Renaudot's attempt to set up a Free Medical School and his relations with the men of his era. Allow me to say that you could do a great deal to revive the memory of this important citizen of Loudun; could we not— and you are well placed to judge—start a movement in favor of Renaudot and replace the portrait on display in our town hall with a depiction that is more accurate and more tangible? My book has been sent to the newspapers in Poitiers, which I hope will review it. I think, furthermore, that the historical, political, and literary press in Paris will begin writing about the famous scientist and philanthropist, founder of *La Gazette*. If such is the case, and if a public subscription were set up, I would be at your disposal, following preliminary agreement, to give a lecture on Renaudot. You are a much better judge than I about all of these desiderata, and I have sent you my book solely as a sincere gesture of gratitude. I remain yours respectfully, Gilles de la Tourette, 43 rue Monge.

The chairman of the Parisian committee was Gilles de la Tourette's good friend Claretie, and Alphonse Humbert (1844–1922) was the representative from the Paris city council. Several journalists were involved, and the Faculté de Médecine was represented by Paul Brouardel (1837–1906), Jean-Martin Charcot (1825–1893), Victor Cornil (1837–1908), and Alexandre Laboulbène (1825–1898). Gilles de la Tourette, assisted by Marcel Baudouin (1860–1941), was secretary general. In 1892, *"to promote the statue,"* the committee published a brochure containing excerpts from Gilles de la Tourette's book. The committee's address, 14 Rue de Beaune, was Gilles de la Tourette's personal address at the time. Its treasurer was a certain Mr. Delabre, a neighbor who had the exact same address! A sketch of the future statue illustrated the back of the brochure, accompanied by these words: *"It seems that the Gazeteer's day of justice has finally arrived. Ever grateful to its great men, the City of Paris, where he spent nearly all of his life, where he developed his innovations, where he died and was buried, has placed a commemorative plaque at the site where his "Bureau d'adresse" once stood. The City Council has recently supported a movement to honor his memory, and it is our hope that, on the flower market square, where Rue de la Calandre was once located, a monument to journalism and to charity will soon be erected."* On July 20, 1892, the City of Paris authorized erection of the statue and the government granted a subsidy of 10,000 francs. It is no longer known how many donations were made, but Oscar Roty (1846–1911), an engraver of medals and coins who was primarily known for his 1887 work "La Semeuse," wrote a letter that sheds light on how Gilles de la Tourette approached thanking the generous donors:

My Dear Physician and Friend, Thank you a thousand times over for your kind letter. I am also writing to Doctor Gilbert. I cannot accept the principle of a medal for all of the subscribers. I shall make a gesture to them, but when I deem it necessary. I do not want them to think they are entitled to it. I shall make the brochure at my own expense, and I think that is sufficient. I would be very grateful if you could explain to these gentlemen on the committee what I have explained to you, and I authorize you to say what I, myself, would be unable to express. Thank you in advance! Please give my respectful greetings to Mrs. Gilles de la Tourette. I wish good health to your dear children and to you, with all of my heart.

The archives in Loudun contain a receipt for a donation in the amount of one hundred francs, from a certain "de la Tourette" on November 19, 1892.

The committee commissioned the sculptor Alfred Boucher (1850–1934), who had twice been a runner-up for the Grand Prix de Rome and who won the Grand Prix du Salon in 1891 for his work "Piété filiale." Boucher remains well known for his sculptures immortalizing Laennec, Maupassant, and Casimir-Perier. He was primarily a public works sculptor whose career was crowned with the Grand Prix for sculpture at the 1900 World's Fair. Edouard-Ernest Mizard (1842–?) was the architect for the monument, which stood seven meters high and rested on a stone base. The bronze statue went up in the Fourth Arrondissement of Paris on Rue de Lutèce, *"as close as possible to the former Rue de la Calandre, now covered over by the Préfecture de Police grounds. The Bureau d'adresse, where Théophraste Renaudot developed his timeless innovations, stood on Rue de la Calandre, at the outlet of Marché-Neuf under the Grand-Coq sign."* Renaudot was shown seated at his writing desk, quill in hand, on a stone pedestal embellished with a rooster, a reference to the original sign that hung near the Bureau d'adresse. On the pedestal were the words: *"Il faut que en un estat / les riches aydent aux pauvres, / son harmonie cessant lorsqu'il / y a partie d'enflée outre mesure / et les autres demeurant atrophiées; Seulement feray-je une prière aux Princes et aux Estats estranges, de ne perdre point inutilement leur temps à vouloir fermer le passage à mes gazettes, voeu que c'est une marchandise dont le commerce ne s'est jamais pu deffendre et qui tient cela de la nature de torrents qu'il se grossit par la résistance."* (In a nation, it is necessary that the rich help the poor; harmony ceases when one part is unduly swollen and the others remain atrophied. The one request I would make to Princes and foreign nations is that they not waste their time trying to block my gazettes, a kind of merchandise whose commerce has never been overcome because it, like the torrent, grows stronger in the face of resistance.) The statue was dismantled and melted down by the occupying forces in 1941 to recover the copper (Figure 15.3).

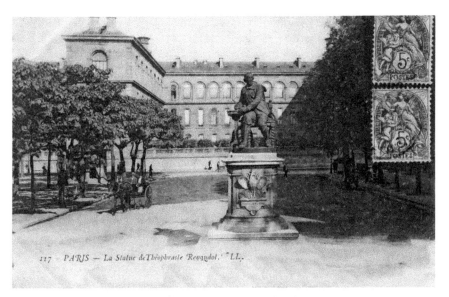

117 PARIS — La Statue deThéophraste Renaudot. ⁓LL.

FIGURE I5.3 A 1910 postcard showing Renaudot's statue in Paris, with Hôtel Dieu hospital in the background.
Private collection of the author.

Another pamphlet, entitled *Inauguration des statues de Théophraste Renaudot, ses principales œuvres—La Gazette—jusqu'en 1893* printed at the Imprimerie de La Gazette de France (rue Baillif) in 1893, was most likely written and published by Hatin. It contained a facsimile of a 1631 issue of Renaudot's *Gazette*, a brief biography of Renaudot, and a history of *La Gazette* up until 1893. The historical section, which discussed the paper's political positions throughout the nineteenth century, was clearly written by someone with Hatin's historical expertise, rather than by Gilles de la Tourette. In addition to the rich illustrations of the main figures referred to, the pamphlet shows an engraving of Boucher's Renaudot, the statue whose erection both Hatin and Gilles de la Tourette worked to bring about, and which represents a kind of truce between two men otherwise opposed by their egos.

Official Inauguration

The official inauguration took place on June 4, 1893; Charles Dupuy (1851–1923), Président du Conseil (head of the French government under the Third Republic) and Minister of the Interior, presided over the event (Figure 15.4). Dupuy gave a speech, as did Claretie: *"Doctor Gilles de la Tourette devoted all of his zeal, all of his generous ardor to a man's memory and has vivified Renaudot's image*

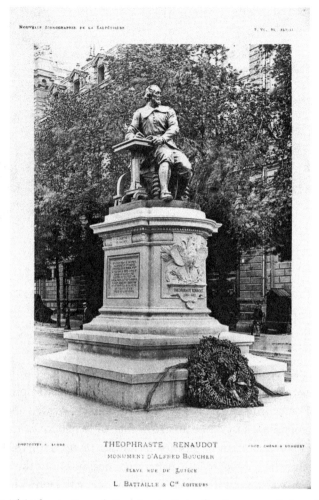

FIGURE 15.4 Théophraste Renaudot's statue in Paris after it was unveiled on July 3, 1893. *Nouvelle Iconographie de La Salpêtrière*, 1893.
Private collection of the author.

through his own erudition. He can be credited with kindling the soul of the sculptor, Mr. Alfred Boucher, with his special enthusiasm for Renaudot, and Mr. Boucher has created a masterpiece of which our city can be proud." There were also speeches by Brouardel and by Humbert (President of the Paris City Council), Eugène Poubelle (1831–1907) (Prefect of the Seine), Ernest Cadet de Gassicourt (1826–1900), and Joseph Grasset (1849–1918). Brouardel stated: *"I am personally happy that a former student, Mr. Gilles de la Tourette, was the one to revive the memory of this great man, who added a glorious page to the history of French medicine."*

On June 3, 1893, the day before the inauguration, Gilles de la Tourette was officially made a Chevalier of the Légion d'honneur. The decoration was bestowed on him by Dupuy, in recognition of his efforts to bring about the statue's erection. Claretie had been his sponsor. Here is how Edouard de Lavarenne (18?–1907) summarized Gilles de la Tourette's ascent: *"With his historical knowledge, and his enthusiasm, he was one of the most instrumental proponents for the statue that the City of Paris raised to the famous Théophraste Renaudot, founder of journalism, philanthropist, and also the first to have the idea of creating free services for the poor. By the zeal with which he pursued this campaign, also evident in his book about our great ancestor, Théophraste Renaudot, Gilles de la Tourette came to the attention of public officials and, at quite a young age, was decorated with the Légion d'honneur. Good fortune has indeed smiled upon him."*[14] After the glorious heights reached in June, the second half of 1893 was to be extremely difficult for Gilles de la Tourette.

Georges Guinon (1859–1932) set aside his resentment to pay his colleague this homage in *La Nouvelle Iconographie de La Salpêtrière*: *"The statue of Théophraste Renaudot, sculpted by the skillful Alfred Boucher, was inaugurated on June 4, Rue de Lutèce. This event, of interest to the entire medical field and all physicians, is a reparation that, while it comes too late, restores dignity to a man of principle whom his peers unjustly disparaged. It is also a personal triumph for Dr. Gilles de la Tourette, who fought long and hard to see this reparation accomplished. In 1884, he took it upon himself to study unpublished documents about Théophraste Renaudot and to tell the story of this man and his work, the source of many far-sighted innovations. His book was both a surprise and a success."*[15]

A letter addressed to Montorgueil that dates from a few years later (January 23, 1897) shows that Gilles de la Tourette's interest in Renaudot was an enduring one and that he very likely provided notes for an article in *L'Eclair*:

My dear friend, I shall be very happy to see you about Renaudot. I looked for the volumes we discussed, which I mention in my book (page 94) based on Hatin's writings. I was less fortunate than Hatin, who also published them or at least included excerpts. Richelieu collaborated even more actively and, especially, more secretly, pages 203-207. I shall be at your disposal if you have trouble with my notes. In any event, see you Saturday. Cordially yours.

In his book, Gilles de la Tourette mentioned a source from Hatin's book and copied certain passages. For example, he stated that he had not been able to find the three-volume history published by Griffet in 1758.[16] Henri Griffet (1698–1771) was a Jesuit and historian, former student of rhetoric at the Collège Louis Le Grand de Charles Porée (1675–1741), as was Voltaire. In his history of King Louis XIII, Griffet claimed that Louis XIII himself, and also Richelieu, wrote the articles that Renaudot published in his *Gazette*, in which case it would have been more an instrument of propaganda than a newspaper.

Renaudot and Gilles de la Tourette

Isn't it possible to compare these two men? Aren't all of the qualifiers used to portray Renaudot also applicable to Gilles de la Tourette? Both were dynamic and ambitious, had inventive and innovative minds, and lived lives full of various activities and interests.

In 1899, Gilles de la Tourette helped André Bégué (1873–?), one of his *internes*, prepare a thesis on the history of medicine, focusing on *"Renaudot's charitable consultations."*[17] This sort of service still exists today. Charitable organizations such as Doctors Without Borders and the Red Cross continue to offer free medical care for those in need. Renaudot was *"indefatigable; he organized free medical consultations that brought in not only hosts of sick patients, but also many students eager to learn about therapeutic innovations such as antimony and other chemical remedies that Renaudot spoke highly of and that were condemned by the medical school. Surrounded by a group of learned physicians, he founded the Conférence du Bureau d'adresses, a sort of unpretentious Academy of Sciences whose reports are still very worth reading."*[3] As for Gilles de la Tourette, he was always interested in trying new treatments, in teaching, and in the activities of learned societies. It isn't surprising, then, that he took Renaudot as a model and praised him highly.

Finally, Théophraste Renaudot is remembered every fall during the season of literary awards in France. Since 1925, the Prix Renaudot has been awarded by a jury of journalists at the same time as the Prix Goncourt.[18]

Notes

1. Le Gendre P. Gilles de la Tourette 1857–1904. *Bulletins et Mémoires de la Société Médicale des Hôpitaux de Paris.* 1905;21(3):1298–1311.
2. Gilles de la Tourette G. *Théophraste Renaudot d'après des documents inédits.* Paris: E. Plon, Nourrit et Cie. 1884.
3. Chéreau Ach. Théophraste Renaudot. *L'Union Médicale.* 1878;25(3):25–29; (7):73–78; (13):145–150; (19):217–223; (22):253–257.
4. "Polychreston cures diseases that have no other remedy, such as paralysis, turning, apoplexy, falling sickness, melancholy, catarrhs and swelling, cough, colic, stones, suffocation of the mother, contagious diseases, fevers, gouts, and infinitely more." Made up of more than eighty plants, this is one of the first placebos.
5. *Discours sur le scelet, c'est a dire sur les os de l'homme. Avec une leçon anatomique faicte en suitte sur le mesme scelet.* Loudun: Quentin Mareschal, 1620. A remarkably rare work as only one copy is known to exist and is held by the medical library at Northwestern University (Chicago, Illinois, 60611, United States).
6. Renaudot Th. *La Présence des absens, ou Facile moyen de rendre présent au médecin l'estat d'un malade absent, dressé par les Drs en médecine consultans charitablement à Paris pour les pauvres malades. Avec les figures du corps humain. Ensemble l'instruction.* Paris: Bureau d'adresse. 1642.

7. Emery M. *Renaudot et l'introduction de la médication chimique, étude historique d'après des documents originaux*. Thèse. Montpellier: Imprimerie Centrale du Midi Hamelin. 1888.

8. Gilles de la Tourette wrote to Montorgueil on May 22, 1894: "At my age you are not yet venerable unless you are in a Masonic lodge, where incidentally I never got beyond the level of apprentice."

9. Hatin E. *Histoire du journal en France*. Paris: G. Havard. 1846.

10. Hatin E. *Histoire politique et littéraire de la presse en France: avec une introduction historique sur les origines du Journal et la bibliographie générale des journaux depuis leur origine (La Presse littéraire aux XVIIᵉ et XVIIIᵉ siècle. La Presse politique)*. Paris: Poulet-Malassis et de Broise. 1859.

11. Hatin E. *Enfin! Théophraste Renaudot aura-t-il la statue qu'il mérite à tant de titres! L'absolue vérité sur sa vie et ses œuvres*. Paris: H. Champion. 1892.

12. Chéreau Ach. Théophraste Renaudot. *L'Union Médicale*. 1878;25 (3):25–29; (7):73–78; (13):145–150; (19):217–223; (22):253–257.

13. Gilles de la Tourette G. *La vie et l'œuvre de Théophraste Renaudot. En vente au bénéfice de la statue*. Paris: Edition du comité. 1892.

14. de Lavarenne E. Gilles de la Tourette. *La Presse Médicale*. 1893;1(45):353–354.

15. Guinon G. Renaudot médecin. *La Nouvelle Iconographie de La Salpêtrière*. 1893;6(4);358–364.

16. Griffet H. *Histoire du règne de Louis XIII, roi de France et de Navarre*. Paris: Chez les Libraires associés. 1758.

17. Bégué A. *Les consultations charitables de Théophraste Renaudot*. Thèse no. 137. Paris: JB. Baillière. 1899.

18. Georges Charensol (1899–1995), co-founder of the Prix Renaudot, explained how the journalists who met at the Drouant restaurant created the Prix Renaudot. Waiting together for hours to hear who had won the Prix Goncourt, the most prestigious French literary award, the journalists decided to create their own literary prize and to usefully occupy the long wait with their own deliberations. They announced the winner of the Prix Renaudot immediately after the announcement of the winner of the Prix Goncourt.

$$\sim 16 \sim$$

Commentator for *La Revue Hebdomadaire*, 1892–1900

La Revue Hebdomadaire

"Gilles de la Tourette wrote regularly for a literary journal, Le Revue Hebdomadaire, *as a scientific commentator starting in 1892,"* noted Paul Le Gendre (1854–1936), his friend and biographer. *"This, for him, was a form of relaxation that complemented his purely medical work."*[1] *La Revue Hebdomadaire* was published from May 1892 to February 1939, and aimed *"to give the most complete overview of contemporary intellectual movements."* It printed episodes from the novels of famous authors before they were published as books, for example *Rose et Ninette* by Alphonse Daudet (1840–1897), *Aziyadé et Fantôme d'Orient* by Pierre Loti (1850–1923), and *Le Docteur Pascal* by Emile Zola (1840–1902). Each issue brought readers the latest in culture, with literary and theatrical reviews by Louis Ganderax (1855–1941) and music reviews by Paul Dukas (1865–1935). The journal also featured poetry, travel logs, and historical commentary by Ernest Lavisse (1842–1922), Paul Bourget (1852–1935), and Anatole France (1844–1924).

Gilles de la Tourette authored a total of thirteen "scientific chronicles" from 1892 to 1900, most of them between 1892 and 1893, with less frequent contributions from 1894 to 1900. Seven he wrote using the pen name "Paracelse" and six under his own name. Since only his first chronicle was truly scientific, the title *Chronique scientifique* under which his commentary appeared seems somewhat inappropriate. Two of the articles were historical biographies, of Marguerite Bottard and Jean-Martin Charcot, while the others were the equivalent of "opinion pieces," with Gilles de la Tourette tackling sociological or public heath issues, or reviewing successful theater productions and press coverage of courtroom cases in the style of a pamphleteer. In each article, Gilles de la Tourette analyzed the manner in which authors or legal specialists represented the mentally ill, positioning himself as defender of the medical-psychological theories of the Salpêtrière School, particularly with regard to hysteria and heredity.

There is no documented explanation for why Gilles de la Tourette chose the pen name "Paracelse," but it is nonetheless fitting. Paracelsus, born Philippus Theophrastus Aureolus Bombastus von Hohenheim (1493–1541), was an alchemist, astrologist, and physician who rebelled against the aphorisms of Galen and Avicenna—what constituted the dogma of his day—and wrote his own observations of patients and their diseases, along with the methods he tried to treat them: *"Who can ignore the fact that most physicians today have failed shamefully in their mission, by exposing their patients to the gravest risks? They have attached themselves to the dictums of Hippocrates, Galen, and Avicenna with extreme pedantry. . . . I will teach practical and theoretical medicine two hours every day. . . . Experience, in its wisdom, is our supreme teacher and the master of my own work. Thus experience and reason, rather than the authority of Hippocrates, Galen, and Avicenna will guide me when I attempt to prove something."*[2] The portrait of Paracelsus by Walter Pagel (1898–1983)—which highlights Paracelsus's perpetual effervescence and his violent, critical mind, carried by a strong voice[3]—could have been inspired by Legendre's portrait of Gilles de la Tourette in 1881: *"A jovial and exuberant boy, with the gift of the gab and a presumptuous tone . . .; very enthusiastic, but rather impatient, he was not one to let those who contradicted him exhaust their arguments little by little, then refute them point by point."*[1]

Gilles de la Tourette's Chronicles

Jacques Inaudi: A Human Calculator

On July 9, 1892, for his first chronicle, Gilles de la Tourette related the astonishing feats of the young Italian, Jacques Inaudi (1867–1950) (Figure 16.1): *"A singular little fellow, this Jacques Inaudi, veritable human calculator! He is both the star of a show at the Concert Parisien and a subject under study at the Académie des Sciences. At the Académie, his talents were most interestingly on display. I defer to Mr. Charcot and Mr. Darboux,[4] who recently wrote a substantial report on this phenomenon. . . . In 1879, at the age of twelve, he was already famous. Broca presented him to*

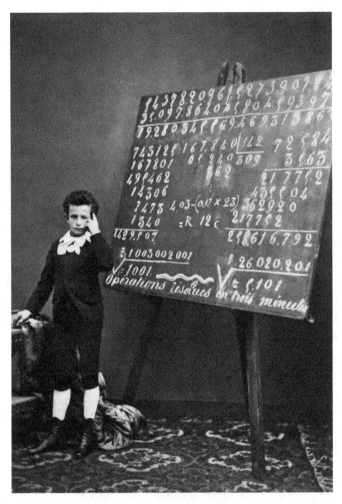

FIGURE 16.1 Jacques Inaudi (1867–1939), Italian mathematical prodigy as a child, around 1875. Copyright Adoc-photos, with permission.

the Société d'Anthropologie. After analyzing his processes of calculation, Broca noted that he can neither read nor write; he has the numbers in his head, but does not write them down."[5] While Paul Broca (1824–1880) concluded his expert assessment by denying the existence of any specific cerebral organ for calculation, in contrast to the phrenologists, he was the first to note that Inaudi had an extraordinary nonvisual memory for numbers.

Uncritically reporting the surprising words of his teacher Charcot with regard to the adolescent and seeming to lend credence to the phrenology of the German anatomist Franz Joseph Gall (1757–1828), Gilles de la Tourette started by describing Inaudi's skull: *"He is plagiocephalic, and even more striking, his slanted skull has a central crest and two abnormal bumps, one on the right, the other on the left. He's got two math bumps[6]!"* Was this humor? Gilles de la Tourette also presented the concepts of Charcot, inspired by the work of Théodule Ribot (1839–1916), on the existence of multiple memories: *"The mental faculty vulgarly known as memory is merely an assembly. According to the specialists, the latest analysis indicates there are only partial memories, specialized and localized, each relatively independent. One of these memories can be singularly exaggerated, most often at the expense of the others; Inaudi exemplifies such a case. All of the interrogations and experiments he underwent show that his memory of colors, shapes, events, places, pieces of music, and so forth does not exceed normal average performance and is even inferior, while the partial memory of numbers is extraordinarily developed."* Charcot examined Inaudi on February 27 and on March 1 and 3, 1892, at La Salpêtrière and confirmed that his ability to calculate was based solely on auditory memory. Gilles de la Tourette noted: *"Numbers for him have neither front nor back, right nor left. He can as easily repeat his 400 numbers starting with the last on the left, as with the last on the right, since for him, there is no difference. He hears numbers so well he has only to translate them into ordinary language. And here is what astonishes scientists: excessive development of the partial memory for numbers is already remarkable, but this degree of memory operating by the senses, and more specifically the auditory center, is very remarkable indeed."* Gilles de la Tourette had a true talent for presenting specialized material in an accessible manner. In this passage, without specifically indicating as much, he was following the thinking of his teacher Charcot, who was working on a model for aphasia, the famous bell model composed of multiple memories or "centers."[7,8]

Gilles de la Tourette as Sociologist

"Guillotine and electricity"—now there's a subject for a "scientific chronicle"![9] Taking his cue from the previous week's news, during which three condemned men were guillotined in France, Gilles de la Tourette adopted a darkly humorous tone to compare the humaneness of the death penalty, as it existed at that time, in France and the United States. He started with a detailed biography of the physician Joseph-Ignace Guillotin (1738–1814), former member of the Commission du Magnétisme appointed by Louis XVI and nonetheless deputy for the Third Estate after the Revolution. Guillotin was in favor of prohibiting execution by hanging: *"Louis XVI had abolished torture, but punishments remained inequitable: the gentleman was beheaded, the commoner hanged. . . . On December 1, 1789, he had the National Assembly adopt a measure whereby, for the same crime, the punishment would be the same regardless of the criminal's station in life. Moreover, anyone condemned to death would be beheaded. And he proposed the use of a machine*

that would dispatch the condemned man without undue suffering." Gilles de la Tourette noted that the surgeon Antoine Louis (1723–1792) made the punishment *"practical by ensuring the immobilization of the head and by calling for a slanted blade, instead of the crescent-shaped blade originally planned. Cut, mortals, do not crush!"* Gilles de la Tourette did not neglect to cite the thesis defended by Paul Loye (1861–1890) before Paul Brouardel (1837–1906), who had also been Gilles de la Tourette's teacher. Loye confirmed that loss of consciousness and death were immediate with the guillotine.[10] He had built a guillotine in the courtyard of the Sorbonne and beheaded some one hundred dogs to prove cessation of brain activity; he did note, however, that the heart could continue to beat for a few minutes. In his chronicle, Gilles de la Tourette did not hesitate to describe a few ghastly scenes occurring in the United States where the person condemned to electrocution did not immediately die. *"A punishment is, in my opinion, a direct reflection of the nation using it,"* he noted. *"The guillotine is clear and incisive like the French mind; the axe is suitable for heavy Germany. . . ."* He concluded: *"Thank you, it is a statue and not merely a bust that I ask now for Doctor Guillotine."* At no point in his article did Gilles de la Tourette question the legitimacy of the death penalty.

Gilles de la Tourette as Sanitarian

On October 8, 1892, Gilles de la Tourette was moved to write of the *"detestable sanitary conditions of the Penmarch and Bay of Audierne fishermen* [Brittany], *decimated by alcoholism, tuberculosis, small pox, and typhoid fever. On their behalf, I call for an intervention of the Director of Public Health."*[1] Gilles de la Tourette described his visit:[11] *"In this region, alcoholism and superstition walk hand in hand. In 1883, I saw a Pardon pilgrimage, near Audierne, the men walking in long lines, a candle in one hand, and a bottle of brandy in the other. What songs they sang! At night, the ditches along the road were full of drunkards who had fallen while fighting and lay asleep on the ground."* He was also alarmed by the infant mortality rate: *"Their large families would be even larger were the infant mortality rate not so high. . . . Many young children die of tuberculous pneumonia. Even more suffer from osseous manifestations of scrofula that they survive. How many children are left crippled for life! One Pardon day, I counted more than twenty women limping as a result of untreated coxalgia."* But this could also have been congenital hip dysplasia, a familial pathology whose high incidence in Brittany Gilles de la Tourette seemed unaware of. As an atheist, he lamented *"another cause of mortality: when a child is born, he is locked in a cupboard or box until his baptism, to prevent the devil from stealing his soul."* To better the crude conditions in which these poor people lived, Gilles de la Tourette recommended improving diet, personal hygiene, and cleanliness of the home. He set his highest hopes on education: *"The law on schooling has affected the fishermen in their livelihood. Henceforth, all thirteen-year-old shipboys that join the crew know how to read. It goes without saying that education can do much to change the social conditions of these sailors."* He observed, however, that *"once they return from sea, they forget the most basic notions of hygiene. Very discouraging indeed."*

Gilles de la Tourette also took a sanitarian's view in his chronicle of January 28, 1893, which examined military hygiene. *"In peacetime, the soldier complains about hardtack, which is unpleasant and hard to digest. There is no remedy; old supplies must be used up. . . . Soldiers refuse hardtack not only because it is difficult to digest, but because it is spoiled. And in almost all cases, the spoilage is not very perceptible; no rot, mold, or the like. Only once the soldier has bitten into the biscuit does he realize it is full of worms."* Gilles de la Tourette then described caterpillars swimming in broth, the life cycle of the *Ephestiae elutella* moth, its development and formation of galleries in hardtack, and so forth. He concluded by recommending that hardtack be kept free of all contamination by improving hygiene during preparation. He also called for replacing the poor wooden packaging used at the time with tin boxes.[12]

Apparently concerned about the state of national defense, Gilles de la Tourette devoted his November 14, 1896, chronicle to the impact of mobilization on hospital care: *"Overnight, hospitals will find themselves without their chief physicians, at a time when the number of wounded is sure to rise sharply, doubling the usual hospital load."* Aware that prefects and other administrators were required to perform their usual duties and not respond to the mobilization order, Gilles de la Tourette suggested that this prerogative also apply to hospital physicians and surgeons.[13]

Gilles de la Tourette as Alienist

On July 23, 1892, Gilles de la Tourette covered the subject of *"the criminally insane"* in relation to his teaching of legal medicine (he passed the *agrégation* exam in 1895).[14] François Koënigstein (1859–1892) was an anarchist known as "Ravachol" or by the nickname "Rocambole de l'anarchisme." He was guillotined on July 11, 1892, after being condemned to death for various crimes and attempted crimes (Figure 16.2). *"Albeit a criminal, Ravachol was no less insane."* Ravachol, who had worked as a counterfeiter, was *"accused of five assassination attempts, the desecration of graves, and the attempted bombing of two six-story buildings—incidentally home to honest magistrates. He could not be more proud of his feats, to the point of bragging about them. Readers will recall that this is what led to his arrest. . . . A criminal like his grandfather, who was*

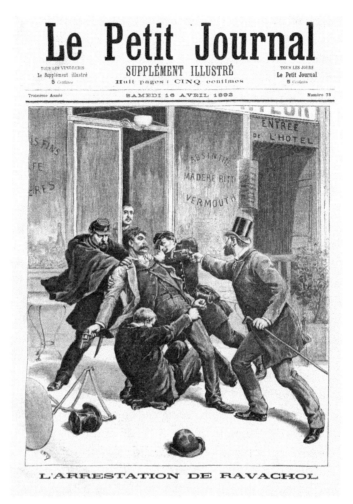

Le Petit Journal

TOUS LES VENDREDIS
Le Supplément illustré
5 *Centimes*

SUPPLÉMENT ILLUSTRÉ
Huit pages : CINQ centimes

TOUS LES JOURS
Le Petit Journal
5 *Centimes*

Troisième Année · SAMEDI 16 AVRIL 1892 · Numéro 73

L'ARRESTATION DE RAVACHOL

FIGURE 16.2 Ravachol arrest, March 30, 1892.
Private collection of the author.

hanged, and perhaps like his father, Ravachol has been guillotined. What a perfect thesis subject for alienists who concur with the theories of Mr. Lombroso, head of the Italian School, who first conceived of the born criminal!" Irony aside, Gilles de la Tourette adhered to the ideas of Cesare Lombroso (1835–1909), as did everyone in the medical community at the time: *"I say in all sincerity, Ravachol was a hereditary lunatic; he presented the most accentuated characteristics of ambitious delirium common to degenerates."* Gilles de la Tourette took this occasion to criticize French legislation, which *"absolutely refuses to consider that lunatics can be criminals."* At that time, the criminally insane were sent to asylums for varying periods, then released, and often recidivated. *"I shall say it again, we should look to England where the criminally insane are definitively sent to special asylums and can thus do no more harm."* The concept of heredity, or congenital determinism, to which Gilles de la Tourette subscribed, reveals his philosophical affiliation with Prosper Lucas (1808–1885)[15] and Bénédict-Augustin Morel (1809–1873),[16] who developed the concept of "degeneration" only two years before the publication of *On the Origin of Species* by Charles Darwin (1809–1882). Another of Charcot's students, Charles Féré (1852–1907), dealt with degeneration in his book, *La famille névropathique*, published in 1894.[17]

Like Charcot, Gilles de la Tourette enjoyed the theater milieu, as Claretie has written: *"Very involved with the theater, Gilles de la Tourette began a series of articles that he published in fragments in* La Revue Hebdomadaire. *He intended to make them into a book on madness in dramatic works:* La folie au théâtre. *To this end, he studied* Hamlet *and* La Reine Juana *(Joanna the Mad) from both a scientific and moral perspective. He even studied* Froufrou, *which he saw as a case of hysteria in fashionable society. Nothing surpassed these monographs in originality. Gilles de la Tourette, the psychologist and psychiatrist, saw cases all around him. He set out to show, and would perhaps have succeeded, that Orestes's furor in* Andromaque *is the result of hallucination. The 'thick night' is congestion, the snakes of the Furies are a hallucinatory phenomenon, as are Coupeau's rats; this is where the desperate lover resembles the alcoholic. How the melancholic and tender love of Colardeau differs from these macabre endings!"*[18]

He was especially interested in seeing and comparing works that featured deviant behaviors, for example the plays of Alphonse Daudet (1840–1897), such as *L'Arlésienne*, practically a standard of medical truth: *"I know of nothing better than* L'Arlésienne, *as nothing is truer. From the very first scenes, the situations are so compelling and so strongly expressed that one has an immediate foreboding of how the play will end."*[19] *"Alphonse Daudet, in* L'Arlésienne, *offers poignant examples of cerebral decline through hereditary determinism."*[1]

Gilles de la Tourette sought to dissect the characters' mental state in the plays he reviewed. As Legendre noted: *"He was harsh with authors who borrowed bits and pieces from medical theories, without fully understanding them, to create conventional characters."* The focus in theater productions on "madness" was intensified by press coverage of Charcot's lessons at La Salpêtrière. One way the Master sought to demystify hysteria was to invite philosophers and writers to his lessons, attended by Jules Claretie (1840–1913), Octave Mirbeau (1848–1917), Joris-Karl Huysmans (1848–1907), and Jules Lermina (1839–1915).[20]

When the play *Froufrou* by Henri Meilhac (1831–1897) and Ludovic Halévy (1834–1908), originally produced in 1869, was restaged, Gilles de la Tourette wrote in his November 29, 1892, chronicle that this drama *"is as young as it ever was and will remain so, for the authors have instilled* Froufrou *with a reality: morbid nervous heredity, and have analyzed a type of mental alienation with exceptional talent.*"[21] Froufrou "*is brainless, physically charming, incapable of focusing her mind on a serious idea; she thinks only of frivolities.*" Froufrou's mother is dead, her father is loving but inconstant, and her sister is "*wisdom itself.*" "*The two sisters grew up seeing the same scenes and spent time in the same company. One became wise, the other mad, because their brains were congenitally molded from different clay, because morbid heredity weighed heavily on one while sparing the other.*" In reality, the play presents a banal case of adultery in which it is difficult to identify "madness" or "mental degeneration," but only disregard for the social conventions of the time.

While *Froufrou* met with Gilles de la Tourette's satisfaction, he criticized Alexandre Parodi (1840–1901), author of *Reine Juana* [Joannna the Mad],[22] for not highlighting "*the historically well-characterized degeneration of his heroine, daughter of a royal household in which madness was hereditary, all while portraying her with symptoms of hysterical delirium in the conventional, cliché way madness is usually theatricalized.*"[1] Jeanne, as she is known in French, inherited from her mother, Isabella the Catholic, the throne of Castile that her father, Ferdinand, tries to usurp by forcing her to abdicate. "*She jealously watches over the coffin of her husband, refusing to allow his inhumation, even a year after his death. A strange idea for one sane of mind!*" Jeanne is locked away, even though she is not mad; the play focuses on the venal hypocrisy of the physician, formerly a monk, who attests to her madness. After seven years in a convent, she is forced to meet the man who poisoned her husband. Her son, now in power, orders the meeting to worsen her mental state. "*This is the last straw. She goes irremediably mad, with hallucinations of red dogs. While it may be news to Mr. Parodi, this is perfectly characteristic of hysterical delirium, rather than real madness, which is the historical reality. But there you have it. The audience always demands delirium, always the same delirium; they understand nothing else and neither do the authors, probably. . . . This is the truth, fiction aside. Jeanne was veritably mad, and the indefinite conservation of her husband's cadaver was the first episode of her real madness—I would add, her hereditary madness, because the family tree of the house of Spain, although real, was even more demonstrative of hereditary madness than the Rougon-Macquart family tree.*" Gilles de la Tourette then went through the family members one by one to support his hypothesis that hereditary madness is deterministic.

Seven years later, Gilles de la Tourette would return to this subject. "*The other evening, these thoughts came back to me at the Opéra-Comique as I listened to the musical portrayal of the Polish Jew—a true drama of madness—which I had once promised myself I would analyze for the readers of* La Revue Hebdomadaire."[23] The play, by Émile Erckmann (1822–1899) and Alexandre Chatrian (1826–1890), was a masterpiece in Gilles de la Tourette's estimation: "*This drama of madness gives us to witness, with implacable logic, one man's fight against morbid determinism, which he first uses in full cognizance of its implications and without regret, to procure wealth and admiration, before ultimately succumbing to it. His entourage and the public believe an accident is to blame and continue to consider him, even after his death, a perfectly honest man. . . . The door opens and we see a Polish Jew. Because he is wearing the traditional Jewish dress, he could easily be mistaken for the man Mathis killed. Mathis's emotion is overwhelming. He feels dizzy, his ears buzz, reminding him of the bells that were tinkling at the collar of his victim's horse. He teeters and falls, losing consciousness. We see clearly here the gradual worsening of symptoms, as one would say in medicine. . . . This is not merely a crafty peasant, astute in his affairs, trying to get away with something; he is a veritable madman, an unscrupulous and savagely selfish lunatic who won't hesitate to commit a crime to enlarge his fortune. The moral madness at the root of his mental state is still held in check by the force of reason, allowing him to keep up appearances. One day, however, by the very laws of its development, this madness will explode utterly beyond his control, leading to his perdition and ultimately to the grave. While awake, Mathis has much to be happy about: he is admired by his fellow men, appears reasonable, rigorously honest, and can even oblige others to pardon his good fortune. But at night Mathis loses all control. He has nightmares in spite of himself during which he speaks aloud; his will, led astray by hypnagogic hallucinations, cannot prevent their manifestation. . . . Mathis has actual auditory hallucinations, symptoms of ever growing madness. . . . This drama has been staged by the authors in the clearest fashion, with laudable understanding of the madness that grows day by day in Mathis, with his delirious interpretations, his auditory hallucinations, and his torments. They have portrayed a criminal madman, whom everyone considers to be a perfectly honest man, and in whom the lethal brain congestion of the final paroxysm is naturally attributed to overwork and a little Hünevig white wine that he shares too liberally with his guests. And yet, Mathis is undeniably a madman: his madness, for those perceptive enough to see it, is evident with every step. It progressively affects his normal development, and while the final congestion that closes the drama is perhaps more in keeping with the laws of the theater than with the facts of mental pathology, it is no less acceptable in the medical domain."* Gilles de la Tourette went on to conclude: *"It is a true drama, true to life, with a natural progression, very different from the laboriously composed dramas of the Norwegian School, borrowed from bits and pieces of mental pathology books, and hence outside of any lived reality."*[20]

It should be noted that, in his chronicles, Gilles de la Tourette was not very rigorous with the terms he used. For example, he mentions the *"hysterical delirium"* of Reine Juana, whereas his constant goal was to distinguish hysteria, which is not delirium and thus not madness, from true madness, a fate without remedy whose victims cannot escape their implacable heredity.

Furthermore, Gilles de la Tourette's comments should in no way be seen as anti-Semitic,[24] given that he undoubtedly shared the Dreyfusard opinions of his friend Jean-Baptiste Charcot.[25]

Cauvin Affair

In 1896, Gilles de la Tourette took an interest in a young criminal involved in a legal case known as *"L'Affaire Cauvin."* An old woman had been strangled by her fifteen-year-old servant, Marie Michel, who had acted in a fit of rebellion against her employer's domestic tyranny. *Fait accompli*, Michel had sought out her neighbor, Louis Cauvin. The doctor pronounced death by strangulation. After having initially confessed, Marie Michel withdrew her statement and accused Cauvin of the crime, claiming that she had been nothing more than an unwilling accomplice. Despite his repeated declarations of innocence and the absence of any proof, Louis Cauvin was condemned to forced labor for life, a sentence that was upheld in an appeal. Marie Michel was acquitted. Over the years that followed, she was placed in various institutions for illegitimate children. One day, she heard a sermon that left her horrified and realized the grave consequences of her deceit, not only for herself and "her soul," but also for Cauvin. She confessed her crime, stating that she could no longer live with the guilt of knowing she had let an innocent person be condemned. After several legal twists and turns, she was found guilty of perjury; Cauvin would be cleared of all wrongdoing. Gilles de la Tourette noted: *"The radical inconsistency of Michel who, after accusing Cauvin, incriminated herself, rightfully led to an examination of her psychic faculties. Who was assigned this examination? Two Navy physicians (the affair is being judged in Toulon), certainly very knowledgeable about tropical diseases, but it is readily apparent they are in no way qualified for this case. . . . Here, incidentally, are their conclusions: Marie Michel is neither mad, nor a hysteric. . . . She is a latent hysteric. She is the victim of self-suggestion, causing her to incriminate herself. . . . I have not examined Marie Michel, but in my opinion her mental state should be interpreted in an entirely different manner than that of the Toulon experts. First of all, what is latent hysteria? And if the hysteria is latent, why does it produce self-suggestion? Marie Michel, according to these experts, is a self-incriminator: what are self-incriminators, from a mental standpoint? Hysterics? This is doubtful, to say the least. Hysterics accuse others; take, for example, the Roncière-le-Noury affair, which also ended with an undeserved condemnation. But do these subjects accuse themselves? There are no scientific facts to confirm this. Moreover, in hysterics, self-suggestion or extrinsic suggestion is fleeting—mobile, like their very minds—when it does not have a real basis, such as desire, or the need to proclaim one's innocence.*

It would have been necessary to demonstrate that Marie Michel was a hysteric—and this, the experts were unable to do. . . . Does Marie Michel belong to the category of self-incriminating lypemaniacs? Who would dream of asserting this? In reality, what she says is logical, perfectly coordinated. She may be infantile, moronic, but she is not a madwoman who takes the fable of her delirium for reality. . . . Marie Michel is not a real criminal, a born criminal as Lombroso would say. She is a criminal by accident: she killed in a moment of rage, and very likely did not intend to cause death." What Gilles de la Tourette did not say in his chronicle was that, on his own initiative, he contacted Cauvin's famous lawyer, Félix Decori (1860–1915) (Figure 16.3), a friend of Raymond Poincaré (1860–1920), and provided him a medical certificate in support of his defense arguments.

The Loudun archives contain a letter written by Gilles de la Tourette on March 6, 1896, on medical school letterhead (Figure 16.4):

Paris, March 6, 1896, Dear Sir and Colleague,

I have been following with great interest the Cauvin Affair insofar as it provides material for psychological observation. However, I must admit that the expert

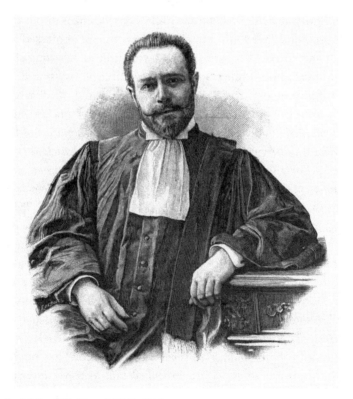

FIGURE 16.3 Maître Félix Decori (1860–1915).
Private collection of the author.

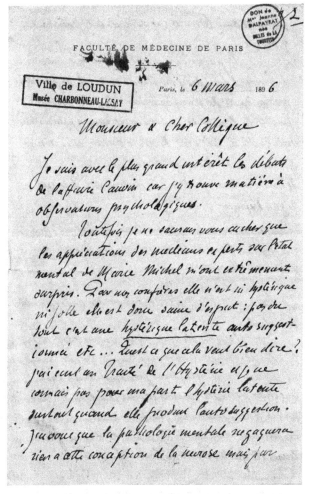

FIGURE 16.4 Gilles de la Tourette's initial letter to Decori.
Copyright Musée Charbonneau-Lassay, Ville de Loudun, with kind permission.

physicians' evaluation of Marie Michel's mental state surprises me in the extreme. For our colleagues, she is neither hysterical nor mad, and thus sound of mind. But wait, she is a latent hysteric demonstrating self-suggestion, and so forth. What, precisely, is the meaning of this? Though I authored a treatise on hysteria, I am unfamiliar with latent hysteria, especially latent hysteria with self-suggestion. I must say that mental pathology will gain nothing from this conception of neurosis; on the contrary, your client does have something to lose.

In mental pathology as in the courtroom, situations must be made clear beyond the shadow of a doubt, and I am taking the liberty to send you my assessment of this affair, exclusive of direct examination, of course, which I could not make. Incidentally, I think it would confirm what I shall point out to you. My colleagues say: Marie Michel is under the influence of self-suggestion, which causes her to accuse herself. There are but two categories of patients—and note that I speak of patients, not sane people— liable to such self-suggestion: 1) hysterics, but with them, self-suggestion is never so persistent, or so consistent; it is instead a passing phenomenon, as mobile as their minds. Furthermore, in my opinion, it remains to be demonstrated that Marie Michel is a hysteric, for what, after all, is latent hysteria? 2) The second category includes melancholics with ruinous and self-incriminatory ideas, but these patients are not la- tent, I can assure you; no error is possible in their case. Moreover, they keep to their asylums and would be incapable of making an appearance in court. How to under- stand Marie Michel's mental state? There is no reason to rack one's brain to prove the existence of an imaginary neurosis. In my opinion, Marie Michel is sincere and speaks the truth, and the examination of her mental state will establish as much this time. During an argument, in a fit of anger, she grabbed her employer by the neck. The lady resisted, Marie tightened her grip, and since the lady was getting on in years, the larynx was already ossified and fractured easily. A fifteen-year-old girl accustomed since childhood to peasant labor is perfectly capable of breaking an old woman's neck. I have performed enough autopsies to confirm as much with certitude. At the old lady's age, the larynx is very fragile. Once Michel had killed her employer, she thought only of exonerating herself, so she accused Cauvin and a series of unfortu- nate circumstances led to a conviction—a judicial error similar to that in Dr. Lafitte's case, in which I was recently involved. Now, how did the accuser come to play the role of self-incriminator? In my opinion, Marie Michel is not a born criminal—that is, she does not exhibit the kind of mental insanity whereby all of her morals could be contained in a teacup. Such criminals, the true type and most frequent of all, would not hesitate to accuse their neighbor, but would never incriminate themselves. For the simple reason I have just explained, namely that crime for them is a natural cerebral function, and remorse or regret for the acts committed are words that do not exist in their vocabulary. . . . [The last sheet seems to have disappeared from the archives.]

A brief message sent to Georges Montorgueil (1857–1933) at the news- paper *L'Eclair* shows how Gilles de la Tourette discreetly informed the press of his secret activities: *"Thank you for the article. Here is the report I gave to Decori, which you may use once he reads it to the jury. Before then, it might compromise Cauvin. Thank you once again."*[26]

A letter from Decori (23 Bd Poissonnière), dated March 27, 1896, indicates how useful Gilles de la Tourette's spontaneous assistance had been for strengthening his arguments:

Dear Sir and Colleague,

I apologize sincerely for taking so long to thank you for the opportune and helpful assistance you so generously provided in the Marie Michel case. Had I not been so pressed for time when I returned to Paris, and were I not obligated to leave for several days next week for the Easter holiday, I would have come to thank you personally. The certificate you provided and your high scientific standing certainly convinced the jury that a fifteen-year-old peasant girl was capable of breaking an eighty-year-old woman's neck. The only argument of the prosecution was that this was not, in fact, possible. The unequivocal opinion of the physicians on this matter had led the prosecution to seek an accomplice and resulted in Marie Michel's fabrication. However, after reading your letter, the physicians were much less sure of themselves, where previously they had been categorical, and they began to contradict their position. This poorly disguised change in strategy had a strong impact on the jury. Thank you once again for your decisive aid. I shall not fail to consult you on this matter if it goes any further. I remain yours most sincerely, Felix Decori.

Because of the media's coverage of the affair and Cauvin's acquittal, Decori had his defense speech printed. The Loudun archives contain a copy with a handwritten dedication: *"To Mr. Gilles de la Tourette, Many thanks for his spontaneous and generous assistance, Félix Decori, August 1896"* (Figure 16.5). Gilles de la Tourette's chronicle had appeared four months before this date.[27]

Gilles de la Tourette as Polemicist

The dramatist Eugène Brieux (1858–1932) *"more inspired in* Les Remplaçants *and* Les Avariés, *made an attempt to ridicule the supposed 'failure of science' and of physicians in* L'Evasion."[1] Gilles de la Tourette continued: "L'Evasion, *a play in which hypochondria is hereditary, left me in a melancholy mood. I was desperate to learn why the audience, at least in part, seemed to delight in the tirades against science, delivered with compunction by puppets contrived by Mr. Brieux. How could it be laudable to vilify science, and especially medicine, at the end of a century filled with the most incredible discoveries? Those for whom science did not produce what they wanted may find reasons, but I intend to show the error of their demands. . . . Mr. Brieux portrays Dr. Bertry, a member of the Académie de Médecine, if you please, and a professor of neuropathology, as a charlatan who secretly mocks the science to which he owes his reputation and all of its advantages. 'I have a problem,' Belleuse says to him, 'a patient I can't seem to help.' The doctor's ingenuous response? 'That happens.' 'Of course, but . . . he wants to go to Lourdes.' 'Let him.' Belleuse, dismayed: 'You don't think . . . what if it cures him?' 'You can always find some scientific explanation.' 'Suggestion!' 'By George, the answer for everything.' "*[28] Gilles de la Tourette, the progressive, was visibly insulted by the mockery made of science, his own ideal. What was even worse, although unstated in Gilles de la Tourette's article and in the play was the implied mockery of Jean-Martin Charcot, who had died

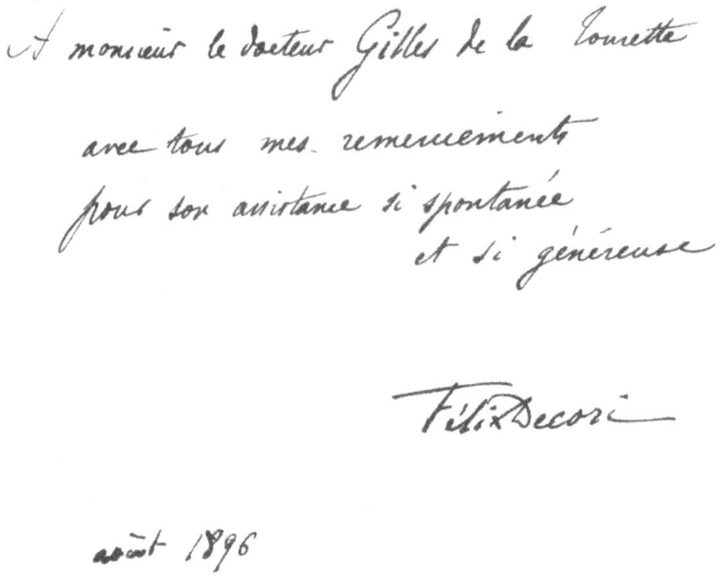

À monsieur le docteur Gilles de la Tourette

avec tous mes remerciements
pour son assistance si spontanée
et si généreuse

Félix Decori

août 1896

FIGURE 16.5 Print version of Decori's defense speech dedicated to Gilles de la Tourette.
Copyright Musée Charbonneau-Lassay, Ville de Loudun, with kind permission.

three years before the play premiered at the Comédie Française: "*Dr. Bertry is the author of works on heredity, maintains that psychic diseases are hereditarily transmissible, and prides himself, wrongly or rightly, on establishing the laws of heredity in such cases.*

"*In this march toward progress with all of the marvelous discoveries made along the way, each branch of human intellectual activity wanted its part in the glory. Literature was clamoring for its share, and so adopted a new formula, a scientific formula. The watchword was documentation, owing to the principles of the universally triumphant experimental method. . . . The psychologists of the novel and the play, legion in number, were also willing converts. . . . Rather than going profoundly within so as to 'deepen' their minds in the manner of Montaigne, the adepts of the new 'scientific' school attended the classes given by alienists. Philosophy has become psychophysiology; in the laboratories of the psychic sciences, there is only talk of reaction time, of a reduction in the field of consciousness. The most widely read works discuss at great length the diseases of memory, intelligence, or will. The learned societies of hypnology include among their members more doctors of philosophy than medical professors. The physicians pulled out before the invaders arrived. And the upshot of all of this? Words, words, said Shakespeare, who had no need to dissect brains to become a great philosopher. . . . The scapegoat, it turns out, is medicine, which has failed the hopes of all of these feeble philosophers, these novelists lacking in imagination, these untalented playwrights in need of human subject matter. So they set out to destroy what they had so recently idolized. Medicine, a science? Ha! It left us with nothing but disillusionment. Their stones began to rain down on physicians. . . . Physicians have led our consciences astray; they believe in neither God nor Lourdes, says Mr. Brieux, with their fatalism and false laws of morbid heredity, 'their laws that rob us of all hope, making more men crazy and vicious than heredity itself.' They are 'the ministers of this goddess of disappointment they call science.' On the contrary, Mr. Brieux, science has not failed, and at the risk of being guilty of every form of pride exemplified by Bertry, I intend to prove it to you, assuming this is even necessary."* Gilles de la Tourette cited the work of Pasteur on rabies, the progress of asepsis in obstetrics and surgery, the reduction in deaths by infection, and so forth. If Mr. Brieux were to contract rabies, he noted, he would hasten to vaccinate himself, or *"if croup caused his throat to swell shut, he certainly wouldn't seek out a shaman to cure his ills."*

Isn't this debate still relevant? In his study exploring whether medicine is art or science,[29] Jacques Poirier concludes in the best way possible: *"Like the old Chinese proverb says, medicine 'must walk on both of its legs': the rational and the supernatural, the technical and the human, skill and humanity, Science and Art. That said, medicine is neither an exact science nor a fine art. Sadly, physicians who are not scientists are not artists; they are charlatans (crooked or naive, depending on the case), or they are incompetent or incapable. And those who do not bring human values to bear on their scientific medical practice, are simply not physicians."*

Gilles de la Tourette as Biographer

In 1893, after the death of his revered master Jean-Martin Charcot, Gilles de la Tourette publishes an hagiographic and respectful eulogy in *La Nouvelle Iconographie de La Salpêtrière*.[30] He reproduces the same one in *La Revue Hebdomadaire*.

Hospitals in Paris underwent considerable change at the end of the nineteenth century. As they moved from providing accommodation to care, their mission shifted from helping to healing. The glorification of scientific progress, as opposed to religious obscurantism, affected all of French 'Republican' society, in particular a significant part of the medical profession, led by figures such as Désiré-Magloire Bourneville (1840 –1909), former interne (house officer) under Charcot and also his publisher. Bourneville helped bring about the creation of nursing schools and the gradual replacement of religious orders by educated secular nurses. Marguerite Bottard (1822 –1906), Charcot's chief nurse made famous by André Brouillet's painting *Une leçon clinique à La Salpêtrière*, would be glorified and decorated as a model for this movement. In 1898, Gilles de la Tourette illustrates for *La Revue Hebdomadaire* this progressive current of thought and revisits the struggle to secularise hospitals under the Third Republic in France. At the same time, it renews interest in the exemplary career of a nurse whose name was recently given to a building at La Salpêtrière Hospital.[31]

Chronicles Written by Gilles de la Tourette

1. Paracelse. Le calculateur Inaudi. *La Revue Hebdomadaire*. July 9, 1892;(2)303–308.
2. Paracelse. Guillotine et électricité. *La Revue Hebdomadaire*. July 16, 1892;1(3):302–309.
3. Paracelse. L'état mental de feu Ravachol. *La Revue Hebdomadaire*. July 23, 1892;1(4):625–629.
4. Paracelse. Les pêcheurs de Pen'March et de la baie d'Audierne. *La Revue Hebdomadaire*. October 8, 1892;1(5)296–311.
5. Paracelse. L'état mental de Frou-Frou. *La Revue Hebdomadaire*. November 26, 1892;1(6):624–629.
6. Paracelse. Hygiène militaire. Les parasites des biscuits de troupe. *La Revue Hebdomadaire*. January 28, 1893;2(4):618–627.
7. Gilles de la Tourette G. La folie de la Reine Juana. *La Revue Hebdomadaire*. August 19, 1893;2(8):461–470.
8. Gilles de la Tourette G. Le Professeur Charcot. *La Revue Hebdomadaire*. August 26, 1893;2(8):608–622.
9. Paracelse. A propos du procès Cauvin. L'état mental de Marie Michel. *La Revue Hebdomadaire*. April 4, 1896;5(4):118–131.
10. Gilles de la Tourette G. Le service des hôpitaux et la mobilisation. *La Revue Hebdomadaire*. November 14, 1896;6(11):305–310.
11. Gilles de la Tourette G. A propos de l'évasion de Monsieur de Brieux. *La Revue Hebdomadaire*. January 30, 1897;6(1):687–703.
12. Gilles de la Tourette G. Mademoiselle Bottard. *La Revue Hebdomadaire*. January 22, 1898;7(1):562–565.
13. Gilles de la Tourette G. L'état mental du juif polonais. *La Revue Hebdomadaire*. August 11, 1900;9(8):266–279.

Notes

1. Le Gendre P. Gilles de la Tourette 1857–1904. *Bulletins et Mémoires de la Société Médicale des Hôpitaux de Paris.* 1905;21(3):1298–1311.

2. Paracelse Bombast Ph. Théophile. *Les XIV livres des Paragraphes, où sont contenus en Epitome ses secrets admirables, tant physiques que chirurgiques, pour la curation très-certaine & methodique des maladies estimées incurables. Traduicts du latin en françois, avec explications et annotations très amples. Par C. de Sarcilly, Escuyer, sieur de Montgautier, Cauville, Culey, Canon, &c. très-expert en la doctrine Paracelsique. Oeuvres non encor veus, & très nécessaires à tous Médecins, Chirurgiens, Apothiquaires, & à tous gens curieux de leur santé.* Paris: Chez Hervé du Mesnil, ruë S. Jacques, à la Samaritaine. 1631.

3. Pagel W. *Paracelsus: An Introduction to Philosophical Medicine in the Era of the Renaissance.* Basel and New York: S. Karger. 1958.

4. Gaston Darboux (1842–1917), mathematician.

5. Paracelse. Le calculateur Inaudi. *La Revue Hebdomadaire.* 9 juillet 1892;1(2)303–308.

6. In contemporary French, a popular saying for a person highly talented in mathematics is that he or she has "a bump for math"—an expression directly inherited from phrenology.

7. Charcot JM. Physiologie psychologique. Un calculateur prodige: Inaudi. *Le Progrès Médical.* 1892;15:78.

8. Nicolas S, Guida A, Levine Z. Broca and Charcot's research on Jacques Inaudi:the psychological and anthropological study of a mental calculator. *J Hist Neurosci: Basic and Clinical Perspectives.* 2014;23(2):140–159.

9. Paracelse. Guillotine et électricité. *La Revue Hebdomadaire.* 16 juillet1892;1(3):302–309.

10. Loye P. *Recherches expérimentales sur la mort par décapitation.* Thèse no. 268 Paris. Chateauroux: A. Majeste. 1887.

11. Paracelse. Les pêcheurs de Pen'March et de la baie d'Audierne. *La Revue Hebdomadaire.* 8 octobre 1892;1(5)296–311.

12. Paracelse. Hygiène militaire. Les parasites des biscuits de troupe. *La Revue Hebdomadaire.* 28 janvier 1893;2(4):618–627.

13. Gilles de la Tourette. Le service des hôpitaux et la mobilisation. *La Revue Hebdomadaire.* 14 novembre 1896;6(11):305–310.

14. Paracelse. L'état mental de feu Ravachol. *La Revue Hebdomadaire.* 23 juillet 1892;1(4):625–629.

15. Lucas P. *Traité philosophique et physiologique de l'hérédité naturelle dans les états de santé et de maladie du système nerveux, avec l'application méthodique des lois de la procréation au traitement général des affections dont elle est le principe.* Paris: JB. Baillière. 1847–1850.

16. Morel AM. *Traité des dégénérescences physiques, intellectuelles et morales de l'espèce humaine.* Paris: JB. Baillière. 1857.

17. Féré Ch. *La Famille névropathique.* Paris: Alcan. 1894.

18. Clarétie J. La Vie à Paris. *Le Temps,* 1904;44(15 885):2–3.

19. Paracelse. L'état mental de Frou-Frou. *La Revue Hebdomadaire.* 26 novembre 1892;1(6):624–629.

20. Poirier J, Philippon J. Theater in Professor Charcot's galaxy. *Front Neurol Neurosci.* 2013;31:215–224.

21. Paracelse. L'état mental de Frou-Frou. *La Revue Hebdomadaire.* 26 novembre 1892;1(6):624–629.

22. Gilles de la Tourette. La folie de la Reine Juana. *La Revue Hebdomadaire.* 19 août 1893;2(8):461–470.

23. Gilles de la Tourette. L'état mental du juif polonais. *La Revue Hebdomadaire.* 11 août 1900;9(8):266–279.

24. Raphaël F. Présence du juif dans l'oeuvre d'Erckmann-Chatrian. In F Raphaël, R Weyl (eds.), *Regards nouveaux sur les juifs d'Alsace*. Strasbourg: Éditions des Dernières Nouvelles d'Alsace. 1980.

25. Goldtsein J. The wandering Jew and the problem of psychiatric anti-semitism in fin-de-siècle France. *J Contemporary Hist*. 1985;20(4):521–552.

26. Archives Nationales 428AP/2 Correspondance Montorgueil-Gilles de la Tourette.

27. Paracelse. A propos du procès Cauvin. L'état mental de Marie Michel. *La Revue Hebdomadaire*. 4 avril 1896;5(4):118–131.

28. Gilles de la Tourette A propos de l'évasion de Monsieur de Brieux. *La Revue Hebdomadaire*. 30 janvier 1897;6(1):687–703.

29. Poirier J. *La médecine est-elle un art ou une science? Mémoire de la science, 4*. Paris: Académie des Sciences. 2004.

30. Gilles de la Tourette G. J.-M. Charcot. *Nouvelle Iconographie de La Salpêtrière*. 1893;6(3):240–250

31. Walusinski O. Marguerite Bottard (1822–1906), nurse under Jean-Martin Charcot, portrayed by G. Gilles de la Tourette. *Eur Neurol*. 2011;65(5):279–85.

Correspondence Between Octave Lebesgue, Known as Georges Montorgueil, and Gilles de la Tourette

F ROM 1892 UNTIL his death, Gilles de la Tourette kept up steady correspondence with a journalist who signed his letters with the name of Georges Montorgueil. This exchange of letters is interesting for the light it sheds on certain aspects of Gilles de la Tourette's activities.[1]

Who Was Montorgueil?

Octave Lebesgue (1857–1933), born in Paris, first worked as a singer/songwriter after his military service. His career as a journalist began at a newspaper founded in 1881, *Le Réveil Lyonnais*. In 1901, in *Les Arts et les Lettres*, a Parisian novelist and politician by the name of Léon Riotor (1865–1946) published a series of "notes," written in 1883 and 1884, which described his early days as a writer in Montmartre. Riotor's memoirs were written in seven parts, including *Les Jeunes,* of interest to us, as well as *Hydropathes, les Hirsutes,* and *Nous Autres. Les Jeunes* describes a cenacle of ambitious young writers who met in an office on Rue de Tournon in Paris. In addition to Riotor, the group included Georges Auriol (1863–1938), Victor Margueritte (1866–1942), Jean Blaize (1860–1943), and Octave Lebesgue. Riotor described Lebesgue as follows: *"Octave Lebesgue is an ardent, indefatigable writer for a daily paper who turns out an article a day on behalf of the disinherited, the weak, and the humble. I met him two years ago in Lyon,* with *Auriol. At the time, he was struggling to get by at* Le Réveil de Lyon *and* La Bavarde.*"*² Lebesgue later wrote for several Parisian newspapers including *Paris, La Bataille, Le Mot d'Ordre, L'Echo de Paris,* and the satirical journal, *Le Courrier français.* Among his many pseudonyms, Georges Montorgueil was the one he most frequently used. Other pseudonyms included Germinal, Brincourt, Jean Valjean, and Caribert. He later became head of the news department for the paper, *L'Eclair,* then editor-in-chief of the major paper, *Le Temps* (1861–1942), from 1900 until the time of his death. Also from 1900 until his death, he was the director of *L'Intermédiaire des chercheurs and des curieux,* one of the first journals on science for the general public. Lebesgue also wrote librettos for three musical dramas: *Mérovig, La Cloche du Rhin,* and *Léone,* working with Pierre-Barthélemy Gheusi (1865–1943) and Emmanuel Arène (1856–1908), with music composed by Samuel Rousseau (1853–1904). Lebesgue-Montorgueil remains best known for his many books on Parisian life, including *Le Café-Concert, La Vie des Boulevards, Les Plaisirs du Dimanche, La Vie à Montmartre,* and *La Parisienne peinte par elle-même,* which were magnificently illustrated with engravings by famous artists of his day, such as Auguste Brouet (1872–1941), Charles Jouas (1866–1942), Paul-Adrien Bouroux (1878–1967), Charles-Jean Hallo (1882–1969), Edgar Chahine (1874–1974), Henry Cheffer (1880–1957), Georges Gobô (1876–1958), and Adolphe Willette (1857–1926). Lebesgue also wrote educational books for children that were highly popular with adults, illustrated by the artist Jacques Onfroy de Bréville (1858–1931), known as JOB. JOB's flair for detail influenced and enchanted generations of children who delighted in his drawings of military dress and of Napoleon and Murat. Montorgueil also explored the world of wine in a series entitled *"Monseigneur le vin."* He wrote several volumes, one on each viticultural region in France. Due to Montorgueil's talent as a writer and the beauty of the illustrations, most of his books are collector's items and are often very valuable.³ Montorgueil was friends with many writers and artists including Charles Cros (1842–1888), Albert Samain (1858–1900), and Fernand Xau (1852–1899). He was also close to Emile Zola (1840–1902). In a letter from 1885, the year *Germinal* was published, Zola wrote to Montorgueil: *"If human beings were perfect, if they were divine, what reason would there be to try and improve their fate? No, people are lowly, ignorant, in the mud, and we must work to lift our fellow man upward."*⁴

A Close Friend

One example of the positive response Montorgueil's illustrated books met with is an undated visiting card, with the following inscription by Gilles de la Tourette: *"Thank you, my dear friend, from your affectionate, devoted reader. Your book is exquisite. It delighted my historian's soul, that part of me fascinated by Renaudot and Gaufridi (my book will soon be published). My daughter cannot put it down, there isn't enough to go around, and I haven't even mentioned the illustrations! Full of good lessons. I hope to see you soon for I need to speak with you, and also ask about the cover of this lovely book. I'm counting on you."* This somewhat enigmatic note indicates that Montorgueil had given his friend one of his beautifully illustrated books on a historical subject that appealed to Jeanne Gilles de la Tourette. The book to be published probably refers to a text Gilles de la Tourette prepared in 1891 with Henry Meige (1866–1940), on the 1611 trial of Gaufridi, a priest in the Accoules district of Marseille. The text, which dealt with possession and exorcism, was never published and has never been found. But in 1936, Meige published a book under the same title without mentioning Gilles de la Tourette.

In his letters, Gilles de la Tourette called his friend "Montorgueil." They wrote each other frequently, a *"mutual exchange of good and loyal services."* Gilles de la Tourette kept Montorgueil informed about research at La Salpêtrière, a subject of great interest to the latter. And, as we shall see, Montorgueil served Gilles de la Tourette's purposes by launching press campaigns. Montorgueil had connections in various ministries. He associated with, and obtained favors from Louis Barthou (1862–1934), a journalist-turned-politician who, from the age of thirty-two, in 1894, held high-ranking government positions. He was successively Minister of Public Works, Minister of the Interior, Keeper of the Seals (Minister of Justice), and finally Président du Conseil (head of the French government under the Third Republic) in 1913. It was known that Gilles de la Tourette benefited from the political backing of Alexandre Millerand (1859–1943), a left-wing member of Parliament and close to Désiré-Magloire Bourneville (1840–1909). What is less well known is that Montorgueil used his influence with Alfred Picard (1844–1913), Commissioner General of the 1900 World's Fair, to sway the nomination of the fair's Chief Physician by one vote.

Though both shared similar left-leaning ideas, they never discussed politics in their letters. Some of Gilles de la Tourette's content, as well as his style, were indicative of megalomania and a degree of disconnection from reality. It is likely that, by 1893, certain signs of his general paralysis were making themselves felt in these letters.

Some of the letters discussed events from everyday life, such as this brief note, dated February 11, 1896, from gilles de la Tourette: *"My dear friend, I am very pleased to inform you of the birth of my son, François, who I hope will be a good one! Everyone is fine and I am, too. Affectionately yours."*

Brief exchanges testified to their genuine friendship, as well as documenting daily matters in their respective social lives. On June 22, 1898, Gilles de la Tourette referred to his family life: *"My dear friend, . . . I was supposed to go see a house near Caen on July 3, to inquire about renting it during the summer holidays. In case the site wasn't suitable, I had asked that the house where I have vacationed in St Vaast la Hougue for the past three years be reserved for me . . . ."*

On December 5, 1899, Gilles de la Tourette congratulated Montorgueil on becoming a father and also tried to further his efforts to obtain the Légion d'honneur medal for Marguerite Bottard: *"My dear friend, All our sincerest congratulations for the good news you have just shared with us. I hope that all goes well, that Mrs. Montorgueil is back on her feet in no time, and that your little daughter brings you joy as she thrives. . . . Incidentally, I have seen Mr. Barthou who was very amenable for Miss Bottard, as was Mr. Lebon,[5] whom I saw in the company of Jean Charcot. If Mr. Humbert could find the right moment, a word to Mr. Barthou would be very helpful. I hope to see you and speak again in the near future. I send, my dear friend, my cordial regards."*

Epistolary archives do not always reveal the circumstances and contexts in which the exchange took place. One example is this short note dated January 14, 1893: *"My dear sir, I really do not know how you do it, how you write your articles so well and so accurately with so little information. I am going to give you some information here: I wanted to use this for my scientific column in the* La Revue Hebdomadaire *but I do not have the time just now and I'm afraid it will no longer be current. Can you hypnotize someone against his will? The answer is no; everything else you hear is folly. Can we convince you? I beg of you to be so kind as to dine with us Friday, January 20, at 7:30 (informally). Among other friends present, Auvard and Caubet, who recently published a treatise on surgical and obstetrical anesthesia. I shall round out the evening with a general statement of the conditions for hypnotizing someone in spite of himself (or in spite of one's self; I am at odds with the Académie). And we shall drink to the health of Théophraste Renaudot who owes so much to you. I do hope you will come. Cordially, Gilles de la Tourette."* The key to appreciating Gilles de la Tourette's compliment to his friend is missing. Perhaps one of Montorgueil's articles had referred to a lesson given at La Salpêtrière on the subject of hysteria and hypnosis. While Gilles de la Tourette did write articles for *La Revue Hebdomadaire*, he never wrote one on hypnotism. The other guests, Alfred Auvard (1855–1940) and Edmond Auguste Caubet (1863–1920), had published *Traité d'anesthésie chirurgicale et obstétricale* in the "Bibliothèque Charcot Debove" collection in 1892.[6] The debate over the possibility of hypnotizing someone against his or her will recalls the Eyraud-Bompart affair in 1890. Gilles de la Tourette had defended the position of the Salpêtrière

School, that free will is maintained under hypnosis and that it is impossible to hypnotize someone against his or her will. We will never know what Gilles de la Tourette wanted to tell his friend about hypnosis without consent. As for Théophraste Renaudot, he was one of the idols in Gilles de la Tourette's journalistic hall of fame.

Gilles de la Tourette's Blunder

Gilles de la Tourette, who had just taken the exam to become a hospital physician, was afraid he had made a mistake and sought to remedy the situation with the help of his friend:

"May 4, 1893, Dear Sir and Friend, The examination for hospital physicians has just come to an end for me. I was 4 points ahead. Last Monday I was in the first session for the last test, and I passed. I am very happy to let you know.

Yesterday evening, walking along the boulevards, I ran into our friend, Alphonse Humbert, and two of your associates. I gave them the very recent good news. They immediately said: 'That's worth printing in *L'Eclair.*' A nice gesture, of course, but I had to insist and refuse their kindness. The exam is only officially over next Sunday or Monday, and before then no one must know anything. So, if Humbert or someone else announces the news to you, please don't make anything public. Once the examination is officially over, I shall inform you through the mail. The world of physicians is a strange one, with all of its reticence. But so it is, if you want to be part of the profession . . . you also have to accept the drawbacks. I am very happy. For the last ten years, I have done nothing but work, and at last I am free. I am going to start on the 2nd volume of my treatise on hysteria, so as to give it to you.

Sincères salutations, Gilles de la Tourette.

P.S.: If, despite my request (but I doubt this will happen), a notice were to appear in the paper, please, I beg of you, see to its removal. The consequences could be disastrous for me."

How could Gilles de la Tourette know he had passed when the tests were not even finished yet? Was he so sure of himself that he couldn't resist the urge to brag? This is a possibility, given his temperament, but his illness may have been manifesting itself already. Or did an unscrupulous jury member inform him he had passed? Clearly, a premature announcement in the press would do nothing but harm. Gilles de la Tourette regretted his disclosure, especially that he told journalists. He turned to Montorgueil to help him avoid any negative impact. His letter's postscript expresses deep concern about his blunder, but, under different circumstances, Gilles de la Tourette would have been pleased to see himself in the paper. Alphonse Humbert (1844–1922), a disciple of Auguste Blanqui (1805–1881) and an "internationalist," wrote for the republican newspapers that criticized Napoleon III (1808–1873). During the Paris Commune (1871), he was active at *La Renaissance* and became an editorialist at the *Le Père Duchêne*, which he renamed *le Fils du Le Père Duchêne*, in reference to a newspaper of the same name started in 1789, then again during the Revolution of 1848. His revolutionary engagement led to his deportment to Nouméa in New Caledonia. Georges Clemenceau (1841–1929) pardoned him in 1879. Shortly thereafter, he was elected to the Paris city council and became a member of Parliament representing La Seine from 1893 to 1902.[7] The phrase "our friend Alphonse Humbert" confirmed the progressive outlook that Gilles de la Tourette and Montorgueil shared; both also had anti-clerical views.

A Hectic Life

A letter dated November 30, 1894, is full of interesting details:

My dear friend, The agrégation examination starts in 15 days: I shall be playing my last chip. I am overworked, plus I am correcting the proofs for Volume II while at the same time reviewing nephritis, colitis, and other fascinating subjects like a madman! My friend Michault, who was our secretary for Renaudot in Loudun, is terribly eager to enter the Ordre des palmes académiques! I got Claretie to sign; please ask Mr. Alphonse Humbert to sign! I shall sign afterward as secretary general and also Risler and then he will get his ribbon. I shall have the office boy bring the paper to *L'Eclair* tomorrow. Many thanks to you and to Mr. Humbert; my apologies that I did not come to see you personally, but I am so busy I hardly know where to start. Cordially.

Gilles de la Tourette was working on several important tasks at once. He was preparing his second attempt at the *agrégation* examination. He was correcting the proofs for the second volume of his hysteria treatise, which Charcot had read and prefaced just before his death. Michault was a friend from Loudun who must have been involved with a local committee on the erection of a Théophraste Renaudot statue. Gilles de la Tourette was probably trying to help him enter the Ordre des palmes académiques (for distinguished professors and figures in the world of culture) by leveraging his network of relations. Charles Risler (1848–1923), mayor of the Seventh Arrondissement, was Gilles de la Tourette's landlord and friend, a member of the board for the public hospital system in Paris, and also on the Paris Renaudot committee. Gilles de la Tourette led the effort to get this statue erected, and, thanks to Jules Claretie (1840–1913), he was himself awarded the Légion d'honneur medal. Michault was awarded the decoration he sought, as well.

On November 26, 1895, Gilles de la Tourette wrote: *"Next Friday at 5:15 on the dot, I am giving a lesson on stigmata and hysteria at Hôpital Cochin. Perhaps this would be of interest to you? At any rate I would be delighted to see you. Cordially yours."* Charcot, of course, had courted the press, and Gilles de la Tourette was also pleased when a journalist was present at his lessons.

This note of thanks is undated: *"Thank you my dear friend. This morning I was reading* Le Petit Havre *and saw one of your articles, in which your admiration for me was clear. My wholehearted thanks to you. All is well and we shall see many more."*

A Mediator and Advertiser

Gilles de la Tourette also introduced Montorgueil to professional and cultural contacts who might interest him, as this undated invitation shows: *"Paris Saturday, On Monday (23, 7:30) you are going to have to dine somewhere. So, join me for an informal meal. I shall be in the company of a compatriot of Ibsen and Bjørnstjerne Bjørnson who is an alienist in Christiania. I am sure he will illuminate us on how his fellow countrymen think. In a jacket, as a comrade and friend. If I do not hear from you, it means we agree cordially. We shall wait for you until 7:45."*

Oslo, the capital city of Norway, was called by the name of Christiania from 1624 to 1924. Gilles de la Tourette had a physician friend there who was passing through Paris. He thought that by citing two of the most famous Norwegian writers, Henrik Ibsen (1828–1906) and also Bjørnstjerne Bjørnson (1832–1910), who would receive the Nobel Prize for literature in 1903, he could spark Montorgueil's curiosity.

A further invitation on May 15, 1894: *"My dear friend, It was perfect. . . except for your absence. I did not remain inactive. The old mayor of Loudun, the one who disparaged me, wanted the red ribbon; he is still chasing after it. Please be so kind as to come to dinner on Friday, the 18th, 7:30, formal attire. A few of your friends will be in attendance. I am writing a note to our dear President Alphonse Humbert who has yet to attend one of my dinners. I hope all is agreed. Thank you again and here's to Friday."* Whatever had been perfect remains a mystery. Gilles de la Tourette clearly did not care for Alphonse Dumereau (1834–?), mayor of Loudun between 1880 and 1896. Indeed, before a statue of Théophraste Renaudot was erected in Paris, he was opposed to the idea of having one in Loudun.

On March 28, 1899, Gilles de la Tourette sent a telegram to Montorgueil: *"I just presented a talk at the Académie de Médecine. So, you may publish something when you like, if our new procedure of cranial exploration is of interest to you, in which case you will surely find an interesting way to present it to your readers. We do not palpate the skull like Lavater, but we do tap to feel for lumps and that is the key point. Thank you, yours cordially."* Gilles de la Tourette and the surgeon Antony Chipault (1833–1920) published the text from this presentation shortly afterward in *La Gazette des Hôpitaux: "With respect to operations on the skull, it would be desirable to be able to identify as accurately as possible, prior to the operation, the thickness of the skull wall to be operated on. Anatomical research, such as that done by Péan in particular, has established the normal thickness of these walls according to skull region. But this work only applies to normally constituted skulls and does not help us determine whether, for a given case, the walls are thinner or thicker than the normal state. We believe that we have found the means to solve this problem, at least in part, by methodically tapping on the skull, using a small hammer or, preferably, tapping directly with the finger. The finger perceives the elasticity and resistance that are complementary and correlative to the sound produced. The patient must always keep his mouth closed during this procedure; the results vary greatly depending on whether the mouth is open or closed. . . . Percussion performed as we have described enables recognizing the comparative tone of the skull: clear in children, dull in adults, especially in males, and less dull in elderly persons. The tone in the frontal and parietal regions is clearer than in the occipital region. From these facts, we can already conclude that the tone varies with the thickness of the wall, since children have thinner skulls than adults, and since the parietal region is thinner than the occipital region."* They then gave a few examples of their work. In actual matter of fact, this approach provides only a rough estimation of the thickness of the skull bone and is of limited use for the surgeon.[8] Radiography would eliminate all of these ineffective clinical examinations. Even in its day, their publication garnered no interest.

Satirical Documents on Mesmer

In 1889, when Gilles de la Tourette was *chef de clinique* (senior house officer or resident) under Charcot, he published an article entitled *Documents satiriques sur Mesmer*[9] in *La Nouvelle Iconographie de la Salpêtrière*. He appears to have given a lecture on the same subject shortly thereafter, then sent the manuscript he had prepared for his speech to Montorgueil, accompanied by this undated letter:

My dear friend, I would like to thank you in advance for your initiative, always excellent. I wrote out my lecture, which will appear in La Revue Internationale. At least this way it was ready, though of course I did not read it. I used the notes in the margins, which I needed for the dates.

I am sending it to you as is, with most of the images I projected. If you do something with this, you will most certainly do it this evening. So I shall come for my manuscript tomorrow afternoon; please place it in an envelope with my name on it and leave it with the office boy.

To sum up, I tried to depict Mesmer from the time of his arrival in Paris in 1778 until his departure in 1785. I traced his career using caricatures and satirical allegories from the period. I demonstrated that this German, who claimed he was a philanthropist, was in fact a shameless scoundrel; in 6 years, after having unsettled an entire population, he left France with 600,000 pounds, an enormous sum at the time. I demonstrated that, if he was such a success, after failing pitifully in Vienna, it was because he found in Paris not only a people forever inclined to the marvelous, but also the overture to tragic circumstances. Minds were abuzz with what I shall call 'this nervous shiver, the prelude to revolution. . . .

Affectionately, Gilles de la Tourette.

The first chapter of Gilles de la Tourette's 1887 book, *L'hypnotisme et les états analogues au point de vue médico-légal,*[10] contained an expanded version of this article, without the etchings of the version published in *La Nouvelle Iconographie de La Salpêtrière*. We can assume that Gilles de la Tourette wanted Montorgueil to report on his lecture in *L'Eclair*, and that, as Montorgueil had not been able to attend the lecture, the preparatory manuscript would enable him to write it up. A torn, undated newspaper clipping gives an idea of the article Montorgueil likely wrote: *"Where do they come from? What is a somnambulist? and is a somnambulist truly sleeping? We asked Doctor Gilles de la Tourette these questions, and he kindly answered us with his usual perspicacity. 'Somnambulists,' he told us, 'are most often neurotics who are accustomed to sessions held by magnetism societies. The magnetizer recognizes, through their behavior, that they are neurotic. He publicly puts them to sleep and they fall into a state of somnambulism. The magnetizer cultivates this ability, which at first flatters them. It seems to confer a mysterious aura on them, which they later try to take advantage of.' 'They will then have the office of their dreams, decorated with a skull annotated with "Gall's system," a Kabbalah table, and a framed diploma that comes with their subscription to the 'magnetic chain'. . . . For your studies and your work, Doctor, you spent time within the world of somnambulists. Do you feel that this industry should not be tolerated? 'Do not ask me to be judge and jury. . . I said, I admit it, that in our legal code, there are articles that cover this commerce and the more dangerous commerce of hypnosis by charlatans, and that we would do well to apply these codes.'"*

Hypnosis Practices

Montorgueil was likely planning a further article on the controversial subject of public hypnotism. He had probably discussed with Gilles de la Tourette his idea of going to meet Hippolyte Bernheim (1840–1919), head of the Nancy School. In November 1897, Gilles de la Tourette replied to Montorgueil: *"My dear friend, One last point. By stating that there is no hypnotism, that is, no patholog-ical phenomenon, that there is nothing but a natural occurrence, all dangers that may be inherent in hypnosis practices are dismissed. Clients come in droves and they come with no fear. On the contrary, we maintain that accidents are legion and that impru-dent hypnosis practices are dangerous. Our precautionary stance encourages potential clients to keep their distance. This sums it up. You cannot, of course, say this. But you can refer Mr. Bernheim to the chapter of my book that describes hypnosis accidents, the danger of rogue hypnosis, and observations borrowed from many other authors. With affection. Gilles de la Tourette."*

"Hypnosis is a precious ally in the treatment of certain phenomena and in several complications of hysteria. . . ," wrote Gilles de la Tourette. "There is an enormous difference between hypnosis practiced by physicians who understand its properties and take its risks into account, and maneuvering done not only by charlatans but also by well-intentioned individuals, including physicians totally unaware of proper hypnosis practices who court dangers they do not understand."[11] Here, too, Gilles de la Tourette remained loyal to Charcot's views and never deviated from them, at a time when hypnosis practices were taking over fairs and perfor-mance halls.[12] He always came back to his arguments, which were based on Mesmer's practices and on the report from the commission appointed by Louis XVI. This commission, tasked with *"examining animal magnetism,"* in-cluded members from the Royal Academy of Sciences: Jean-Sylvain Bailly (1736–1793), Antoine Lavoisier (1743–1794), Gabriel de Bory de Saint-Vincent (1720–1801), Benjamin Franklin (1706–1790), and Jean-Baptiste Le Roy (1719–1800). The commission concluded that there was no evidence of a fluid called "animal magnetism" and called attention to the dangers associated with this belief: *"Touching, imagination, imitation—these are the true causes of the results attributed to this new agent known by the name of animal magnetism, the fluid said to circulate in the body and to be passed from one individual to another. . . . We must examine the attacks and convulsions produced by the processes of this so-called mag-netism in the gatherings around the baquet, to understand if they can be useful and can heal or relieve illness. The effect is solely understood through general experimen-tation and has not been determined by any positive experiments, but it would appear there is no room for doubt. It is often said in medicine that faith can save the pa-tient; such faith is the fruit of the imagination, and the imagination operates by gentle means: by establishing overall peace and quiet, by restoring order to the functions, by rekindling hope. Hope is life; whomsoever gives hope revitalizes. However, when the imagination produces convulsions, it uses violent means and these means are almost always destructive. Only in very rare cases are such means useful at all—in desperate cases that require total upheaval to enable renewal. Medicine should apply these dangerous disruptions like it would a poison. Necessity is the driver and frugality the rule. The need is momentary, the shock must be used once only. Far from repeating it, the intelligent physician occupies himself with the means for repairing the necessary harm it produced. However, with public treatment using magnetism, the attacks are provoked day after day. They are long, violent, and harmful. Habitually inducing these attacks can only have disastrous consequences.*"[13] Gilles de la Tourette's arguments to Montorgueil closely resemble the commissioners' findings. One hundred years later, he was trying to make the same point.

All of the letters that these two men exchanged reflect their complicity and the progressive ideology they shared.

Lafitte Affair

Gilles de la Tourette's interest in journalism, which began in adolescence, continued during his career as a physician, as his close ties to Montorgueil demonstrate. Gilles de la Tourette invested a great deal of time and energy in a press campaign to help a physician unjustly and severely sentenced, as his correspondence indicates.

In the fall of 1894, debate over a controversial court ruling filled the pages of the medical journals, then spilled into the general press. In his article dated September 12, 1894, in the newspaper *La Presse*, journalist Emile Willème (1864–?) described the case: *"For the past month, the good people in Rosny-sur-Seine and in Mantes have been up in arms over the judgment handed down against Doctor Lafitte, a physician in Rosny. Doctor Lafitte was sentenced to three years imprisonment on July 24 by the Versailles criminal court for abortion practices, but it is claimed there was no proof. The medical journals have protested vehemently against the court's ruling, which, they claim, places physicians 'at the mercy of anyone seeking to do them harm.'"* Following an accusation in an anonymous letter, an investigation of Dr. Lafitte was initiated to determine if he had performed an illegal abortion. The conclusions of the experts named to examine the patient were ambiguous since they were unable to determine whether the abortion had been spontaneous or induced. The experts believed Dr. Lafitte would be cleared of any wrongdoing, given the lack of substantial proof, but the court sentenced him to prison, which led several members of the medical profession to launch a press campaign aimed at liberating their colleague. Dr. Lafitte was viewed as a devoted practitioner, and many in his town protested his sentence. Responding to the journalist, the deputy mayor stated: *"To sentence such an honest man based on the testimony of a girl like that! Both of them are known here.*

What can I say about the girl. . . . She has condemned herself, now is not the time to heap criticism on her, but I can tell you that she had already been accused of having three abortions, and no one is surprised. As for the physician, when I saw him taken away by the gendarmes, who handled him roughly, tears came to my eyes. I told the gendarmes they could have shown a bit more consideration for such a man, that I had seen them be gentler in the past. They replied that they had strict orders. Everyone here is ready to testify on Lafitte's behalf, for he is an honest man."

A report substantiating a petition for individual amnesty, filed by Dr. Lafitte's lawyers, Georges Haussman (1847–1902) and Albert Gauthier de Clagny (1853–1927), was sent to the President of France, Jean Casimir-Perier (1847–1907),[14] in office since June 27, 1894. The Medical Press Association, founded by Auguste Cézilly (1833–1903) in 1889, and its representatives, Victor Cornil (1837–1908) and Félix de Ranse (1834–1904), played a key role in galvanizing the medical profession, which was beset by frequent liability trials against physicians. The Association assigned Marcel Baudouin (1860–1941), a physician and journalist (editorial secretary at *Le Progrès Médical*), and Gilles de la Tourette, with the task of preparing Dr. Lafitte's dossier. The President received Baudouin and Gilles de la Tourette on October 22, 1894. The close relationship between Gilles de la Tourette and Montorgueil is clearly revealed in this letter from the former, dated Sunday, October 21, 1894:[15] *"My dear friend, Tomorrow we shall see Mr. Casimir-Perier. Please highlight the following: 'The delegation from the Medical Press Association and its President, etc.' The important thing is that Cornil has drafted a very significant report, and there is more I need to tell you. So please, tomorrow evening, Monday, find time to meet me at 6:30 pm at L'Eclair, if you can. I shall bring you many documents and this time we shall see!"*

And the next day: *"Monday, 6 o'clock. You are a good friend with an honest heart. Your article, positioned squarely in the center of the page, is superb. I hope that doors will open for Dr. Lafitte, whom I had never heard of before, as I told you. I shall immediately send your article to Dr. Cézilly, President of the Medical Press Association. Cézilly, as I have seen in the papers, is concerned about our colleague, who has been victimized. Our thanks also to Mr. Henri who was willing to see me. Affectionately, until tomorrow."*

On October 27, 1894, a detailed article was published in *Le Progrès Médical*.[16] The legal proceedings were meticulously analyzed to underscore every flaw. The young woman's name was given, "the Chevalier girl," herself the victim of an anonymous declaration. The article included the report sent to the French President, and its conclusions were clear: *"This was a premature birth; however, no one saw the fetus. It is certain that the Chevalier girl made attempts to abort, but it has not been proven that these attempts, or other procedures by third parties, had the result she sought. . . . However, let us assume for a moment that the Chevalier girl did abort following criminal procedures. What are the charges against Dr. Lafitte? We have only the allegations made by the Chevalier girl, who consistently lied, and about whose past we have no information whatsoever. The fundamental question that sums up the entire case, is this: Was the abortion the result of criminal procedures by Dr. Lafitte? We formally reply in the negative. Indeed, analysis of the trial documents shows that there is no valid evidence that Dr. Lafitte tried to perform an abortion on the Chevalier girl. In Dr. Lafitte's defense, we shall not refer to his highly honorable antecedents. We shall not bring up his record in the Navy and in the colonies; we shall not speak of his five children and his mother, reduced to poverty due to his imprisonment. We shall simply ask, what motive could have driven him to criminal action? The prosecution was unable to find one. It clearly was not financial gain, since it has been proven that, for the five visits, the special bandages, and the medicine prescribed (iron pills, tannins for injection, quinine wine), he received from his patient a sum total of 33 francs. In conclusion, Mister President, we state our conviction that Dr. Lafitte is innocent, and we respectfully request that you exercise, on his behalf, your right to grant a pardon. We request total amnesty for an innocent man. Paris October 22, 1894."*

Gilles de la Tourette probably sent this issue of *Le Progrès Médical* to Montorgueil.

[No date]

My dear friend, I am sending you a new article in Le Progrès Médical *written by M. B. (Marcel Baudoin) on behalf of our unfortunate colleague, Dr. Laffitte,[17] a widower and father of five children. I do not know him; I had never heard of him before. But he is innocent. I am speaking from a human vantage point and not to support my profession; you know to what extent I am outside the world of physicians. Do something for him. I am also sending you the issue of* La Médecine Moderne *that came out today, Saturday. It contains an article on Wagner's music and its psychological effects, about which you will certainly write an article, as you have expressed interest in doing. I do not know the author of the article. Could you send me back my two issues for my collections; I shall send you others when I find something of interest. Kind regards to Mr. Humbert and Mrs. Humbert. Cordially.*

Gilles de la Tourette's intentions are clear here. He counted on his friend to launch a press campaign in support of the approach taken by the Medical Press Association. This brief message was dated October 27, 1894: *"My dear friend, Your article was perfect in every way. I wanted to tell you immediately, but I waited to have the copies of the report I had ordered. This took a while but finally, here they are. The report will be published in its entirety by all newspapers, or at least many of the medical journals. It is not easy reading, but you will see what I mean. Cordially."*

This is a perfect example of Gilles de la Tourette's lobbying his friend. On September 1, *L'Eclair* reported on Dr. Lafitte. *"Where does this affair stand* now? *The medical press, which holds its meetings in Mr. Marguery's establishment, will examine Dr. Lafitte's case this evening. Group action has been taken to establish Dr. Lafitte's innocence. The entire medical world is watching those leading the protest. The Court of Cassation is to examine Dr. Lafitte's case next Thursday."* Nicolas Marguery (1834–1910) had a restaurant, La Sole Marguery, next to the Gymnase theater on Boulevard de Bonne-Nouvelle in Paris. On September 2, 1894, *L'Eclair,* which would later be known for its support of Captain Dreyfus, ran a large headline on the front page: *"Innocent man in prison. Doctor Lafitte before his peers in the medical press."* This was the result of Gilles de la Tourette's efforts to get Montorgueil involved in Dr. Lafitte's case.

On September 2, 1894, Georges Patinot (1844–1895) wrote an editorial that appeared in the publication he directed, *Le Journal des débats politiques et littéraires.* His article revealed the latent conflict of ideologies in this affair: *"Miscarriage of justice? In the past few years, there have been many alleged cases of legal error that have been zealously whipped into sensations by the press. . . . Now we have the case of Dr. Lafitte who, last July, was sentenced to three years in prison by the High Court in Seine-et-Oise, for abortion. Some people, including Dr. Lafitte's colleagues, believe that the jury in Seine-et-Oise was wrong, or that, at the very least, it convicted the physician without sufficient proof. Such is the opinion of the medical press, whose members met two evenings ago at Marguery's restaurant. They decided that Dr. Cornil and Dr. Gilles de La Tourette would contact the officials at the Court of Cassation on their behalf, before the ruling next Thursday on the appeal lodged by Dr. Lafitte. These gentlemen are not tasked with discussing the appeal cases that might be brought up. They will focus solely on the innocence of their colleague and the situation that physicians in France would face if they found themselves exposed to the litigation and sentencing conditions that Dr. Lafitte faced. Their resolution is curious indeed, as is the underlying approach. First of all, Court of Cassation judges, and all judges for that matter, must analyze the cases they are called upon to judge based on the arguments presented during the trial. It is unthinkable that they should ever receive delegations who come on behalf of certain parties. Secondly, the medical press representatives intend to call the attention of Court of Cassation officials to the purported innocence of Doctor Lafitte. This is an issue that these magistrates are forbidden to examine, insofar as they must exclusively consider any procedural defects or legal errors. It is our opinion, therefore, that the judges at the Court of Cassation are duty-bound to close their door to the representatives of the medical press."*[18]

A few days later, on September 13, 1894, a journalist at the newspaper *Le Temps* wrote: *"Juries are no longer in fashion these days. Dr. Lafitte's conviction was criticized from the start and today, it is already being appealed. The radical papers are seeking the physician's rehabilitation. We do not quite understand their involvement, unless it is aimed at once again undermining our faith in the legal system, with which they are not on particularly good terms."* On September 14, 1894, *"after fairly long deliberations in an emotionally tense atmosphere, the Court of Cassation handed down its ruling that there were no grounds to the legal arguments raised and due process of law had been respected. They thus dismissed the appeal lodged by Doctor Lafitte."*[19]

Gilles de la Tourette was outraged by the article in *Le Temps* and stunned by the Court's ruling. He responded in a letter dated September 14 and addressed to *Le Temps* (Figure 17.1):

To the Editor-in-Chief, Allow me, as a representative of the Medical Press Association, to protest against the way your staff writer distorted the motivations that have

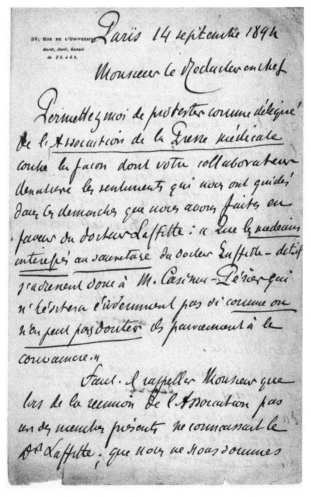

FIGURE 17.1 Letter written by Gilles de la Tourette to the journal *Le Temps* on September 17, 1894.

guided us in our initiatives on behalf of Dr. Lafitte. "Physicians concerned with saving Dr. Lafitte," he writes, "should indeed turn directly to Mr. Casimir-Perier, who will not hesitate if they succeed in convincing him, as we feel certain they will." Must I remind you, dear Sir, that not one of the members present at the Association meeting even knew Dr. Lafitte, that we took our stand only after a meticulous investigation conducted by our representative, Dr. Cézilly, which, in addition to the testimony from the expert himself, Dr. Vibert, irrefutably proved the innocence of our colleague.

Furthermore, Dean Brouardel, professor of forensic medicine, in response to our request, sent three letters to our association, which I submitted to Mr. Sallantin, President of the Court of Cassation; Mr. Sevestre, counselor; and Mr. Melcot, attorney general. These letters left no doubt whatsoever concerning Dr. Lafitte's innocence. The court, which rules solely on form, preferred to follow Mr. Sevestre's arguments rather than Attorney General Melcot, who eloquently asserted that the form had been defective. Let us hope that the court is not troubled by its verdict! Presently we have no choice but to request that amnesty, normally reserved for the guilty, be applied to an innocent man. Dr. Lafitte is a widower. His aged mother, who is seventy-six years old, is raising his five children; they have been reduced to poverty. Though the writer at *Le Temps* is not, as we are, convinced of the innocence of this poor man, he could at least respect the humanity shown by those looking after this unfortunate family, rather than insinuate that they are exploiting the case. I dare to hope, dear Editor-in-Chief, that in your fairness, you will publish this letter. Sincerely yours, Gilles de la Tourette, Hospital Physician, Chevalier de la Légion d'honneur.

Gilles de la Tourette crossed out the last line of his letter: *"Former assistant in legal medicine at the medical school,"* but he did not hesitate to refer to his former teacher, Brouardel, to add weight to his remarks. Gilles de la Tourette sent one copy to Montorgueil, and he continued to solicit his friend: *"I am sending this letter to Hébrard. I leave tomorrow night. If he does not publish it, or if there is nothing in* Le Temps, *I shall send you a telegram. Publish it, you know what I mean. You can add a little sauce.* Le Temps *has conducted a vicious campaign. Why? They irritate everyone and refuse to publish the rectifications and also* [illegible word] *at Mr. G. de la Tourette's request for an article. Such louts! You are masterful in these situations. Cordially."*

At the time, *Le Temps* was run by Adrien Hébrard (1893–1914). The September 22, 1894, issue of *Le Progrès Médical* published the letter Gilles de la Tourette had sent it. Bourneville, editor-in-chief of *Le Progrès Médical*, preceded the article with this comment: *"Despite the efforts undertaken by many associations and medical societies, the appeal lodged by Dr. Lafitte was dismissed. Almost all of the daily papers, regardless of their orientation, rued the decision handed down by the Court of Cassation, and added that the appeal's rejection might even be due to the insistence of the entire medical corps. This, to a certain extent, is also our opinion, aware as we are of the habits and jealousies of judges; here was an opportunity to disparage physicians and wield judicial power. However, if we could all start anew, our initiatives at the Medical Press Association would be the only course of action. Despite this glaring failure, for which the reporting judge is almost entirely responsible, we must not lose time with idle discussion. There is still action to be taken. A colleague at the newspaper* Le Temps *gave us the following advice: 'Nowadays,' he said, 'there is only one entity that has not always been with us. Non-existent during the French Revolution, and during the Directoire, that entity is amnesty. We all know that Lesurques, whose innocence was thoroughly proven, was executed because he could not appeal. The power that amnesty bestows upon the President of France draws its purpose and morality straight from our impossibility to deal with exceptional cases such as this one. Physicians concerned with saving Dr. Lafitte should indeed turn directly to Mr. Casimir-Perier, who will not hesitate if they succeed in convincing him, as we feel certain they will.' We must heed this advice and waste no time, even though this newspaper is reputedly hostile to the campaign undertaken by the medical press, to 'save' our unfortunate colleague. The words used in* Le Temps *are awkward and reveal their position, which our friend Gilles de la Tourette responds to emphatically in the letter below."* Then, following the text by Gilles de la Tourette, Bourneville concluded: *"For the time being, there is nothing more to say. As we have already stated, we shall return to the question of responsibility in this affair once Dr. Lafitte is released. And he will be released, at some point."*[20]

The journalist at *Le Temps* whom Bourneville mentioned had referred to Hugues Nicolas Joseph Lesurques, a financier born in Douai on April 1, 1763, and guillotined on October 3, 1796, in Paris, victim of one of the most infamous miscarriages of justice in the history of France, known as the "Courrier de Lyon" case. Bourneville used his journal to make a call for donations, appealing to the solidarity of the medical corps. He also launched a petition in favor of a pardon for Dr. Lafitte.[21] The October 1, 1894, issue of *L'Eclair* told its readers: *"And so, poor Dr. Lafitte is in prison because judicial formalism in France does not allow us to release innocent men who have been wrongly convicted. What will become of him? We are receiving very alarming news. He is not eating. He cannot sleep. His nights are tortuous. He is deeply anemic and his anemia is very painfully affecting his intellect, once so lively and spirited. If we do not give him freedom, sunshine, fresh air, and return him to his family, he will soon be lost to us, as a physician who recently visited him reported."* Gilles de la Tourette was the physician who had visited the prisoner, and, needless to say, he gave Montorgueil a full report. Gilles de la Tourette must have thought that his description of the physical and mental deterioration of Dr. Lafitte would make the public, informed by Montorgueil, more compassionate. He wrote this letter on October 15, 1894:

My dear friend, We haven't exactly triumphed yet, but we are close. So the issue is ripe. I have seen certain documents, I am writing to you to get the other document, and I shall give you everything very rapidly, I hope. I would like [illegible]. Thank you for the Lafitte case. Here is the latest. Madame Casimir-Perier recently hosted my wife in a very friendly fashion. My wife gave her a petition from Dr. Lafitte's little twin girls. Naturally this remains between the two of us. Nothing for the paper. I have more than enough with the exposure in good old Renaudot's gazettes. If amnesty does not work, I shall be giving you the most superb article. . . . In that case, we shall hold nothing back. The behavior of the court in S. & O. is unspeakable; and of course, they are the ones who will perform the counter-investigation required by the Amnesty Committee, the State's Council etc., etc. We are leaving it to the accuser to judge. . . those who committed this ignominious act are being asked if, by chance, the convicted person is perhaps not guilty. You see the reply. Let us hope the outcome is the right one! Otherwise. . . .

P.S.: Do not mention my wife's meeting with Mrs. Casimir-Perier to any of your colleagues, as they may lack your discretion.

Baudouin was pleased to announce the following to the readers of *Le Progrès Médical:* "*On Wednesday, October 31, 1894, at six o'clock, the President of France signed the total remission of the sentence that had been handed down against Dr. Lafitte. Thanks to one of our friends, we were immediately informed and in turn informed the concerned parties. We would like to express our deep gratitude to all those who encouraged and helped us in this campaign to rehabilitate an innocent man who had been sentenced in truly extraordinary circumstances. Above all, we wish to express our profound gratitude to our colleagues in the political press who, generally speaking, came to the defense of Dr. Lafitte and added their clear, strong voices to the more modest voice of the medical press . . . .*"[22]

La Foi qui guérit

In 1882, Bourneville launched "La Bibliothèque Diabolique," a collection of books he hoped would play a major role in disseminating secular republican ideas. Bourneville's ambition was that these books, whose medical and historical content was based on irrefutable scientific premises, would help overcome superstition. In his preface to Charcot's work, *La Foi qui guérit* (Faith-healing), Bourneville wrote: "*One of the driving forces that led us to publish the Bibliothèque Diabolique was a desire to expose our contemporaries to the strangest documents that had been published on 'magicians,' 'witches,' and hysterical-demonopathic epidemics, along with the simple, moving stories behind individual cases. We also wanted to show that the unfortunate individuals at the center of these dramas were sick, and not criminals, that they required medical treatment backed by science, and not courts, magistrates, and executioners. Such a demonstration—initiated by Jean Wier and continued in this century by Calmeil, Littré, Charcot, Axenfeld, Valentiner, and by ourselves and other physicians whose number grows daily—will ultimately prove the truth to all minds free from the preconceived notions and superstitions that, for too long, have cast their shadow over human intelligence. In his book,* La Foi qui guérit, *Mr. Charcot has summarized his teaching on cases deemed miraculous, which, in fact, come within the definition of hysteria. His thorough description based on in-depth study of irrefutable facts, is of a nature to convince even the most exigent."*[23]

Gilles de la Tourette added: *"On this subject we must re-read one of his last works, a sort of philosophical testament produced in collaboration with* La Revue Hebdomadaire.*"*[24] Bourneville integrated Charcot's text as a new volume in his collection, but only did so in 1897, four years after the Master's death. The first publication, in French, *"a scathing attack on Lourdes and the Church's teaching on the subject of miracles,"*[25] appeared in December 1892, in *La Revue Hebdomadaire,* then was reprinted in *Les Archives de Neurologie* in 1893.[26] The original text had been written in English and was to be published in November 1892 in *The New Review* of London, but it did not appear there until January 1893, one month after being published in French.[27] In her 1994 article, Jacqueline Lalouette raised the question: Did Charcot, who read and spoke English, write his text himself, or had it been translated? A letter to Montorgueil from Gilles de la Tourette on October 20, 1892, provides the answer (Figure 17.2): *"Dear Sir, Upon returning home, I found a letter from England. Apparently, the article arrived in London too late; it was not possible to do the translation in time. It will therefore come out on December 1, and not on November 1. As of the morning of December 3, you can use it as you please, since* La Revue Hebdomadaire *comes out on Friday and the 3rd is a Saturday. It is only a matter of time.*

As it would be disastrous for me (for the reasons I have already explained) if you were not informed on time, I have taken the liberty of enclosing a post card, to avoid any delay. . . . Gilles de la Tourette."

La Revue Hebdomadaire began its article as follows: *"The New Review of London has published, in its December 1 issue, an outstanding article by Professor Charcot, entitled 'Faith-Healing—La Foi qui guérit.'* La Revue Hebdomadaire *is pleased to have reached an agreement with the English periodical that enables it to provide its readers with an important scientific document that is very relevant today. Therein the eminent head of the Salpêtrière School gives his well-founded opinion on a problem whose solution is highly controversial."* It is clear here that the agreement

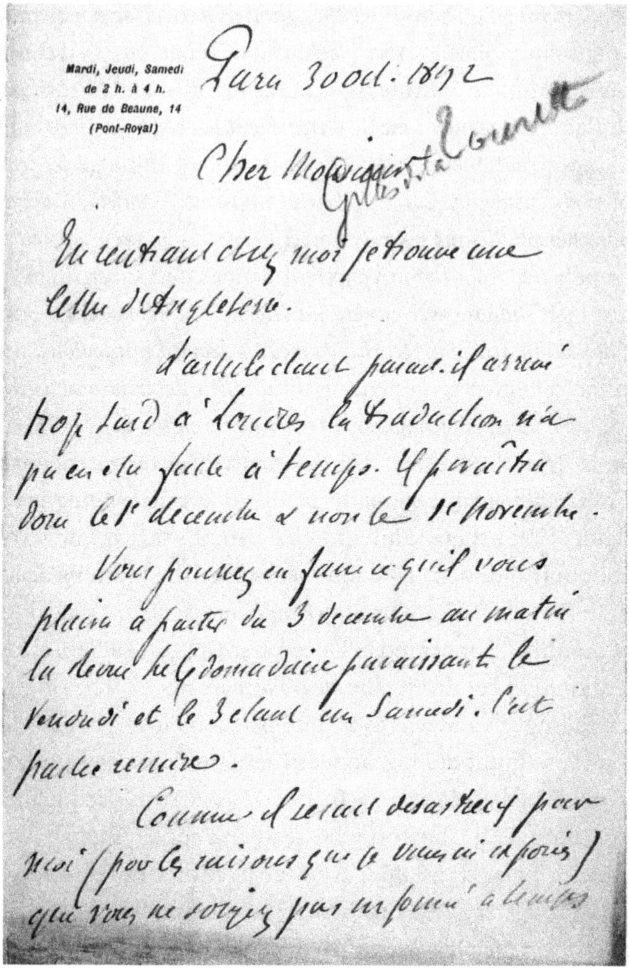

FIGURE 17.2 Letter to Montorgueil from Gilles de la Tourette on October 20, 1892.
Copyright Archives Nationales, Paris, with kind permission.

reached between the two periodicals was not respected due to the delay with the translation and that the French text appeared before the text in English.

This letter also indicates that Gilles de la Tourette had asked his friend Montorgueil to wait one month before publishing his article, for which Montorgueil doubtlessly provided much of the material himself. Even though *The New Review* had, in fact, not yet published anything, on December 4, 1892, Montorgueil ran the following headline in his paper, *L'Eclair*: *"Breaking news: The miracles at Lourdes assessed by Mr. Charcot."* The subhead stated: *" 'Faith-healing', a sensation-causing article. Hysterical contractions. The influence of volition. Phenomenon of suggestion. Determinism of miracles."* In his article, Montorgueil referred to Zola by name, even though Charcot himself had never referred to Zola.

Furthermore, Charcot's text in *La Revue Hebdomadaire* began as follows: *"In the context of a famous writer's recent journey to a religious sanctuary . . .*, The New Review *asked me for my opinion on faith-healing."* Whereas, one month later, *The New Review* published the following from Charcot: *"The journey of a celebrated man of letters to a religious shrine and the discussions that have risen with regard to it roused so much interest that they afford me an opportunity for offering my opinion on the faith cure."* Had Charcot's opinion been sought, or did he spontaneously offer it? In his *L'Eclair* article, Montorgueil explicitly stated: *"The English asked Mr. Charcot for a consultation on faith-healing. The event that prompted their request was Mr. Zola's visit to the pools in Lourdes. They wanted to know what the illustrious physician at La Salpêtrière thought about the healings that had been reported in the shrines. Charcot had to reply both to non-believers who denied such healing, and to those who pronounced the events miracles. Lourdes and La Salpêtrière are identical with respect to the pathological phenomena we may be given to see.* The New Review *was the first to publish this article, and now* La Revue Hebdomadaire *is providing the translation."* Unfortunately, the information that Montorgueil had received first-hand, directly from Gilles de la Tourette, ended up confusing things. Montorgueil had been sure of his information and had not taken the trouble to find out whether the December issue of the English periodical had actually contained the article by Charcot. Furthermore, Montorgueil explicitly gave its supposed title, "Faith-healing," whereas the article that appeared in *The New Review* in January 1893 was entitled "Faith-cure." Was publication in London postponed to January 1893 due to a conflict between the two editorial boards following the untimely publication in Paris? Charcot himself probably did not monitor the editorial path the article took, and he may well have assigned the task to Gilles de la Tourette.

Notes

1. Montorgueil G. Archives Nationales. Cote 428AP/2. Correspondance Montorgueil-Gilles de la Tourette.
2. Riotor L. *Les Arts et Letters*. Paris: A. Lemerre. 1901.
3. http://fr.wikipedia.org/wiki/Octave_Lebesgue
4. Private archives.
5. André Lebon (1859–1938), teacher, later a politician and minister. He turned to racketeering in France's African colonies and instigated the shameless exploitation of natives reduced to slavery in French Equatorial Africa.
6. Auvard A, Caubet E. *Anesthésie chirurgicale et obstétricale*. Paris: Rueff. 1892.
7. http://www.paris15histoire.com/humbert.htm

8. Gilles de la Tourette G, Chipault A. De la percussion méthodique du crâne, contribution au diagnostic cranio-encéphalique. *Gazette des Hôpitaux civils and militaires.* 1899;71:342.

9. Gilles de la Tourette G. Documents satiriques sur Mesmer. *Nouvelle Iconographie de La Salpêtrière.* 1889;2:59–64 / 103–106.

10. Gilles de la Tourette G. *L'hypnotisme and les états analogues au point de vue médico-légal.* Paris: E. Plon-Nourrit. 1887.

11. Gilles de la Tourette G. *L'hypnotisme and les états analogues au point de vue médico-légal.* Paris: E. Plon-Nourrit. 1887.

12. Gordon RB. From Charcot to Charlot: unconscious imitation and spectatorship in French cabaret and early cinema. *Critical Inquiry.* 2001;27(3):515–549.

13. Bailly, Lavoisier, Bory de Saint-Vincent, Franklin, Leroy. *Rapport des commissaires chargés par le Roi de l'examen du Magnétisme animal. Imprimé par ordre du Roi.* Paris: Imprimerie Royale. 1784.

14. Jean Casimir-Perier (1847–1907) was the sixth President of France, succeeding Sadi-Carnot who had been assassinated.

15. On October 15, 1894, Captain Dreyfus was arrested on orders from Commander Mercier du Paty de Clam, following an expert appraisal of handwriting after the French secret service accused him of having written a *"bordereau"* sent to the German Embassy. This was the beginning of the Dreyfus affair.

16. Haussmann, Gauthier de Clagny, Cornil, Cézilly, De Ranse, Marcel Baudouin, Gilles de la Tourette. L'affaire Lafitte; mémoire remis à M. le Président de la République à l'appui de la demande de grâce. *Le Progrès Médical.* 1894;20(43):273–276.

17. The incorrect spelling used by Gilles de la Tourette is respected.

18. Patinot G. *Erreur judiciaire? Le Journal des débats politiques and littéraires.* 2 Septembre 1894. 106è année.

19. Anonyme. Rejet du pourvoi du Dr Lafitte en cassation. *Le Progrès Médical.* 1894;20(37):179.

20. Bourneville DM. Le cas du Dr Lafitte. *Le Progrès Médical.* 1894;20(38):190.

21. Bourneville DM. Affaire Lafitte. *Le Progrès Médical.* 1894;20(40):227.

22. Baudouin M. L'affaire Lafitte. *Le Progrès Médical.* 1894;20(44):299.

23. Charcot JM. *La foi qui guérit.* Paris: Aux Bureaux du Progrès Médical, Felix Alcan. 1897.

24. Gilles de la Tourette G. Le Professeur J.-M. Charcot. *La Revue Hebdomadaire.* 26 August 1893;2(8):608–622.

25. Lalouette J. Charcot au cœur des problèmes religieux de son temps. *Le Revue Neurologique.* 1994;150(8–9):511–516.

26. Charcot JM. La foi qui guérit. *Archives de Neurologie.* 1893;25:72–89.

27. Charcot JM. Faith-cure. *The New Review.* 1893;8(1):18–31.

Gilles de la Tourette the Poet?

O NE OF THE surprises in the Loudun archives is the poetry written by
Gilles de la Tourette. The first poem is dated May 27, 1890, and written
on paper from the Hôtel Schweizerhof de Lucerne in Switzerland. Gilles de
la Tourette may have been on holiday, more inclined to romantic and literary inspiration. A few introductory words precede Gilles de la Tourette's
verses.

> Described as mad or fou, and also as gentlemanly, the Fou de Bassan [northern
> gannet] is a large bird of the polar regions that lives amid the storms, flying
> high, looking everywhere, as if he had lost his mind. . . . (Joussenel, *Le monde
> des Oiseaux*)

The humor of this poem is heightened in French because the name of the
northern gannet contains the word "fou," which means "crazy" or "insane."
Gilles de la Tourette can be seen here as mocking himself since he must have
realized that many of his friends and colleagues considered him a little crazy.
From a literary perspective, the poem can be viewed as a pastiche of a La
Fontaine fable. Did Gilles de la Tourette's wife view it as a sign of his affection?

It is difficult to know whether these poems should be taken as initial signs
of Gilles de la Tourette's disease or whether they are a simple manifestation of
his imagination and the pleasure he took in writing.

Reviens!	Come back!
I	I
Savez vous bien ce qu'est un « fou »	Have you ever seen a "fou"
C'est un sauvage oiseau du pôle	That wild bird of the Poles
Jadis fort gai, narguant la geôle	Once full of mirth, not bound by
Comme un pinson joyeux et fou	the earth
Savez vous bien ce qu'est un « fou »?	Like a lark, mad with joy
C'est un sauvage oiseau du pôle.	Have you ever seen a "fou"?
	That wild bird of the Poles.
II	II
Savez vous où cinglait le « fou »	Do you know where the "fou" was off to
Certains jours sombres de nuages	When the storm darkened the sky
Riant du vent et des orages	He laughed out loud, to spite the clouds
Cherchant partout comme un vrai fou	Searched right, then left, as of
Savez vous où cinglait le « fou »	mind bereft
Certains jours sombres de nuages?	Do you know where the "fou" was off to
	When the storm darkened the sky?
III	III
Je sais bien où s'en va le « fou »	I know where the "fou" was headed
Il s'enfuit à grande envolée	He flees with a haste that blinds
Pour retrouver sa bien aimée	For his beloved he has got to find
Blanche mouette au rire fou	White solan with his mad laughter
Je sais bien où s'en va le « fou »	I know where the "fou" was headed
Il s'enfuit à grande envolée	He flees with a haste that blinds
IV	IV
Mais pourquoi donc pleure le « fou »	But why is the "fou" weeping
Tout éperdu, le cœur en rage	His heart broken and blue
Prenant du hibou le ramage	He borrows from the owl his coo
Le triste oiseau qu'est le hibou	That sad song full of rue
Mais pourquoi donc pleure le « fou »	But why is the "fou" weeping
Tout éperdu, le cœur en rage	His heart broken and blue
V	V
Morte la joie! Le voilà fou	Joy is dead! He's mad instead
Il a perdu sa bien-aimée	His beloved he cannot find
Froufou bien loin s'est envolée	Froufou left him for distant skies
La retrouver, il ne sait où!	What is he to do?
Le malheureux le voilà « fou »	Poor boy, now he is "fou"
Il a perdu sa bien-aimée	His beloved he cannot find
Figure 18.1	

Reviens!	Come back!
Envol	Taking Wing
Reviens vite ma douce amie	Hurry back, my sweetheart
Reviens ma Blanchette chérie	Sweet Blanchette, come back to me
Je t'aimerai toute ma vie	Do so and I'll love you for all eternity
Vite reviens, Blanche Froufou	Hurry back, White Froufou
Toi, Blanchon, ma mie, reviens ou	Blanchon, dear heart, come back, or else
Comme le triste oiseau du pôle	Like the sad bird of the Poles
Pour toujours muré dans la geôle	Locked forever in chagrin's gaol
Du chagrin qui l'a nommé « fou »	That chagrin that made him "fou"
Ton pauvre ami deviendra fou	Your poor love will end up mad
Comme le triste oiseau du pôle	Like the sad bird of the Poles
Chanson	Song
Connais-tu la belle, connais-tu l'Amour	What do you know, my Beauty, what do
Je l'ai connue Belle et tu l'es toujours	you know of Love
Pourquoi son cœur n'est-il pas fidèle	I have known it to be Beauty, like yours
Le mien l'est toujours	eternally
Quel esprit d'amour t'anime encore	Why is that heart not faithful
ma belle	When mine forever is
Est-ce pour jouir du plaisir des cieux	Oh Beauty, what sense of love still
Ou bien c'est encore pour l'aimer	fills you
toujours	Do you wish to relish paradise?
Que je veux chanter	Or is it to love her forever
Notre bel amour	That my heart sings
Il est gai, il est bon, il est douceur	Our sweet love
Il est parfumé, il sent bon	So gay, so good and gentle
Plus que toute la terre	And it smells of sweet perfume
Il est équitable et bon	More than all the world
Je termine, ma mie dorée, mon amour	It is fair and good
et venir vite, amie adorée	I'll close, my treasure, my love
27 mai 1890	Hurry to me, dearest darling
Figure 18.2	

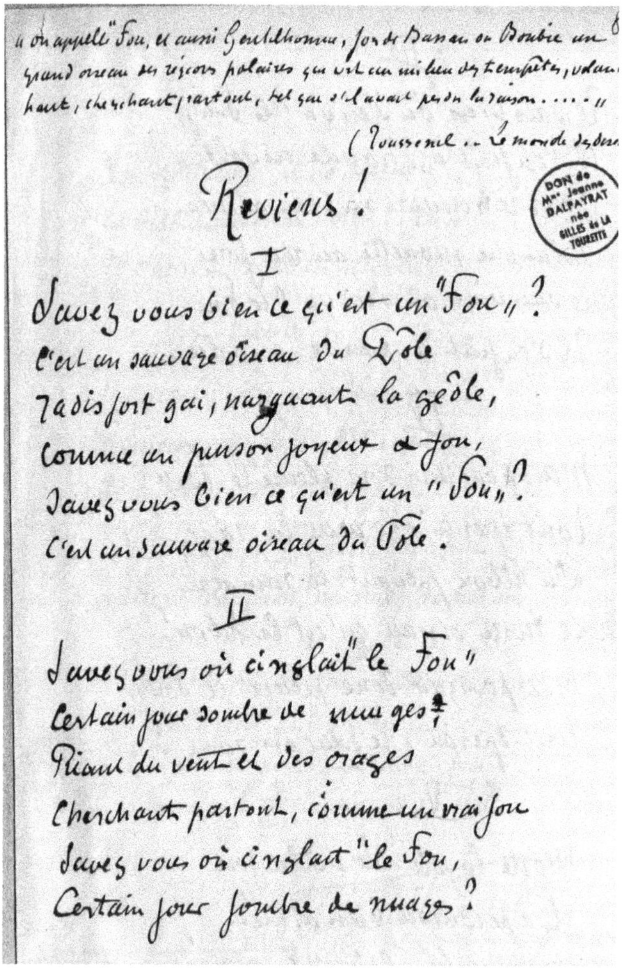

FIGURE 18.1 A poetry by Gilles de la Tourette.

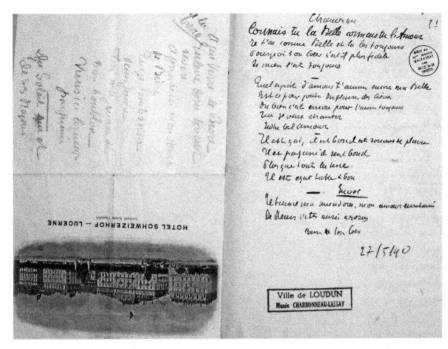

FIGURE 18.2 This poem is dated May 27, 1890, and written on paper from the Hôtel Scweizerhof.
Copyright Musée Charbonneau-Lassay, Ville de Loudun, with kind permission.

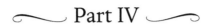

Part IV

Bibliography

$$\sim\!\!\sim 19 \sim\!\!\sim$$

Recapitulative List of All Gilles de la Tourette's Publications

GILLES DE LA Tourette was a precocious and prolific author. His first articles were written in 1881, when he was an *externe* and, later, a temporary *interne*. His first text, in *Le Progrès Médical*, concerned a state of apparent death in which certain Hindus, called "fakirs," immobilize themselves, undergoing training that Gilles de la Tourette described in detail. He already seemed fascinated by the study of paranormal behaviors, as he would be of hypnotism. For his second publication, once again in *Le Progrès Médical*, he translated articles from the *Medical Record* of August 20, 1881, and the *Philadelphia Times*. The subject was the health of the twentieth president of the United States, James Abram Garfield (1831–1881); the articles followed his assassination. Gilles de la Tourette read American newspapers not as divertissement, but to maintain his English language skills. (This worked in his favor for his nomination as Chief Physician for the 1900 World's Fair in Paris.) In November 1881, he translated the *New York Medical Record* to provide readers with details, illustrated by many drawings, of Garfield's autopsy. He continued by translating an article in the *Lancet* of May 13, 1882, describing the injuries that Lord Frederick Cavendish and M. Thomas Burke sustained after an anarchist murder in Dublin, Ireland, on May 6, 1882. He also provided a few short, unsigned translations from the *Medical Record* in *Le Progrès Médical*.

Aside from neurological and psychiatric diseases, Gilles de la Tourette wrote about a wide variety of subjects, including liver cancer, syphilitic psoriasis, varicose ulcers, clubfeet, the physician's emergency medical kit, a visit to the Saint-Hans asylum near Copenhagen, and the moving of the

Paris morgue to a new location. Some of his articles have titles that today seem shocking, such as *De la menstruation compensatrice par le conduit auditif externe,* which was a translation of an article by a certain Dr. Field, to which Gilles de la Tourette added his commentary. The article discussed compensatory menstruation via the outer ear canal and appeared in the *Medical Press* of February 8, 1882. Ignorance of the physiology of the menstrual cycle at the time led to every sort of speculation. One of the young amenorrheic women described probably had otitis resulting from a cholesteatoma. She bled periodically from the ear canal, and this symptom could not be explored with the technical means available at the time. Using simplistic logic, the physicians proposed that menstrual blood was being evacuated through the ear (demonstrating that there has always been a simple but false explanation for all diseases). Another young woman bled regularly from the veins in her face. The same explanation of "compensatory menstruation" was given. Was it superior vena cava syndrome, with periodic bleeding in the swollen veins of the face (possible compression of the superior vena cava due to mediastinal lymph node tuberculosis)?

From 1882 to 1901, Gilles de la Tourette regularly provided bibliographies—that is, reports on his readings in French and other languages. He did not limit himself in the way of subjects—covering everything from medical history to "medical geography"—in newspaper articles, doctoral theses, and books.

His biographies were remarkable for their form, their polished literary style, and their substance, which offered a generous wealth of historical information. The first, written in 1882 on François-Germain Lemercier (1818–1882), a physician and disciple, then a colleague of Louis Thomas Jérôme Auzoux (1797–1880), described these artisans of ingenious anatomical models.[1] The second covered the life and work of Adolphe Wurtz (1817–1884), a professor of biological and organic chemistry originally from Alsace who isolated organic alkaloids, glycols, and formaldehyde. This brief work revealed Gilles de la Tourette's considerable knowledge of chemistry. Wurtz was the dean of the Faculté de Médecine from 1865 to 1875 and played an important role in defending the rights and freedoms of university professors and students facing the inquisitorial measures of the imperial police before the Franco-Prussian War. Gilles de la Tourette took evident pride in relating Wurtz's conduct with the highest praise.[2] His third biography was on Amédée Blondeau (1848–1884), who was, like himself, from Loudun. Blondeau was a hero of the battles of Loigny-Poupry and Patay in 1870, and he had been mentioned by Louis Blanc (1811–1882) and Désiré-Magloire Bourneville (1840–1909). Like them, Blondeau had both the spirit of a powerful orator and a taste for journalism. He authored a thesis inspired by Bourneville and defended it before Charcot, on *"permanent bradycardia with syncopal and epileptoid attacks."*[3] Blondeau became an editor at *Le Progrès Médical,* a hothouse of progressive republicans where he and Gilles de la Tourette became friends.[4] The last two biographies, more so than the earlier works, reflect a high degree of genuine emotional involvement because they concern two of Gilles de la Tourette's beloved teachers, François Damaschino (1840–1889)[5] and Charcot,[6] who were his hospital colleagues as well as close friends.

Born to a family originally from Corfu, Damaschino was a brilliant student, *interne* in 1861, then *agrégé* in 1867. He was named to the Chair of Internal Pathology in 1874 after the premature death of Alexandre Axenfeld (1825–1876). Damaschino was a brilliant speaker and teacher, and his lessons demonstrated his *"profound erudition and the lucidity of his method of presentation."* His *Leçons sur les Maladies des voies digestives*[7] was considered a reference work for more than fifteen years. Gilles de la Tourette was his *interne* in 1883 and became a close friend; Damaschino was a witness at his wedding. Gilles de la Tourette had nothing but good things to say about him. In addition to presenting his neurological work, Gilles de la Tourette highlighted the fact that he was an innovator: *"The open-minded Damaschino was one of the first to follow the path of microbial research."*

Charcot wrote twenty-one prefaces in his lifetime, and Gilles de la Tourette was the only author who had the privilege of three of them. The first preface was for *Sœur Jeanne des Anges, supérieure des Ursulines de Loudun* (1886), written with Gabriel Legué (1857–1913). The second was for the German version of Gilles de la Tourette's treatise on hypnotism (1888): *Der Hypnotismus und die verwandten Zustände vom Standpunkte der gerichtlichen Medicin*; the French version was prefaced by Paul Brouardel. Finally, the third preface was for Gilles de la Tourette's 1891 *Traité clinique et thérapeutique de l'hystérie.*[8]

In 1888, Gilles de la Tourette, along with Paul Richer (1849–1933) and Albert Londe (1858–1917), founded *La Nouvelle Iconographie de La Salpêtrière,* under the direction of Charcot. Gilles de la Tourette's publications appeared in numerous journals—*Le Progrès Médical, Les Archives de Neurologie, La Nouvelle Iconographie de La Salpêtrière,* and *La Semaine Médicale*—which often featured identical articles. Some of the articles were made into booklets. It is likely that his name, like that of Charcot or Babiński, was taken as a sign of quality work and respectability when it appeared in the list of authors or editors for a medical journal; it evidently figures on the first page of *La Nouvelle Iconographie de La Salpêtrière,* but also on that of *Le Progrès Médical* and *Les Archives de Neurologie,* as well as the Belgian *Journal de neurologie et d'hypnologie* headed by Jean Crocq (1868–1925) and Xavier Francotte (1854–1931).

Theses

Gilles de la Tourette was only an *agrégé* and thus did not have the rank of a professor for overseeing thesis work. Here is a list, which may not be exhaustive, of the theses he inspired.

Alexandre Athanassio (1863–?)

> Athanassio A. *Des troubles trophiques dans l'hystérie*. Thèse no. 162. Paris: H. Jouve. 1890

Jacques Catrou (1865–?)

> Catrou J. *Etude sur la Maladie des Tics convulsifs*. Thèse no. 129. Paris: H. Jouve. 1890.

Jacques Artières (1863–1892)

> Artières J. *Etude des névralgies hystériques, en particulier de la névralgie faciale*. Thèse no. 335. Paris: H. Jouve. 1891.

Lucien Hudelo (1863–1955)

> Hudelo L. *Contribution à l'étude des lésions viscérales dans la syphilis héréditaire, Lésions du foie*. Thèse no. 120. Paris: G. Steinheil. 1890.

Arsène Bardol (1863–?).

> Bardol A. *De l'hystérie simulatrice des maladies organiques de l'encéphale chez les enfants*. Paris: L. Battaille et Cie. 1893.

André Bégué (1873–?)

> Bégué A. *Les consultations charitables de Théophraste Renaudot*. Thèse no. 137. Paris: JB. Baillière. 1899.

Georges Gasne (1868–1910)

> Gasne G. *Localisations spinales de la syphilis héréditaire*. Thèse no. 7. Paris: G. Steinhel. 1897. (Reviewed by J-B. Charcot in *Archives de Neurologie*. 1897;9(17):417–418).

Armand Schwanhard (1872–?)

> Schwanhard A. *Contribution à l'étude de la forme pseudo-tabétique de la myélite syphilitique*. Thèse no. 51. Paris: Carré et Naud. 1897.

As a co-author of articles, Gilles de la Tourette's name is associated with:

Paul Blocq (1860–1896)
Angelo Bolognesi (1857–?)
Fernand Bottey (1858–1900)
Henri Cathelineau (?)
Jean-Baptiste Charcot (1867–1936)
Antony Chipault (1866–1920)
Edouard Damain (1865–?)
Gustave Durante (1865–?)
Adolphe Dutil (1862–1929) (Figure 19.1)
Alfred Fournier (1832–1914)
Georges Gasne (1868–1910)
Lucien Hudelo (1863–1955)
Jean-Charles Kohne (1834–?)
Gabriel Legué (1857–1913)
Louis Magdelaine (1864–?)
Gheorghe Marinescu Georges Marinesco (1863–1938)
Henry Meige (1866–1940)
Aaron Zaguelmann (1860–?)

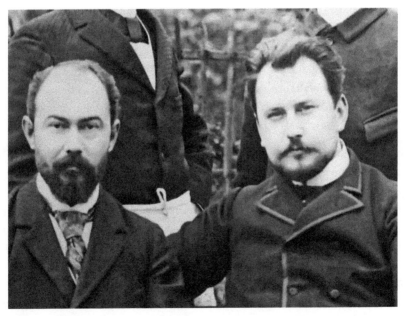

FIGURE 19.1 Pierre Janet (1859–1947), on left; Adolphe Dutil (1862–1929), on right in 1892.
Private collection of the author.

Books Written by Gilles de la Tourette

1884

Gilles de la Tourette G. *Théophraste Renaudot, d'après des documents inédits. La Gazette, Un essai de faculté libre au XVII*ᵉ *siècle, Le bureau d'adresses, Les Monts-de-piété, Les consultations charitables.* Paris: E. Plon, Nourrit. 1884.

1885

Gilles de la Tourette G. *Études cliniques et physiologiques sur la marche, la marche dans les maladies du système nerveux étudiée par la méthode des empreintes.* Thèse no. 84. Paris: Noizette. 1885.

Gilles de la Tourette G. *Études cliniques et physiologiques sur la marche, la marche dans les maladies du système nerveux étudiée par la méthode des empreintes.* Paris: Delahaye et Lecrosnier. 1885.

1886

Legué G, Gilles de la Tourette G. *Soeur Jeanne des Anges, supérieure des Ursulines de Loudun, XVIIe siècle, autobiographie d'une hystérique possédée, d'après le manuscrit inédit de la bibliothèque de Tours. (Préface de M. le Professeur Charcot.)* Bibliothèque diabolique. Collection Bourneville. Paris: Progrès médical et A. Delahaye et Lecrosnier. 1886.

Brouardel P, Gilles de la Tourette G. La mort de Charles IX. In A. Franklin (ed.), *Les grandes scènes historiques du XVI*ᵉ *siècle: reproduction fac-similé du recueil de J. Tortorel et J. Perrissin (1569–1570).* Paris: Librairie Fischbacher. 1886. 8 p.

Brouardel and Gilles de la Tourette discussed the last weeks in the life of Charles IX. They described the fatal progression of his disease, which strongly suggests pulmonary tuberculosis, as confirmed by the autopsy. All of information available to them ruled out the hypothesis of poisoning. They underscored the role of heredity in the death of Charles IX by tuberculosis at twenty-three years of age, citing the death of his grandfather, Henry IV, from syphilis. The historical interest of this chapter lies in its summary and translation of the autopsy conducted by the king's physician, Dr. Mazille, originally written in Latin. These elements give some idea of medical knowledge in the sixteenth century, as well as nineteenth-century interpretations.

1887

Gilles de la Tourette G. *L'hypnotisme et les états analogues au point de vue médico-légal, les états hypnotiques et les états analogues, les suggestions criminelles, cabinets de somnambules et sociétés de magnétisme et de spiritisme, l'hypnotisme devant la loi. (Préface de M. le Dr P. Brouardel.)* Paris: E. Plon-Nourrit. 1887.

1888

Gilles de la Tourette G. *L'ipnotismo e gli stati analoghi sotto l'aspetto medico-legale. Con prefazioni dei Professori Brouardel e Charcot; Versione italiana del Dott. Luigi Bufalini.* Milano: L. Vallardi. 1888.

Gilles de La Tourette G. *Dell'influenza di una intossicazione o di una malattia anteriore sulla localizzazione e sulla forma dei fenomeni isterici. (Clinica delle malattie nervose alla Salpetriere, prof. M. Charcot.)* Napoli-Milano: Dott. Leonardo Vallardi Edit., 1888.

Gilles de la Tourette G, Blocq P, Huet E. *Cinq cas de maladie de Friedreich. (Extrait de la Nouvelle Iconographie de La Salpêtriere.)* Paris: S-L, Imprimerie Réunies. 1888.

1889

Gilles de la Tourette G. *Der Hypnotismus und die verwandten Zustände vom Standpunkte der gerichtlichen Medicin. (Préface de JM. Charcot.)* Hamburg: Richter. 1889.

Gilles de la Tourette G. *L'Hypnotisme et les états analogues au point de vue médico-légal. (Préface de M. le Dr P. Brouardel.)* 2e édition. Paris: Plon-Nourrit. 1889.

Gilles de la Tourette G. *François Damaschino.* Paris: Lecrosnier et Babé. 1889.

Richer P, Gilles de la Tourette G. L'hypnotisme. In A. Dechambre, L. Lereboullet (eds.), *Dictionnaire Encyclopédique des Sciences Médicales.* Paris: Asselin et Houzeau, G. Masson. 1889.

1890

Gilles de la Tourette G, Cathelineau H. *La nutrition dans l'hystérie.* Paris: Le Progrès médical. 1890.

Charcot JM. *Œuvres complètes—T III. Leçons sur les maladies du système nerveux, recueillies et publiées par Babiński J, Bernard A, Féré Ch, Guinon G, Marie P et Gilles de la Tourette G*. Paris: Bureaux du Progrès Médical; A. Delhaye & E. Lecrosnier. 1890.

1891

Gilles de la Tourette G. *L'Épilogue d'un procès célèbre (affaire Eyraud-Bompard)*. Paris: E. Lecrosnier et Babé. 1891.

Gilles de la Tourette G. *Traité clinique et thérapeutique de l'hystérie d'après l'enseignement de la Salpêtrière. (Préface de M. le Dr JM Charcot.)* 1, Hystérie normale ou interparoxystique. Paris: Plon. 1891.

Gilles de la Tourette G, Meige H. *Le procès criminel de Gaufridi, curé des Accoules à Marseille, 1611. Manuscript of 500 pages 1891, now missing, but Henry Meige publishes a book with the same title in 1936, without naming Gilles de la Tourette: Meige H. Gaufridy, le curé des Accoules.* Paris, Gallimard. 1936.

1892

Gilles de la Tourette G. *Exposé des titres et travaux scientifiques du Dr Gilles de La Tourette*. Paris: Impr. de Plon-Nourrit. 1892.

Gilles de la Tourette G. *La vie et les œuvres de Théophraste Renaudot fondateur du journalisme et des consultations charitables. En vente au bénéfice de la statue*. Edition du Comité. 1892. (Figure 19.2)

Gilles de la Tourette G. *Un essai de Faculté libre au XVIIᵉ siècle. Théophraste Renaudot*. (Association française pour l'avancement des sciences (1872–1892). 13 février 1892. Organisation du congrès. Paris: Imprimerie Chaix. 1892.

1895

Gilles de la Tourette G. *Traité clinique et thérapeutique de l'hystérie, d'après l'enseignement de la Salpêtrière. (Préface de M. le Pr. J.-M. Charcot.)* 2, Hystérie paroxystique. Paris: E. Plon-Nourrit. 1895.

1897

Gilles de la Tourette G, Chipault A. *Le traitement de l'ataxie par l'élongation vraie de la moelle*. Paris: Rueff. 1897.

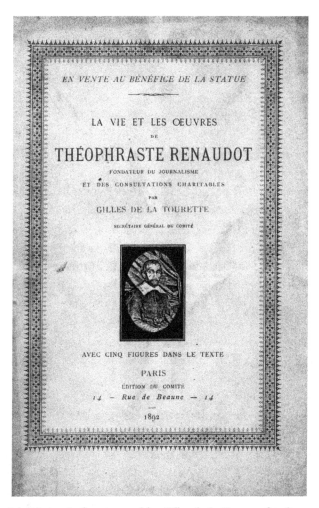

EN VENTE AU BÉNÉFICE DE LA STATUE

LA VIE ET LES OEUVRES
DE
THÉOPHRASTE RENAUDOT
FONDATEUR DU JOURNALISME
ET DES CONSULTATIONS CHARITABLES
PAR
GILLES DE LA TOURETTE
SECRÉTAIRE GÉNÉRAL DU COMITÉ

AVEC CINQ FIGURES DANS LE TEXTE

PARIS
ÉDITION DU COMITÉ
14 — Rue de Beaune — 14

1892

FIGURE 19.2 Subscription leaflet proposed by Gilles de la Tourette for the erection of the Renaudot memorial in Paris.
Private collection of the author.

1898

Gilles de la Tourette G. *Leçons de clinique thérapeutique sur les maladies du système nerveux: hémorragie cérébrale, états neurasthéniques, épilepsie, hystérie, tic douloureux et migraine, morphinomanie, vertige de Ménière, pieds bots, myélites syphilitiques, ataxie locomotrice.* Paris: E. Plon-Nourrit. 1898.

Gilles de la Tourette G. *Les états neurasthéniques, formes cliniques-diagnostic-traitement.* Paris: JB. Baillière. 1898.

Gilles de la Tourette started by mocking the name of the disease in question: *"Ever more comprehensive,* [neurasthenia] *is too often used to mask diagnostic errors."* In a brief historical overview, he criticized George Beard (1839–1883) for his lack of familiarity with French authors, especially Jean-Louis Brachet (1789–1858), and highlighted, as he always did, Charcot's important role in the dissemination of knowledge. After describing the neurasthenic headache, Gilles de la Tourette covered insomnia and gave a rather detailed description of what is today isolated as restless legs syndrome. *"They were prey to a thousand sensations, each more bothersome than the next. They were agitated, tossing and turning in their beds, with trouble notably in their lower limbs: flashes of pain, tingling sensations, prickly sensations, and generalized itching. And they always ended up feeling numb, which was very distressing to them. . . . Many of them, when moving from wakefulness to sleep, experienced sudden jerking in their lower limbs."* A little later, using the term "vertigo," he described what was probably orthostatic hypotension: *"It is a sensation of cerebral blankness accompanied by weakness in the lower limbs, which tend to collapse under the body's weight. A veil forms before the eyes; everything is gray and dull. In the visual field, there are black spots, flying specks, and nearby or distant objects blend into the same plane. These last phenomena are related to marked accommodative asthenopia, which seems to favor this vertiginous state."* Gilles de la Tourette reviewed all of the functional, digestive, cardiac, urinary, and sexual symptoms. Paradoxically, he did not devote much description to the psychological state; his hope was to distinguish and isolate a particular hereditary form, for which he said his inspiration came from Charcot. For Gilles de la Tourette, neurasthenia *"was an etiological classification, strictly speaking."* Constitutional neurasthenia is noteworthy for the absence of a life element triggering the disease, and, in Gilles de la Tourette's description, it strangely resembles hypochondria. Finally, it is interesting to read the chapter on differential diagnosis in which he mentions general paralysis —*"the role of syphilis is still debatable, at least in the etiology of true general paralysis"*—to which he would succumb five years later. Treatment for neurasthenia included hydrotherapy (i.e., *"cold showers on the trunk using a jet shower head"*); static electricity and potassium bromide in small evening doses; diet, of course; and, finally, *"moral treatment,"* which might involve *"travel to a Mediterranean French colony."*

1899

Gilles de la Tourette G. *Formes cliniques et traitement des myélites syphilitiques.* Paris: JB. Baillière. 1899.

This book is the reproduction of chapter IX of his book Leçons de clinique thérapeutique sur les maladies du système nerveux, published in 1898. "It is essentially a practical question; I am certainly underestimating in stating that, of any ten spinal conditions one sees, more than half of them have syphilis as their immediate cause. I do not include tabes in this count; doing so would singularly increase the proportion." He was thus referring to a disease in which the diagnosis of acquired syphilis is certain and requires anti-syphilitic treatment, "contrary to tabes." This subject had been thoroughly studied by others before him, notably Henri Lamy in his 1893 thesis[9] and Jules Ladreit de Lacharrière (1833–1903).[10] Gilles de la Tourette reviewed the clinical aspects of acute and chronic myelitis and syphilitic Brown-Séquard syndromes. He cited the syphilitic spasmodic spinal paraplegia described by the German physician Wilhelm Heinrich Erb (1840–1921) to point out that his teacher, Charcot, had already isolated it in 1880,[11] even though Charcot had clearly noted the contribution of Erb! Gilles de la Tourette did not fail to mention the thesis of his student, Armand Schwanhard (1872–?), and he finished with a discussion of the use of mercury in treatment.

1900

Gilles de la Tourette G. *Les états neurasthéniques, formes cliniques, diagnostic, traitement.* 2ème ed., revue et augmentée. Paris: JB. Baillière. 1900.

Gilles de la Tourette G, Charcot JB. *Le syndrome de Benedikt.* Paris: La Semaine Médicale. 1900.

In 1900, Gilles de la Tourette and Jean-Baptiste Charcot published an article on Benedikt syndrome in the journal *La Semaine Médicale* that was separately published as a booklet shortly thereafter. After summarizing the three observations initially described by Moriz Benedikt (1835–1920), Gilles de la Tourette and Charcot noted that, on February 24, 1893, Jean-Martin Charcot gave a lesson *"in which, reviewing the observations of the Viennese physician, he described oculomotor nerve palsy, accompanied by crossed hemiplegia with shaking, under the name of Benedikt syndrome. He presented his students with a man suffering from this syndrome. This case, the fourth to date to our knowledge, has remained almost completely unknown, since nothing was published about our Master's lesson but a short summary in* La Médecine Moderne. *Noting the similarity between this manifestation and Weber's syndrome, which he had already helped describe, Charcot identified its place among crossed palsies. . . . We have in our possession the many documents collected by Professor Charcot for this lesson, and we drew extensively from them to prepare this work."* Charcot's son was *chef de clinique* (senior house officer or resident) under Prof. Raymond at La Salpêtrière at that time and was treating two patients with the syndrome (Figure 19.3). In these two new cases, for which they gave the observations in this article, Gilles de la Tourette and Charcot looked for the plantar reflex, but did not name it the Babiński sign. Charcot had coined the eponym "Benedikt syndrome"[12] to pay tribute to his friend Benedikt, who published the first case in French in 1889 in *Le Bulletin Médical*.[13] *"At his clinical lesson on February 21, Professor Charcot presented a patient exhibiting a set of symptoms for which he proposed the name of Benedikt syndrome."*[14]

In his library, Charcot kept thirty-eight offprints from works published by Benedikt. This was a sign of their regular exchange, as Charcot did not have as many offprints from any of his other foreign correspondents. When Freud introduced himself to Charcot on October 20, 1885, he came with a letter of introduction that Charcot at once recognized as written by Benedikt from the address on the envelope. Finally, in 1889, Charcot agreed to write a preface for the very controversial book on cranial-cephalic anthropometry

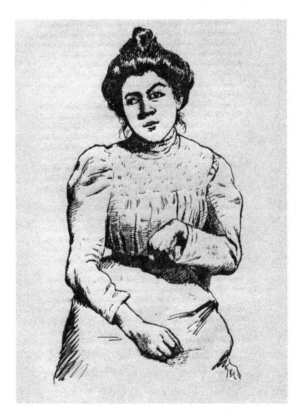

FIGURE 19.3 Benedikt syndrome or paramedian midbrain syndrome; drawing by Paul Richer (1849–1933).
Private collection of the author.

written by Benedikt.[15] Benedikt syndrome is rare and currently almost always secondary to an ischemic cerebrovascular accident, whereas several of the observations presented by Gilles de la Tourette and Charcot were the result of tuberculomas in children. In addition to the discussion of paralysis, the book provides an interesting discussion of the cause of the shaking. Considered *"as intermediary between shaking in hemichorea and hemiathetosis,"* this shaking *"seems always to be exaggerated in voluntary movement,"* which led Gilles de la Tourette and Charcot to compare it, and rightly so, to shaking in multiple sclerosis, but they noted it was caused by *"damage to the pyramidal tract"* rather than to cerebellar pathways. Babiński did inaugural work on the cerebellum, but cerebellar syndrome would not be isolated until 1904, by Gordon Morgan Holmes (1875–1963),[16] and in 1911, by André Thomas (1867–1963).[17]

1901

Gilles de la Tourette G. *Le traitement pratique de l'épilepsie, dose suffisante de bromure, signe de la pupille.* Paris: JB. Baillière. 1901.

The book's introduction attempted to explain epilepsy. This section situates the concepts of the day, of which Gilles de la Tourette wrote: *"One might think that the cerebral lesion liable to result in epileptic convulsions must have a particular quality to produce the seizures. This is possible in certain cases, but I think it preferable to adopt another interpretation, more applicable, in my opinion, to the generality of the facts. It is true that there are still many unknowns in this question of cerebral pathogenesis. What is certain is this: children or adults, following a difficult delivery, infantile convulsions, or arteritis, can suffer brain lesions (as evidenced by persistent hemiplegia in certain cases), but many of them do not have and will never have epileptic seizures, whereas other subjects with similar lesions, or for whom it is possible to suppose as much, will immediately or at a later time become epileptic. In these conditions, the particular quality liable to produce seizures must be attributed to the cerebral substance itself. We are familiar with this quality. In the normal state, the habitual movements of our muscles are dependent upon the excitatory-motor function of the brain. When there is exultation without appreciable lesions, in hysteria for example, or during experimental maneuvers in animals and humans, or when spiked scar tissue forms, followed by epilepsy, this function generates convulsive accidents. Epileptic seizures in these circumstances must therefore be attributed to the exaggeration, the exaltation of the excitatory-motor function of the brain, to its hyperexcitability; in reality, the various causes that we have just cited only play the role of triggering agents."* If epilepsy is due to "hyperexcitability," then reducing it would prevent seizures. The reference treatment at that time was potassium bromide: *"That is what must be applied with perseverance."* Gilles de la Tourette recommended prolonged treatment over several years—regular usage without omission—*"in a family environment"* to ensure compliance, since it is *"a little repugnant"* and often poorly tolerated. Gilles de la Tourette insisted on precisely measuring the dose for each administration (Figure 19.4). He even suggested a graduated glass and gave the name of the pharmacist who sold it. The dose must be *"sufficient,"* which is to say high, with gradual increase in dosage. Gilles de la Tourette proposed *"the sign of the pupil,"* believing he was the first to describe it (a possible symptom of megalomania from his disease); the sufficient dose is obtained if the pupil is dilated with response to light and accommodation. This dose, close to intoxication, is then reduced until *"a lazy reaction in the pupil"* is obtained. Finally, Gilles de la Tourette discussed secondary effects, especially intoxication—during which the patient *"smells like bromide"*—and bromic acne. Status epilepticus called for bromide enemas. Considering his approach particularly effective, he recommended it, after testing it, with other indications: Ménière's disease, disabling migraine, and trigeminal neuralgia. The Loudun archives contain a letter from Henri Lamy

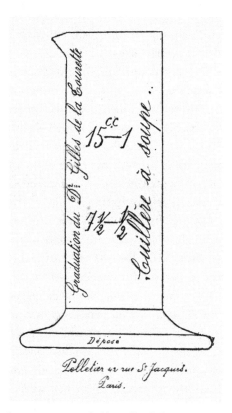

FIGURE 19.4 Bromine dosing recommended by Gilles de la Tourette.
Private collection of the author.

(1864–1909) responding to a request Gilles de la Tourette had sent to Lamy's father-in-law, Charles-Émile François-Franck (1849–1921):

Dear Mr. Gilles, You asked my father-in-law for bibliographic information regarding his research on arterial pressure variations in epilepsy. Since he was busy at the time, and since I am familiar with this bibliography, he asked me to answer you. I have been away. There was a meeting. I admit I have been remiss in responding to you. I believe you will find all of what you are looking for in his 1884–1885 Collège de France lessons[18] (Doin), in particular lessons 19.21. They contain what is important to know on the cardiac and vasomotor effects and on perfusion (I agree with you, no external convulsions). Please feel free to ask if you need more detailed information. Best regards, Paris, August 18, 1900.

1902

Gilles de la Tourette et Gasne. Hystérie, Hypnotisme. In P. Brouardel, A. Gilbert, J Girode. *Traité de médecine et de thérapeutique. Tome 10, Maladies des nerfs périphériques.* Névroses. Maladies des muscles par MM. Pitres, Vaillard, Gilles de la Tourette, Gasne, Grasset, Rauzier, Triboulet, Lannois, Lamy, Sainton, Brissaud, Marinesco. Paris: JB. Baillière. 1902.

1985

Gilles de la Tourette G. Legué G. *Sœur Jeanne des Anges. Suivi de Jeanne des Anges par Michel de Certeau.* Montbonnot-Saint-Martin: J. Millon. 1985.

1990

Gilles de la Tourette G. Legué G. *Autobiographie, Soeur Jeanne des Anges. (Préface de J.-M. Charcot.)* Suivi de Jeanne des Anges, par Michel de Certeau. 2ᵉ éd. corrigée. Grenoble, J. Millon. 1990.
Unpublished manuscripts (cannot currently be found). *La folie dans le Théâtre antique et moderne et le crime passionnel contemporain.*

Articles Published in Journals Other Than *Le Progrès Médical* and *La Nouvelle Iconographie de La Salpêtrière*

1881

Gilles de la Tourette G. Cancer primitif du foie. *Bulletin de la Société Anatomique de Paris*. Mars 1881;56:254–257.

During his temporary *internat* with Landouzy at Hôtel Dieu, Gilles de la Tourette treated a fifty-eight-year old woman, mother of fourteen children (two surviving; all of the others had died at a young age) suffering from anorexia, weight loss, pain in the right hypochondrium, then icterus, refractory constipation, and continual vomiting. The examination revealed a large mass that could be felt under the ribs on the right. After a fever, she died. Gombault's anatomical-pathological results pointed to non-epitheliomatous cancer.

Gilles de la Tourette G. Rotation et déviation conjuguées de la tête et des yeux du côté droit; hémiplégie et hémianesthésie droite; contracture du bras gauche, sans anesthésie. Absence de lésion cérébrale, cérébelleuse et médullaire. Petit faisceau de sclérose bulbaire d'ancienne date. *Bulletin de la Société Anatomique de Paris*. 1881;56:618.

Gilles de la Tourette G. Gomme syphilitique de la 1ère circonvolution frontale gauche empiétant légèrement sur le lobule paracentral avec hémiplégie droite sans hémianesthésie. Rotation et déviation conjuguée de la tête et des yeux. Aphasie. *Bulletin de la Société Anatomique de Paris*. 7 octobre 1881;56:569–571.

A thirty-four-year-old woman hospitalized at Hôpital de la Pitié, under the care of Prof. Cornil.

Gilles de la Tourette G. Deux noyaux séparés, pesant 6 grammes, représentant l'utérus, chez une jeune fille de 18 ans non réglée. *Bulletin de la Société Anatomique de Paris*. 1881;56:619.620.

This young woman with primary amenorrhea died of acute miliary tuberculosis. Gilles de la Tourette autopsied her. He found two normal ovaries, two fallopian tubes, an anterior nucleus representing the cervix, and a posterior nucleus representing the uterine body. He described the syndrome isolated by Karl-Freiherr von Rokitansky (1804–1878),[19] in 1838, and August Mayer (1787–1865),[20] in 1829, which was the cause of primary amenorrhea due to malformation and known as Rokitansky-Mayer-Küster-Hauser syndrome. He did not, however, cite his predecessors. Was this intentional?

1882

Gilles de la Tourette G. Note sur les injections sous-cutanées d'iodure de potassium. *Comptes Rendu hebdomadaires des Séances et Mémoires de la société de Biologie.* 1882;34:853–857.

"When I left Hôpital de Lourcine at the end of November 1882, Dr. Gougenheim, under whom I had been an interne, *suggested to me the idea of subcutaneous injections of potassium iodide, an alternative to oral treatment for syphilis."*

1884

Gilles de la Tourette G, Bottey F. Note sur un cas de sialorrhée d'origine nerveuse. *Comptes Rendus hebdomadaires des Séances et Mémoires de la Société de Biologie.* 1884;36:137–140.

Gilles de la Tourette G, Richer P. Sur les caractères cliniques des paralysies psychiques expérimentales. *Comptes Rendus hebdomadaires des Séances et Mémoires de la Société de Biologie.* 1884;36:198–200.

Gilles de la Tourette G. Un anévrysme de l'aorte ouvert dans une bronche. *Comptes Rendus hebdomadaires des Séances et Mémoires de la société de Biologie.* 1884;36:356.

1885

Gilles de la Tourette G. Présente une pièce osseuse. Ancienne fracture tibia –péroné par balles survenue au cours de la guerre de 1870. Volumineux cal spontanée enchâssant des débris de balles. *Bulletin de la Société Anatomique de Paris.* 1885:60:135.

Gilles de la Tourette G. Young woman; sudden death after miscarriage. Splenic infarct, vegetation masses at the edges of the mitral valves. Infectious endocarditis. *Bulletin de la Société Anatomique de Paris.* 1885:60:155.

Gilles de la Tourette G. Cancer du foie. *Bulletin de la Société Anatomique de Paris.* 1885;60:177.

Session on March 27, 1885, page 177. Liver cancer in a man aged seventy-five; death was the consequence of massive abdominal hemorrhage; presence of pancreatic cancerous mass blocking the ampulla of Vater. A nodule on the posterior side of the liver that was probably metastatic broke, resulting in the mortal hemorrhage.

1886

Gilles de la Tourette G. Traitement du psoriasis syphilitique par les bains locaux de sublimé. *La Semaine Médicale*. 1886;6(28):285.

Gilles de la Tourette G. Le viol dans l'hypnotisme et les états analogues. *La Semaine Médicale*. 1886;6(31):310.

Gilles de la Tourette G. Le viol dans l'hypnotisme. Séance du 2 août 1886. *Bulletin de la Société de Médecine Légale*. 1886–87;9:380–399.

Gilles de la Tourette G. Le viol dans l'hypnotisme et les états analogues. *Annales d'hygiène publique et de médecine légale*. 1886;16(3ᵉ série):445–464.

Gilles de la Tourette G. De la guérison des grands ulcères de jambe par les pulvérisations phéniquées. *Revue de Chirurgie*. 1886;6:575–582.

Gilles de la Tourette G. Contribution à la détermination de la nature microbienne des efflorescences cutanées d'origine syphilitiques, du traitement du psoriasis palmaire et plantaire par les bains locaux de sublimé. Séance du 17 juillet 1886 Société de Biologie. *Comptes Rendus hebdomadaires des Séances et Mémoires de la Société de Biologie*. 1886;38:365–370.

1887

Gilles de la Tourette G, Blocq P. Sur le traitement de la migraine ophtalmique. *Comptes Rendu hebdomadaires des Séances et Mémoires de la société de Biologie*. Séance du 4 juin 1887;39:361–364.

A case of ophthalmic migraine relieved by potassium bromide treatment.

Gilles de la Tourette G. Le viol dans l'hypnotisme et les états analogues. Société de Médecine Légale. Séance du 2 août 1886. *Bulletin Société de Médecine Légale*. 1887;9:380–399.

1888

Gilles de la Tourette G. Des attaques de sommeil hystérique. *Archives de Neurologie*. 1888;15(43):92–107; 1888;15(44):266–300.

Gilles de la Tourette G. Réponse au Dr Vibert. Etude médico-légale sur les blessures produites par les accidents de chemins de fer. Séance du 9 avril 1888. *Bulletin de la Société de Médecine Légale*. 1888–89;10:170–171.

Gilles de la Tourette G. Traumatisme de la moelle par arme à feu. Séance du 11 juin 1888. *Bulletin de la Société de Médecine Légale*. 1888–89;10:175–179

Gilles de la Tourette G. Dangers de l'hypnotisme et interdiction des représentations théâtrales. Séance du 10 décembre 1888. *Bulletin de la Société de Médecine Légale.* 1888–89;10:252–255

Gilles de la Tourette G. Blessures produites par les accidents de chemins de fer. Réponse à Ch. Vibert. *Archives de l'Anthropologie criminelle et des Sciences pénales.* 1888;3:296– 297.

Gilles de la Tourette G. Dell'influenza di una intossicazione o di una malattia anteriore sulla localizzazione e sulla forma dei fenomeni isterici (Clinica delle malattie nervose alla salpetriere, prof. M. Charcot). Il Morgagni. Napoli-Milano, Dott. Leonardo Vallardi Edit. 1888.

1889

Gilles de la Tourette G. Bibliographie. Liégeois J. De la suggestion et du somnambulisme dans leurs rapports avec la jurisprudence et la médecine légale. Paris: O Doin. 1889. *Archives de Neurologie.* 1889;17(49):156–161.

Gilles de la Tourette G. Diminution et cessation de l'usage habituel de la morphine chez deux tabétiques traités par la suspension. *Archives de Neurologie.* 1889;18(52):126–128.

Gilles de la Tourette G. Séance du 9 avril 1888. Réponse à M. Vibert, Etude médico-légale sur les blessures produites par les accidents de chemin de fer. *Bulletin Société de Médecine Légale.* 1889;10:170.

Gilles de la Tourette G. Traumatisme de la moelle par arme à feu. *Bulletin Société de Médecine Légale.* 1889;10:175–179.

Gilles de la Tourette G. Dangers de l'hypnotisme et interdiction des représentations théâtrales. *Bulletin Société de Médecine Légale.* 1889;10:252–255.

Guinon G. Congrès International de Médecine Légale. Paris 19 au 24 août 1889. De l'influence des traumatismes sur le développement des maladies nerveuses. Controverse entre M. Gilles de la Tourette et M. Vibert. *Archives de Neurologie.* 1889;18(53):293–294.

Gilles de la Tourette G. Réponse au Dr. Bernheim. Valeur relative des divers procédés destinés à provoquer l'hypnose et à augmenter la suggestibilité au point de vue thérapeutique. *La Semaine Médicale.* 1889;9:283.

Gilles de la Tourette G. Congres international de Médecine Légale du 19 au 24 aout 1889. Les traumatismes cérébraux et médullaires dans leurs rapports avec la médecine légale. *La Semaine Médicale.* 1889;9:305.

Gilles de la Tourette G. Congrès international de l'hypnotisme expérimental. Paris, du 8 au 12 août 1889. Rapports de la suggestion et du somnambulisme avec la jurisprudence et la médecine légale, la responsabilité dans les états hypnotiques. *La Semaine Médicale.* 1889;9:327.

Gilles de la Tourette G. De la fièvre dans le goitre exophtalmique. *La Semaine Médicale.* 1889;9:450.

1890

Gilles de la Tourette G. L'automatisme ambulatoire au point de vue médico-légal. Séance du 11 mars 1889. *Bulletin Société de Médecine Légale.* 1890;11:37.

Gilles de la Tourette G. Ecchymoses spontanées état mental des hystériques. Séance 10 mars 1890. *Bulletin de la Société de Médecine Légale.* 1890;11:306–310.

Gilles de la Tourette G, Cathelineau H. La nutrition dans l'hystérie. Séance 14 avril 1890. Compte-rendu de la séance de l'Académie des Sciences. *La Semaine Médicale.* 1890;10:136.

1891

Gilles de la Tourette G. Les zones hystérogènes de l'œil et la migraine ophtalmique d'origine hystérique. *Annales d'oculistique.* 1891;54:266–274.

Gilles de la Tourette G. Une Bibliographie de *"Anatomie artistique— Description des formes extérieures du corps humain au repos et dans les principaux mouvements"* de Paul Richer. Paris: Plon & Nourrit. 1890. *Archives de Neurologie.* 1891;21(61):148–150.

Gilles de la Tourette G, Cathelineau H. Le sang dans l'hystérie normale. Séance du 14 février 1891 de la Société de Biologie. *La Semaine Médicale.* 1891;11:65.

Gilles de la Tourette G. *De l'utilité de l'examen des urines avant la trépanation pour phénomènes d'épilepsie partielle.* Congrès de chirurgie. Paris: Germer-Baillière. 1891.

1892

Gilles de la Tourette G. Hudelo L. Syphilis maligne précoce du système nerveux. *Annales de Dermatologie et Syphiligraphie.* 1892;3(3ᵉ série): 686–689; 705–709.

Gilles de la Tourette G. Syphlis maligne précoce du système nerveux. Société de dermatologie et syphiligraphie. Séance du 9 juin 1892. *La Semaine Médicale*. 1892;12:238.

Gilles de la Tourette G. Note sur un cas de syphilis héréditaire tardive bulbo-médullaire. *Annales de Dermatologie et Syphiligraphie*. 1892;3(3ᵉ série):845–848.

Gilles de la Tourette G. Syphilis nerveuse. Séance du 7 juillet 1892 de la Société de Dermatologie et Syphiligraphie. *La Semaine Médicale*. 1892;12:279.

Gilles de la Tourette G. Des renseignements fournis par l'analyse des urines dans le diagnostic des variétés d'épilepsie partielle. *La Semaine Médicale*. 1892;12:161.

Gilles de la Tourette G. Deux cas de névrose traumatique chez de très jeunes enfants. Réponse à Ch Vibert. Séance du 13 juin 1892. *Bulletin de la Société de Médecine légale*. 1892;12:253–254.

1893

Gilles de la Tourette G, Damain E. Un danseur monomane. Séance du 9 janvier 1893. *Bulletin de la Société de Médecine Légale*. 1893–94;13:13–20

Gilles de la Tourette G, Cathelineau H. La formule chimique de l'attaque hystérique. Séance du 4 février 1893. Société de Biologie. *La Semaine Médicale*. 1893;13:56.

Gilles de la Tourette G, Cathelineau H. La nutrition dans l'hystérie. *Comptes Rendu hebdomadaires des Séances et Mémoires de la société de Biologie*. 1893;45:127–129.

Gilles de la Tourette G. Sein hystérique et tumeurs hystériques de la mamelle. Septième Congrès de Chirurgie du 3 au 8 avril 1893 à Paris. *La Semaine Médicale*. 1893;13:182.

1894

Gilles de la Tourette G. Un cas de paroxysme hystérique à forme de névralgie faciale. Séance du 2 mars 1894. *Bulletins et Mémoires Société Médicale des Hôpitaux de Paris*. 1894;11(13ᵉ série):147–152.

Gilles de la Tourette G. Pourquoi appeler 'pseudo éléphantiasis névropathique' un œdème survenu chez une hystérique confirmée. Réponse à M. Thibierge. Séance du 27 avril 1894. *Bulletins et Mémoires de la Société médicale des Hôpitaux de Paris*. 1894;11(13ᵉ série):267–268.

Gilles de la Tourette G. Réponse au Dr J. Comby. Apoplexie hystérique avec hémiplégie gauche survenue pour la première fois à la suite d'une fulguration; troisième attaque; guérison en moins de quinze jours par le repos et l'électrisation. Séance du 25 mai 1894. *Bulletins et Mémoires Société Médicale des Hôpitaux de Paris.* 1894;11(13ᵉ série):349–350.

Gilles de la Tourette discussed the existence of bulbar hemorrhages after the patient was struck by lightning. Henry Duret (1849–1921) had described these hemorrhages (Duret hemorrhages) in his 1874 thesis, of which Gilles de la Tourette was apparently unaware.

Gilles de la Tourette G, Marinesco G. Note sur l'anatomie pathologique de l'ostéite déformante de Paget. Séance du 15 juin 1894. *Bulletins et Mémoires Société Médicale des Hôpitaux de Paris.* 1894;30:422–427.

Gilles de la Tourette G. L'ulcère rond de l'estomac dans les Hôpitaux de Paris. Pathogénie et statistique. Séance du 15 juin 1894. *Bulletins et Mémoires Société Médicale des Hôpitaux de Paris.* 1894;11(13ᵉ série):393–408.

1895

Gilles de la Tourette G. Chorée récidivante devenue chronique par hérédité similaire. Séance du 5 avril 1895. Société Médicale des Hôpitaux de Paris. *La Semaine Médicale.* 1895;15:15.

Gilles de la Tourette G, Gasne G. Sur l'intoxication chronique par le café. Séance du 12 juillet 1895 de la Société Médicale des Hôpitaux. *La Semaine Médicale.* 1895;15:306.

Gilles de la Tourette G. Diagnostic et traitement de l'épilepsie. *La Semaine Médicale.* 1895;15:437–439.

1896

Gilles de la Tourette G, Chipault A. La phase radiculaire des névrites ascendantes traumatiques. *La Presse Médicale.* 1896;4(46):269–270.

Gilles de la Tourette G. A propos du méningisme. Société médicale des Hôpitaux du 10 janvier 1896. *La Semaine Médicale.* 1896;16:27.

Gilles de la Tourette G. Les troubles trophiques viscéraux dans l'hystérie. Société médicale des Hôpitaux du 29 mai 1896. *La Semaine Médicale.* 1896;16:221.

Gilles de la Tourette G. Diagnostic et traitement du tic douloureux de la face et de la migraine. *La Semaine Médicale.* 1896;16(32):249–252.

Gilles de la Tourette G. Pathogénie et traitement des pieds bots. *La Semaine Médicale.* 1896;16:517–522.

1897

Gilles de la Tourette G, Chipault A. Die wirkliche Dehnung des Rückenmarkes und ihre Anwendung zur Behandlung der Tabes dorsalis. *Therapeutische Wochenschrift.* 1897;4(19):459–462; 1303–1304.

Gilles de la Tourette G. Pathogénie et prophylaxie de l'atrophie musculaire et des douleurs des hémiplégiques. Séance du 9 avril 1897 de la Société Médicale des Hôpitaux. *La Semaine Médicale.* 1897;17:130–131.

Gilles de la Tourette G. De l'élongation vraie de la moelle épinière comme moyen de traitement de l'ataxie locomotrice. Séance du 27 avril 1897 de la Société Médicale des Hôpitaux. *La Semaine Médicale.* 1897;17:149.

Gilles de la Tourette G. Le vertige de Ménière et son traitement. *La Semaine Médicale.* 1897;17:301–306.

Gilles de la Tourette G. Traitement de l'ataxie locomotrice par l'élongation vraie de la moelle épinière. Séance du 7 décembre 1897 à l'académie Nationale de Médecine. *La Semaine Médicale.* 1897;17:452

Gilles de la Tourette G. De l'incontinence d'urines et des matières fécales dans les paraplégies liées aux névrites alcooliques. Séance du 1 décembre 1897 de la Société Médicale des Hôpitaux. *La Semaine Médicale.* 1897;17:461.

1898

Gilles de la Tourette G. Les neurologistes contemporains, Paul Richer. *Archives de Neurologie.* 1898;6(34):347–348.

Gilles de la Tourette G. Diagnostic et pronostic de l'hémorragie cérébrale et des états apoplectiques. *La Semaine Médicale.* 1898;17(32)257–259.

Gilles de la Tourette G. Diagnostic et traitement des états neurasthéniques. *La Semaine Médicale.* 1898;18(16):121–124.

Gilles de la Tourette G. Présente un rapport médico légal du Dr Edgar Gravery. Séance du 12 décembre 1898. *Bulletin de la Société de Médecine Légale.* 1898;15:361.

1899

Gilles de la Tourette G, Chipault A. De la percussion méthodique du crâne; contribution au diagnostic cranio-encéphalique. *Gazette des hôpitaux civils et militaires.* 1899;71:342.

Gilles de la Tourette G. Lèpre et syringomyélie. Séance du 10 février 1899 de la Société Médicale des Hôpitaux. *La Semaine Médicale.* 1899;19:52.

Gilles de la Tourette G. Lèpre et syringomyélie. Séance du 17 février 1899 de la Société Médicale des Hôpitaux. *La Semaine Médicale.* 1899;19:63.

Gilles de la Tourette G. De l'œil tabétique. Séance du 24 février 1899 de la Société Médicale des Hôpitaux. *La Semaine Médicale.* 1899;19:69.

Gilles de la Tourette G. De la percussion méthodique du crane. Séance du 28 mars 1899 à l'Académie nationale de Médecine. *La Semaine Médicale.* 1899;19:108.

Gilles de la Tourette G. La maladie des tics convulsifs. *La Semaine Médicale.* 1899;19(20):153–156.

Gilles de la Tourette G. Diagnostic de l'affection dite chorée des femmes enceintes. *La Semaine Médicale.* 1899;19:305–307.

Gilles de la Tourette G. L'ulcère rond de l'estomac dans ses rapports avec l'hystérie. *La Semaine Médicale.* 1899;19:377–381.

1900

Gilles de la Tourette G. La dose suffisante de bromure et le signe de la pupille dans le traitement de l'épilepsie. *La Semaine Médicale.* 1900;20:331–338.

At the February 1, 1900, session of the Société de Neurologie, Gilles de la Tourette and Babiński had an exchange that was described in *La Revue Neurologique* and *Les Archives de Neurologie;* these descriptions differ significantly. The position defended by Babiński is clear and unequivocal, highlighting Gilles de la Tourette's lack of rigor in establishing his diagnostics. In Gilles de la Tourette's defense, he was already quite sick, as this exchange took place only a year before his hospitalization.

Société de Neurologie, February 1, 1900

Gilles de la Tourette: *"I would like to clarify the precise meaning of an upward response of the hallux. If I have understood correctly, Mr. Babiński attributes this sign to dysfunction of the pyramidal tract. Since he observes it in organic hemiplegia, but not in paralysis and hysterical contractions, this sign would seem to indicate organic damage; one would thus expect it to be absent in conditions of dynamic origin. The patient he presents seems to have a dynamic condition and the upward extension of the hallux is nonetheless clearly present; what then is its diagnostic significance? If this sign is relevant in another way, I would like to know what it is. I can also say that I recently found it absent in a clearly organic syndrome. The patient had*

Benedikt syndrome characterized by oculomotor nerve palsy on the right, and left hem-
iplegia with contraction and one-sided athetotic shaking. The upward extension of the
hallux was absent on both sides or was barely perceptible. The patellar reflexes were
abolished, but the patient very clearly had an organic condition involving the pyram-
idal tract. In contrast, I have seen the upward extension of the hallux in the following
dynamic case. I recently examined, along with Dr. Rouffilange, a twenty-seven-year
old woman who had been in an absolute coma for forty-eight hours. She was a hysteric
with confirmed attacks. Her entire family had had the flu, and she had had slight gas-
tric upset with low temperature at 38 °. This state lasted two days, then she contracted
a violent headache followed almost immediately by coma. Consciousness and general
sensibility were totally abolished; no convulsions, no partial or generalized paralysis
could be detected. This indicated flu-like, spinal, or another sort of meningitis. Due to
her fever, absence of convulsions, and ocular paralysis, and because of her confirmed
hysteria, we diagnosed hysterical coma, then observed a very marked upward exten-
sion of the hallux. As a result, we hesitated and considered an organic lesion causing
excitation of the cortical centers via the pyramidal tract. The hysterical coma diag-
nosis was nonetheless maintained, and rightly so, because after forty-eight hours the
patient awoke, showing the same hysterical stigmata she had had before her patholog-
ical sleep. I wanted to point out these two cases, which indicate that the pathogenesis
of this reflex still needs to be studied and that, while it is often useful in differentiating
between organic and dynamic conditions of the nervous system, it can also lead to
contradictory interpretations."

Babiński: *"Contrary to what Mr. Gilles de la Tourette says, I never maintained*
that the upward extension of the hallux was necessarily indicative of a significant
organic lesion; I even said that this phenomenon could occur temporarily in epilepsy,
during seizures, and in strychnine poisoning. Nor did I claim that this sign existed in
all patients with pyramidal system lesions; I explicitly said that it could be missing in
cases of this type. The idea I expressed, today generally accepted, is that this sign is
linked to dysfunction in the pyramidal system, whether the dysfunction is slight or pro-
found, and that it exists in neither hysteria nor in any subject in which the pyramidal
system is normal. Statistics based on a very large number of cases have confirmed this
way of thinking. Very recently, Mr. Cestan and Mr. Le Sourd published a work on this
subject based on the observation of 300 patients with nervous conditions. In 148 of
them, they witnessed the upward extension of the hallux. And in all of these patients,
without exception, the pyramidal system was affected. In contrast, not one of the 44
hysterics examined presented this sign. These numbers are eloquent and demonstra-
tive. The question is not whether a link exists between this sign and disturbance in the
pyramidal system, since this has been established. All that remains to be determined
is whether this sign can exist exceptionally, in the absence of a disturbance of this
type, for example in pure hysterical paralysis. I do not believe so, and Mr. Gilles de la

Tourette's observation has not modified my opinion, since he did not demonstrate that it was indeed a matter of hysterical paralysis. And not having examined the subject myself, it is difficult for me to discuss the diagnosis. I invite my colleagues to alert the Society to any cases that seem to contradict my way of thinking. The patients can then be examined here, or in the hospital if they cannot be moved, and we shall be able to conduct a fruitful discussion."

Société de Neurologie, February 1, 1900

Gilles de la Tourette: *"Is the diagnostic value of the Babiński sign relative or absolute? One of my patients, twenty years old and a hysteric with very marked convulsive attacks, had a flu with fever and ended up in a coma, which suggested meningitis. The existence of hysteria was the only factor making it possible to hope that her condition was only due to neurosis. The Babiński sign was used to decide the matter; it was positive. Despite this observation, I preferred to maintain the diagnosis of hysteria alone, which her recovery promptly confirmed. And I am able to cite cases of organic lesions where the upward extension of the hallux was absent."*

Babiński: *"I did not maintain that the upward extension phenomenon was necessarily dependent on a significant organic lesion in the pyramidal system; I said that this phenomenon is linked to dysfunction in this system. This dysfunction can be temporary, as in the case of epilepsy; during the seizure, upward extension of the hallux can be observed, while the reflex is normal outside of seizures. In my opinion, Mr. Gilles de la Tourette does not demonstrate that his case involves hysterical motor disturbance. Furthermore, if for no other reason than the fever, the clinical picture in this case is not the classical clinical picture for hysterical hemiplegia. I have never observed this sign in hysteria; I have never observed it in a patient whose pyramidal system can be considered normal. If such cases exist, they must be entirely exceptional. I request that the upward extension of the hallux be kept on the agenda and that all of my colleagues share any observations they might learn of to determine once and for all the absolute characteristic value, or lack thereof, of this sign."*

Compte-Rendu de la séance de la Société de Neurologie du 1 février 1900.
Archives de Neurologie. 1900;9(51):252–253.

Société de Neurologie, June 7, 1900

Chorée de Sydenham and Rheumatism

Gilles de la Tourette refuted the opinion whereby Sydenham's chorea was linked to rheumatism. Of the seventeen cases he observed, he only found rheumatism in one of them, and the onset of the chorea was never before puberty. This indicated that choreas developing after this period, especially during pregnancy, should be linked to hysteria or convulsive tic disorder. Gilles de la Tourette argued that abortion should not be practiced in women with chorea.

Joffroy persisted in positing a certain link between rheumatism and chorea, even though chorea was not always rheumatic in origin. Rheumatism would appear to be an occasional cause, acting simply as an ordinary infectious disease such as measles or flu. Finally, Joffroy had seen cases of chorea in pregnancy that were impossible to link to hysteria or tics.

Compte-Rendu de la séance de la Société de Neurologie du 7 juin 1900. Chorée de Sydenham et rhumatisme. *Archives de Neurologie.* 1900;10(55):65–66.

Gilles de la Tourette G, Charcot JB. Le syndrome de Benedikt. *La Semaine Médicale.* 1900;20:127–133.

Gilles de la Tourette G. Discussion à la Société de Neurologie le 1 février 1900. Double syndrome de Weber, A. Souques. *La Revue Neurologique.* 1900;8(3):148–149.

Gilles de la Tourette G. La localisation cérébrale des troubles hystériques. *La Revue Neurologique.* 1900;8(5):225–227.

Gilles de la Tourette G. Discussion à la Société de Neurologie le 5 avril 1900. Tabes conjugal, A. Souques. *La Revue Neurologique.* 1900;8(7):341.

Gilles de la Tourette G. Des rapports de la chorée de Sydenham avec le rhumatisme, la puberté et la chorée dite des femmes enceintes. *La Revue Neurologique.* 1900;8(12):542–547.

1901

Gilles de la Tourette G. L'application de la méthode de la dose suffisante au traitement de quelques maladies du système nerveux: formes graves et associées de la migraine, vertige de Ménière, névralgie et tic douloureux de la face. *La Semaine Médicale.* 1901;21:33–36.

Articles Published in *Le Progrès Médical,* except for Reports (Comptes Rendus) of Learned Societies

1881

Gilles de la Tourette G. La mort apparente des fakirs. *Le Progrès Médical.* 1881;9(23):454.

Gilles de la Tourette G. Le Président Garfield. *Le Progrès Médical.* 1881;9(37):726.

Gilles de la Tourette G. L'autopsie du Président Garfield. *Le Progrès Médical*. 1881;9(49):963–965.

1882

Gilles de la Tourette G. Les garde-malades. *Le Progrès Médical*. 1882;10(24):401–402.

Gilles de la Tourette G. Empoisonnement à l'iodoforme. *Le Progrès Médical*. 1882;10(12):229–230.

Gilles de la Tourette G. Revue de médecine légale. Les blessures de lord Frederick Cavendish et de M. Burke. *Le Progrès Médical*. 1882;10(21):407–408.

Gilles de la Tourette G. Société anatomique: deux noyaux séparés, pesant 5 grammes, représentant l'utérus chez une jeune fille de 18 ans, non réglée. *Le Progrès Médical*. 1882;10(24):463.

Gilles de la Tourette G. Nécrologie: V.G. Lemercier. *Le Progrès Médical*. 1882;10(28):550–551.

Gilles de la Tourette G. L'autopsie de Guiteau. *Le Progrès Médical*. 1882;10(32):624–625.

Gilles de la Tourette G. De la menstruation compensatrice par le conduit auditif externe. *Le Progrès Médical*. 1882;10(35):668.

Gilles de la Tourette G. Revue de syphilgraphie: Influence des maladies fébriles sur la marche de la syphilis par le Dr Petrowsky; influence de la diathèse rhumastismale sur le lésion initiale de la syphilis par le Dr Lockwood. *Le Progrès Médical*. 1882;10(36):694–695.

Gilles de la Tourette G. Médecine et service militaire. *Le Progrès Médical*. 1882;10(42):815–816.

1883

Gilles de la Tourette G. Des injections sous-cutanées d'iodure de potassium. *Le Progrès Médical*. 1883;11(1):5–6.

Gilles de la Tourette G. Studi e questioni di morologia e Genesi cellulare ed Istogenesi del Sarcoma giganto cellulare par le Dr Luigi Ageno, professeur d'anatomie nomrale à l'Université de Gênes, 1881. *Le Progrès Médical*. 1883;11(4):74–75.

Gilles de la Tourette G. Guy's Hospital Reports publiés sous la direction des Dr Howse et Frédérick Taylor, 3è série, tome25, de 531 pages avec planches; Churchill, Londres, 1881. *Le Progrès Médical*. 1883;11(4):75.

Gilles de la Tourette G. Le choléra et le rapport de M. le Dr Hunter. *Le Progrès Médical*. 1883;11(42):827–829.

Gilles de la Tourette G. Revue de chirurgie. Note sur un cas de spina-bifida traité avec succès pas la ponction aspiratrice et les injections de glycérine iodurée par le Dr Muirhead Little, The Lancet 20 janvier 1883. Passage de 40 pouces d'intestion par le rectum, suivi de guérison par le Dr Saunders, in Maryland Medical janvier 1883. *Le Progrès Médical*. 1883;11(42):833–834.

Gilles de la Tourette G. La Salpêtrière: son histoire de 1656 à 1790, par M. le Dr L. Boucher, 1 vol in-8 de 138 p, aux Bureaux du Progrès Médical. *Le Progrès Médical*. 1883;11(49):998–999.

Blanchard R. Théophraste Renaudot, un essai de Faculté libre au XVIIᵉ siècle. *Le Progrès Médical*. 1883;11(50):1039.

1884

Gilles de la Tourette G. Bibliographie. Histoire de la médecine, d'Hippocrate à Boussais et ses successeurs par M. J. M. Guardia. Paris, 1884. O. Douin. *Le Progrès Médical*. 1884;12(3):55.

Richer P, Gilles de la Tourette G. Clinique nerveuse. Hôpital de la salpêtrière.—M. Charcot. Note sur les caractères cliniques des paralysies psychiques expérimentales (paralysies par suggestion). *Le Progrès Médical*. 1884;12(13):241–242.

Réponse: Bernheim H. des paralysies psychiques expérimentales. Le progrès Médical. 1884;12(14):279.

Gilles de la Tourette G. Bibliographie. La géographie médicale par M. le Dr A. Bordier, Paris 1884. C. Reinwald. *Le Progrès Médical*. 1884;12(19):384–385.

Gilles de la Tourette G. Adolphe Wurtz. *Le Progrès Médical*. 1884;12(20):394–395.

Gilles de la Tourette G. Amédée Blondeau. *Le Progrès Médical*. 1884;12(23):453–454.

Gilles de la Tourette G. L'origine ancienne de la vérole. *Le Progrès Médical*. 1884;12(24):476–478.

Gilles de la Tourette G. Die Medicin in Wien während der Letzen 100 Jahre, par le Dr Th Puschman, professeur d'histoire de la médecine à l'Université de Vienne. Vienne 1884. *Le Progrès Médical*. 1884;12(28):570.

Gilles de la Tourette G. Congrès International de Copenhague. *Le Progrès Médical*. 1884;12(33):662.

Gilles de la Tourette G, Bonnaire J. Compte-rendus des séances du Congrès Internationale de Copenhague. *Le Progrès Médical*. 1884;12(34):680–682.

Bonnaire J, Gilles de la Tourette G. Le Congrès international de Médecine. *Le Progrès Médical.* 1884;12(34):688.

Bonnaire J, Gilles de la Tourette G. Congrès international des sciences médicales. *Le Progrès Médical.* 1884;12(38):764–766.

Gilles de la Tourette G. Présentation au nom du Pr. Charcot d'un album renfermant les photographies de tous les cas intéressants observés à La Salpêtrière et fait une communication: Sur la salivation dans les maladies nerveuses, au point de vue physiologique. *Le Progrès Médical.* 1884;12(39):780–781.

Gilles de la Tourette G. Une excursion à l'asile de St-Hans. *Le Progrès Médical.* 1884;12(39):784–785.

Bonnaire J, Gilles de la Tourette G. Congrès international des sciences médicales. Section de chirurgie. *Le Progrès Médical.* 1884;12(40):800–801.

Gilles de la Tourette G. Les médicaments de garde. *Le Progrès Médical.* 1884;12(42):832–833.

Gilles de la Tourette G. Revue d'histoire médicale: histoire de l'hôpital N.-D. de Pitié, 1662–1882. *Le Progrès Médical.* 1884;12(44):875–876.

Gilles de la Tourette G. Revue de géographie médicale: Essai de géographie médicale de Nosi-Bé, près de la côte Nord-Ouest de Madagascar, par le Dr P.R. Deblenne, médecin de la marine, Paris, 1883, Parent Ed. *Le Progrès Médical.* 1884;12(50):1044–1045.

Gilles de la Tourette G. Société de Thérapeutique. *Le Progrès Médical.* 1884;12(53):1102.

1885

Gilles de la Tourette G. Spiritisme et hystérie. *Le Progrès Médical.* 1885;13–1(4):63–65.

Charcot JM. Leçon recueillie par Gilles de la Tourette G. De l'isolement dans le traitement de l'hysétrie. *Le Progrès Médical.* 1885;13–1(9):161–164.

Gilles de la Tourette G. L'hôpital Laennec, ancien hospice des Incurables (1634–1884). *Le Progrès Médical.* 1885;13–1(18):366–367.

Gilles de la Tourette G. Bibliographie. Histoires, disputes et discours des illusions et impostures des diables des magiciens infâmes, sorcières et empoisonneurs; des ensorcelez et démoniaques et de la guérison d'iceux: item de la punition que méritent les magiciens, les empoisonneurs et les sorcières par Jean Wier. 2 vol. 1 200 pages

réédités sur l'impression de 1579 par Bourneville. Paris, 1885. Aux
Bureaux du Progrès Médical. *Le Progrès Médical*. 1895;13–1(20):401–402.

Gilles de la Tourette G. Le déplacement de la morgue. *Le Progrès Médical*.
1885;13–1(21):417–420.

Gilles de la Tourette G. Revue d'hygiène. *Le Progrès Médical*.
1885;13–2(32):104–105.

Gilles de la Tourette G. Lectures sur l'Histoire de la médecine,
par L. Thomas, sous bibliothécaire à la Faculté de médecine
de Paris. Delahaye et Lecrosnier 1885. *Le Progrès Médical*.
1885;13–2(36):186–187.

Gilles de la Tourette G. Revue de thérapeutique: traitement de la crampe
des écrivains. *Le Progrès Médical*. 1885;13–2(51):524–526.

Gilles de la Tourette G. Traité de zoologie médicale par R. Blanchard,
professeur agrégé à la Faculté de médecine de Paris. JB Baillière,1885.
Le Progrès Médical. 1885;13–2(52):544–545, and *Le Progrès Médical*.
1886;14–2(51):1100.

Criticism of one of the first books on Parasitology.

1886

Gilles de la Tourette G. La biologie aristotélique par G. Pouchet,
professeur d'anatomie comparée au Museum. Alcan, 1885. *Le Progrès
Médical*. 1886;14–1(1):13–14.

Gilles de la Tourette G. Les Fever Hospitals et les hôpitaux flottants pour
la variole à Londres. *Le Progrès Médical*. 1886;14–1(2):22–25.

The need to isolate contagious patients, the example of London.

Gilles de la Tourette G. Société anatomique: présentation d'un
cas de cancer du pancréas étendu au foie. *Le Progrès Médical*.
1886;14–1(3):48.

Gilles de la Tourette G. Revue d'hygiène: Nouveau manuel de la garde-
malade, à l'usage des mères de famille par E. Bérillon, 1885; La santé
publique à Lyon pendant l'année 1884, par J Tessier. *Le Progrès Médical*.
1886;14–1(5):91.

Gilles de la Tourette G. Urbain Grandier et les Possédées de
Loudun par le dr G. Legué, Charpentier 1884. *Le Progrès Médical*.
1886;14–1(11):231–232.

Gilles de la Tourette G. Le laboratoire de biologie. *Le Progrès Médical*.
1886;14–1(24):494–496.

Séglas J. Etudes cliniques et physiologique sur la marche. La marche dans les maladies du système nerveux, par Gilles de la Tourette. *Le Progrès Médical.* 1886;14–1(24):505–506.

Gilles de la Tourette G. Contribution à la détermination de la nature microbienne des efflorescences cutanées d'origine syphilitique. Du traitement du psoriasis palmaire et plantaire par les bains locaux de sublimé (communication à la Société de Biologie du 10 juin 1886). *Le Progrès Médical.* 1886;14–2(30):612–613.

Charcot JM. Cas de mutisme hystérique. Leçon recueilie par le Dr Gilles de la Tourette. *Le Progrès Médical.* 1886;14–2(46):987–991.

Gilles de la Tourette G. Revue d'histoire médicale: Un voyage à travers quelques établissements scientifiques de la France et de l'étranger, par A. Bouchard; Eloge de Lasègue par A. Ritti; Au Tonkin par Challan de Belleval; Histoire de la médecine par Barbillon. *Le Progrès Médical.* 1886;14–2(48):1041.

1887

Bottey F. L'hypnotisme et les états analogues au point de vue médcio-légal par Gilles de la Tourette. Plon, 1887. *Le Progrès Médical.* 1887;15–1(4):75–76.

Aigre D. Sœur Jeanne des Anges, supérieure des Ursulines de Loudun par G. Legué et G. Gilles de la Tourette. Aux bureaux du Progrès médical, 1886. *Le Progrès Médical.* 1887;15–1(6):118–119.

Gilles de la Tourette G. Revue d'histoire médicale: Teignes et teigneux par H. Feulard Thèse 1886; La capitale de l'Equateur au point de vue médico-légale. *Le Progrès Médical.* 1887;15–1(7):139–140.

Charcot JM. Sur le traitement de la migraine ophtalmique accompagnée. Leçon par Gilles de la Tourette et P. Blocq. *Le Progrès Médical.* 1887;15–1(24):476.

Charcot JM. Hystérie et syphilis: de l'influence d'une maladie ou d'une intoxication antérieure sur le mode de localisation et sur la forme des accidents hystériques, leçon résumée par Gilles de la Tourette. *Le Progrès Médical.* 1887;15–2(51):511–512.

Gilles de la Tourette G. Revue d'histoire médicale: La vie privée d'autrefois par A. Franklin, Un grand hôpital parisien en 1886, Lariboisère par L Gallet, La prostitution dans l'antiquité de E. Dupouy, El congresso médico-regional de Navarra en 1886,EFA Vulpian e le sue opere par R. Massalongo. *Le Progrès Médical.* 1887;15–2(52):545–546.

1888

Gilles de la Tourette G, Cathelineau H. La nutrition dans l'hystérie. *Le Progrès Médical* 1888;16(48):445–448.

1889

Charcot JM. Leçon résumée par Gilles de la Tourette G. De la suspension dans le traitement de l'ataxie locomotrice progressive et de quelques autres maladies du système nerveux. *Le Progrès Médical.* 1889;17–1(3):50–51.

Charcot JM. Leçon résumée par Gilles de la Tourette G. De la technique à suivre dans le traitement par la suspension de l'ataxie locomotrice progressive et de quelques autres maladies du système nerveux. *Le Progrès Médical.* 1889;17–1(8):135–137.

Gilles de la Tourette G, Cathelineau H. La nutrition dans l'hystérie. *Le Progrès Médical.* 1889;17–1(18):325–328.

Gilles de la Tourette G, Cathelineau H. La nutrition dans l'hystérie. *Le Progrès Médical.* 1889;17–1(19):349–350.

Gilles de la Tourette G, Cathelineau H. La nutrition dans l'hystérie. *Le Progrès Médical.* 1889;17–2(31):85–87.

Gilles de la Tourette G. Congrès international de Médecine légale. *Le Progrès Médical.* 1889;17–2(34):193–194.

Gilles de la Tourette G. François Damaschino. *Le Progrès Médical.* 1889;17–2(52):592–594

1890

Gilles de la Tourette G, Cathelineau H. La nutrition dans l'hystérie. *Le Progrès Médical.* 1890;18–1(2):19.20.

Gilles de la Tourette G, Cathelineau H. La nutrition dans l'hystérie. *Le Progrès Médical.* 1890;18–1(8):145–147.

Gilles de la Tourette G, Cathelineau H. La nutrition dans l'hystérie. *Le Progrès Médical.* 1890;18–1(9):161–165.

Gilles de la Tourette G, Cathelineau H. La nutrition dans l'hystérie. *Le Progrès Médical.* 1890;18–1(10):188–190.

Gilles de la Tourette G. Revue d'histoire médicale: L'école de Salerne et les médecins salertinains par G. Bécavin,1888; Histoire de la médecine à travers les âges par P. Degnat, 1888; Le moyen-âge médical par E. Dupouy, 1888; Renaudot et l'introduction de la médication clinique, étude historique d'après documents originaux par M. Michel Emery, thèse de Montpellier en 1888; Le Val-de-Grâce histoire du monastère et de l'hôpital militaire. *Le Progrès Médical.* 1890;18–1(16):319.321.

Gilles de la Tourette G, Cathelineau H. La nutrition dans l'hystérie. *Le Progrès Médical* 1890;18–1(17):332–334.

Gilles de la Tourette G. Modifications apportées à la technique de la suspension dans le traitement de l'ataxie locomotrice et de quelques autres maladies du système nerveux. *Le Progrès Médical* 1890;18–1(23):457–459.

Gilles de la Tourette G. Histoire de Bicêtre par Paul Bru. 1890. *Le Progrès Médical.* 1890;18–2(37):202–203.

Gilles de la Tourette G, Cathelineau H. La nutrition dans l'hystérie. *Le Progrès Médical.* 1890;18–2(39):230–232.

Gilles de la Tourette G, Cathelineau H. La nutrition dans l'hystérie. *Le Progrès Médical.* 1890;18–2(43):295–297.

Gilles de la Tourette G, Cathelineau H. La nutrition dans l'hystérie. *Le Progrès Médical.* 1890;18–2(45):394–396.

Gilles de la Tourette G, Cathelineau H. La nutrition dans l'hystérie. *Le Progrès Médical.* 1890;18–2(51):496–497.

1891

Gilles de la Tourette G. L'épilogue d'un procès célèbre. *Le Progrès Médical.* 1891;19.1(5):89–96.

Gilles de la Tourette G, Cathelineau H. Le sang dans l'hystérie nomrale. *Le Progrès Médical* 1891;19.1(7):121–122.

Gilles de la Tourette G. Correspondance: L'épilogue d'un procès célèbre. *Le Progrès Médical.* 1891;19.1(7):135–136.

Raoult A. De la suspension dans le traitement des maladies du système nerveux. *Le Progrès Médical* 1891;19.1(9):165–166.

Gilles de la Tourette G. Notes sur quelques paroxysmes hystériques peu connus: attaque à forme de névralgie faciale, de vertige de Ménière. *Le Progrès Médical.* 1891;19.2(31):73–77.

Gilles de la Tourette G. L'angine de poitrine d'origine hystérique. *Le Progrès Médical.* 1891;19.2(44):305–307.

Guinon G. Bibliographie: Traité clinique et thérapetique de l'hystérie d'après l'enseignement de La Salpêtrière par le dr Gilles de la Tourette, 1891. *Le Progrès Médical.* 1891;19.2(49):445–446.

1892

Gilles de la Tourette G, Cathelineau H. La nutrition dans l'hystérie. *Le Progrès Médical.* 1891;20–1(17):316–317.

Gilles de la Tourette G. Revue d'histoire médicale: Les maladies nerveuses pendant l'antiquité græco-romaine par M. Tournery, 1892; La vue privée d'autrefois, les médecins par A. Franklin, 1892; Saint-Luc patron des anciennes facultés de médecine par Dauchez, 1892; Biographia del doctor José M. de los Rios par J. Manrique, 1891; La syphilis de Ninive et à Babylone par F. Buret, 1892. *Le Progrès Médical.* 1891;20–2(29):48–49.

Gilles de la Tourette G. La médecin vibratoire, application des vibrations rapides et continues au traietement de quelques maladies du système nerveux. Leçon de JM. Charcot. *Le Progrès Médical.* 1891;20–2(35):149–151.

Gilles de la Tourette G, Cathelineau H. La nutrition dans l'hystérie. *Le Progrès Médical.* 1891;20–2(50):481–483.

1893

Gilles de la Tourette G. Damain E. Un danseur monomane. *Le Progrès Médical.* 1893;21–1(2):30–32.

Gilles de la Tourette G, Cathelineau H. La nutrition dans l'hystérie. *Le Progrès Médical.* 1893;21–1(6):100–101.

Guinon G. Attentat contre Gilles de la Tourette. *Le Progrès Médical.* 1893;21–2(49):446.

1894

Haussmann, Gauthier de Clagny, Cornil, Cézilly, de Ranse, Baudouin, Gilles de la Tourette. L'affaire lafitte. *Le Progrès Médical.* 1894;22–1(43):273–276.

1895

Guinon G. Bibliographie: Traité clinique et thérapetique de l'hystérie d'après l'enseignement de La Salpêtrière par le dr Gilles de la Tourette, 1891. *Le Progrès Médical.* 1895;23–2(27):9.

1896

Gilles de la Tourette G. Bibliographie: Clinique des maladies du système nerveux par F. Raymond, 1895. *Le Progrès Médical.* 1896;24–1(14):220–221.

Gilles de la Tourette G. Bibliographie: Le « gros mal » du Moyen–âge et la syphilis actuelle par F Buret, *Le Progrès Médical.* 1896;24–1(15): 234.

1897

Gilles de la Tourette G. Bibliographie: Clinique des maladies du système nerveux par F. Raymond, 1895. *Le Progrès Médical.* 1897;25–1(24):377–378.

1898

Gilles de la Tourette G. Les infirmières décorées, Mademoiselle Bottard. *Le Progrès Médical.* 1898;26–1(2):26.

Plicque AF. Bibliographie: Leçons de clinique thérapeutique sur les maladies du système nerveux. *Le Progrès Médical.* 1898;26–2(51):476.

1899

Gilles de la Tourette G. Revue d'histoire médicale: Un bureau de santé au XVIIᵉ siècle par Dr Langlet, 1898; Récamier et ses contemporains (1744–1852) par P. Triaire, 1898. *Le Progrès Médical.* 1899;27–1(2):26.106–108.

Miraillé Ch. Revue des maladies du système nerveux: Formes cliniques et traitement des myélites syphilitiques par Gilles de la Tourette, 1899. *Le Progrès Médical.* 1899;27–1(10):156–157.

Mallet J. Les états neurasthéniques par Gilles de la Tourette, 1899. *Le Progrès Médical* 1899;27–1(20):326.

Gilles de la Tourette G. Ouverture du cours: Clinique des maladies nerveuses. *Le Progrès Médical.* 1899;27–2(48):436.

1900

Gilles de la Tourette G. Bibliographie: Leçons sur les maladies du système nerveux (année 1897–1898) par le Pr F. Raymond, recueillies et publiées par E. Ricklin, 1900. *Le Progrès Médical.* 1900;28–1(17):266–267.

Banquet Gilles de la Tourette. *Le Progrès Médical.* 1900;28–1(19):304.

Banquet Gilles de la Tourette. *Le Progrès Médical.* 1900;28–1(20):319.

1901

Rellay P. Bibliographie: Traitement de l'épilepsie par Gilles de la Tourette, 1901. *Le Progrès Médical.* 1901;30–2(28):29.

1902

Keraval P. Le traitement de l'épilepsie par Gilles de la Tourette, 1901. *Le Progrès Médical.* 1902;31–1(13): 212–213

Noir J. Bibliographie: Traité de médecine et de thérapeutique, publié sous la direction de MM. P. Brouardel, A. Gilbert & J. Girode, tome dixième: maladies des nerfs périphériques, névroses; maladies des muscles par MM. Pitres, Vaillard, Gilles de la Tourette, Gasne, Grasset, Rauzier, Triboulet, Launois, Lamy, Sainton, Brissaud, Marinesco. *Le Progrès Médical.* 1902;31–2(46): 404.

1904

Nécrologie Gilles de la Tourette. *Le Progrès Médical.* 1904;33–1(22):366.

Articles Published in *La Nouvelle Iconographie de La Salpêtrière*

1888

Gilles de la Tourette G. L'attitude et la marche dans l'hémiplégie hystérique. *Nouvelle Iconographie de La Salpêtrière.* 1888;1(1):1–12.

Gilles de la Tourette G, Blocq P, Huet E. Cinq cas de maladie de Friedreich. *Nouvelle Iconographie de La Salpêtrière.* 1888;1(2): 45–63; *Nouvelle Iconographie de La Salpêtrière.* 1888;1(3): 114–119.

1889

Gilles de la Tourette G. Documents satiriques sur Mesmer. *Nouvelle Iconographie de La Salpêtrière.* 1889;2(1):59–65; *Nouvelle Iconographie de La Salpêtrière.*1889;2(2):103–106.

Gilles de la Tourette G. De la technique à suivre dans le traitement par la suspension de l'ataxie locomotrice progressive et de quelques autres maladies du système nerveux. *Nouvelle Iconographie de La Salpêtrière.* 1889;2(2):85–91.

Gilles de la Tourette G. De la superposition des troubles de la sensibilité et des spasmes de la face et du cou chez les hystériques. *Nouvelle Iconographie de La Salpêtrière.* 1889;2(3):107–129; *Nouvelle Iconographie de La Salpêtrière.* 1889;2(4):170–187.

Gilles de la Tourette G. Le masque de Pascal. *Nouvelle Iconographie de La Salpêtrière.* 1889;2(4):196–202.

Gilles de la Tourette G. Le miracle opéré sur Marie-Anne Couronneau. *Nouvelle Iconographie de La Salpêtrière.* 1889;2(5):241–250.

Gilles de la Tourette G, Dutil A, dessins de Richer P. Contribution à l'étude des troubles trophiques dans l'hystérie, atrophie musculaire et œdème. *Nouvelle Iconographie de La Salpêtrière.*1889;2(6):251–282.

Gilles de la Tourette G, Cathelineau H. Considérations sur la courbe des excrétions dans l'attaque de sommeil hystérique. *Nouvelle Iconographie de La Salpêtrière.* 1889;2(7):290–304.

Gilles de la Tourette G, Cathelineau H. Contribution à l'étude de la nutrition dans l'état normal et dans la fièvre du goitre exophtalmique. *Nouvelle Iconographie de La Salpêtrière.* 1889;2(7):306–310.

Gilles de la Tourette G, Zaguelmann A. Un cas de syringomyélie. *Nouvelle Iconographie de La Salpêtrière.* 1889;2(7):311–317.

Gilles de la Tourette G. L'hystérie dans l'armée allemande. *Nouvelle Iconographie de La Salpêtrière.* 1889;2(7):318–326.

1890

Gilles de la Tourette G. Considérations sur les ecchymoses spontanées et sur l'état mental des hystériques. *Nouvelle Iconographie de La Salpêtrière.* 1890;3(2):49–72.

Gilles de la Tourette G. un dessin inédit d'Adrien Brauwer. *Nouvelle Iconographie de La Salpêtrière.* 1890;3(2):94–96.

Gilles de la Tourette G, Huet E, Guinon G. Contribution à l'étude des bâillements hystériques. *Nouvelle Iconographie de La Salpêtrière.* 1890;3(3):97–119.

Gilles de la Tourette G. Modifications apportées à la technique de la suspension dans le traitement de l'ataxie locomotrice et de quelques autres maladies du système nerveux. *Nouvelle Iconographie de La Salpêtrière.* 1890;3(3):128–133.

1891

Gilles de la Tourette G. Sur un buste d'évêque guérissant les écrouelles. *Nouvelle Iconographie de La Salpêtrière*. 1891;4(2):167–168.

Gilles de la Tourette G. Nouveaux documents satiriques sur Mesmer. *Nouvelle Iconographie de La Salpêtrière*. 1891;4(5):482–484.

1892

Gilles de la Tourette G. Nouveaux documents satiriques sur Mesmer. *Nouvelle Iconographie de La Salpêtrière*. 1892;5(1):55–56.

Gilles de la Tourette G. Sur un tableau perdu de Rubens, représentant la guérison des "possédés." *Nouvelle Iconographie de La Salpêtrière*. 1892;5(2):119.120.

Gilles de la Tourette G. Un bas-relief d'Alfred Boucher. Tobie rendant la vue à son père. *Nouvelle Iconographie de La Salpêtrière*. 1892;5(5):263–234.

Gilles de la Tourette G. Considérations sur la médecine vibratoire, ses applications et sa technique. *Nouvelle Iconographie de La Salpêtrière*. 1892;5(6):265–275.

1893

Gilles de la Tourette G, Hudelo L. Deux observations pour servir au diagnostic des paraplégies syphilitiques. *Nouvelle Iconographie de La Salpêtrière*. 1893;6(1):1–7.

Gilles de la Tourette G. J.-M. Charcot. *Nouvelle Iconographie de La Salpêtrière*. 1893;6(3):240–250.

1894

Gilles de la Tourette G, Magdelaine L. Sur un cas d'ostéite déformante de Paget. *Nouvelle Iconographie de La Salpêtrière*. 1894;7(1):1–14.

1895

Gilles de la Tourette G, Fournier A. La notion étiologique de l'hérédo-syphilis dans la maladie de Little. *Nouvelle Iconographie de La Salpêtrière*. 1895;8(1):23–29.

Gilles de la Tourette G. Le sein hystérique. *Nouvelle Iconographie de La Salpêtrière*. 1895;8(2):107–121.

Gilles de la Tourette G. Marinesco G. La lésion médullaire de l'ostéite déformante de Paget. *Nouvelle Iconographie de La Salpêtrière*. 1895;8(3):205–213.

Gilles de la Tourette G, Bolognesi A. Nature hystérique de la tétanie des femmes enceintes. *Nouvelle Iconographie de La Salpêtrière*. 1895;8(4):277–287

Fournier A, Kohne J Ch, Gilles de la Tourette G. Rapport médico-légal sur un militaire déserteur atteint d'automatisme ambulatoire. *Nouvelle Iconographie de La Salpêtrière*. 1895;8(6):348–353.

1896

Gilles de la Tourette G. La syphilis héréditaire de la moelle épinière. *Nouvelle Iconographie de La Salpêtrière*. 1896;9(2):80–92.

1897

Gilles de la Tourette G. Pathogénie et prophylaxie de l'atrophie musculaire chez les hémiplégiques. *Nouvelle Iconographie de La Salpêtrière*. 1897;10(4):287–293; 1897;10(5):340–346.

Gilles de la Tourette G, Chipault A. Traitement de l'ataxie par l'élongation vraie de la moelle épinière. *Nouvelle Iconographie de La Salpêtrière*. 1897;10(3):144–154.

1898

Gilles de la Tourette G, Gasne G. Le traitement de l'ataxie locomotrice par l'élongation vraie de la moelle épinière. *Nouvelle Iconographie de La Salpêtrière*. 1898;11(1):18–19.

Georges Gasne (1868–1910)

1899

Gilles de la Tourette, Durante G. Un cas de syphilis héréditaire de la moelle. *Nouvelle Iconographie de La Salpêtrière*. 1899;12(2):95–106.

1900

Gilles de la Tourette G. La marche dans les maladies du système nerveux, à propos d'un article de M. Marinesco. *Nouvelle Iconographie de La Salpêtrière*. 1900;13(3):293–295.

Reports of the Société de Biologie, published in *Le Progrès Médical*

Gilles de la Tourette G. Compte-rendu Société de Biologie, séance du 10 mai 1884. *Le Progrès Médical*. 1884;12(20):396–397.

Gilles de la Tourette G. Compte-rendu Société de Biologie, séance du 31 mai 1884. *Le Progrès Médical*. 1884;12(23):455.

And after that issue, each week until:

Gilles de la Tourette G. Compte-rendu Société de Biologie, séance du 22 janvier 1889. *Le Progrès Médical*. 1889;17–1(4):71.

Reports of the Société de Thérapeutique Published in *Le Progrès Médical*

Gilles de la Tourette G. Compte-rendu Société de Thérapeutique, séance du 14 mai 1884. *Le Progrès Médical*. 1884;12(21):418–419.

And after that issue, every two weeks until:

Gilles de la Tourette G. Compte-rendu Société de Thérapeutique, séance du 26 décembre 1888. *Le Progrès Médical*. 1889;17–(4):74.

Notes

1. Gilles de la Tourette G. Nécrologie: V.G. Lemercier. *Le Progrès Médical*. 1882;10(28):550–551.
2. Gilles de la Tourette G. Adolphe Wurtz. *Le Progrès Médical*. 1884;12(20):394–395.
3. Blondeau A. *Etude clinique sur le pouls lent permanent avec attaques syncopales et épileptiformes.*, Thèse no. 246. Paris. Versailles: Cerf et fils. 1879.
4. Gilles de la Tourette G. Amédée Blondeau. *Le Progrès Médical*. 1884;12(23):453–454.
5. Gilles de la Tourette G. François Damaschino. *Le Progrès Médical* 1889;17–2(52):592–594.
6. Gilles de la Tourette G. J-M Charcot. *Nouvelle Iconographie de La Salpêtrière*. 1893;6(3):240–250.
7. Damaschino F. *Maladies des voies digestives: leçons professées à la Faculté de médecine de Paris recueillies par le Dr. M. Letulle*. Paris: F. Alcan. 1888.
8. Goetz CG. The prefaces by Charcot. Leitmotifs of an international career. *Neurology*. 2003;60(8):133–140.
9. Lamy H. *De la méningo-myélite syphilitique*. Thèse no. 433. Paris: Battaille. 1893.
10. Ladreit de Lacharrière J. *Des paralysies syphilitiques*. Thèse no. 56. Paris: Imprimerie Rignoux.1861.
11. Charcot JM. XVIᵉ leçon. Myélites transverses, tabes dorsal spasmodique. *Le Progrès Médical*. 1880;8(18):343–346.
12. Loeb C, Meyer JS. *Strokes due to vertebro-basilar diseases.: infarction, vascular insufficiency and hemorrhage of the brain stem and cerebellum*. Springfield, IL: Thomas. 1965.
13. Benedikt M. Un cas de tremblement avec paralysie croisée. *Bulletin Médical*. 1 mai 1889:547.

14. Londe A. Le syndrome de Benedikt. *La Médecine Moderne*. 1893;4(17):194–195.

15. Benedikt M. *Manuel technique et pratique d'anthropométrie cranio-céphalique (méthode, instrumentation): à l'usage de la clinique de l'anthropologie générale et de l'anthropologie criminelle. Traduction de P. Keraval et préface de JM*. Charcot. Paris: Lecrosnier et Babé. 1889.

16. Holmes GM. A form of familial degeneration of the cerebellum. *Brain*. 1907;30:466–489.

17. André-Thomas. *La Fonction cérébelleuse*. Paris: Doin. 1911.

18. François-Franck Ch-E. *Leçons sur les fonctions motrices du cerveau (réactions volontaires et organiques) et sur l'épilepsie cérébrale*. Préface du professeur Charcot. Paris: Octave Doin. 1887.

19. von Rokitansky KF. Über die sogenannten Verdoppelungen des Uterus. Medizinische Jahrbücher des kaiserl. *Königl. österreichischen Staates Wien*, 1838;26:39–77.

20. Mayer CA. Über Verdoppelungen des Uterus und ihre Arten, nebst Bemerkungen über Harenscharte und Wolfsrachen. *Journal der Chirurgie und Augen-Heilkunde, Berlin*, 1829;13:525–564.

Index